# Feeling Good

# Feeling Good

## The Science of Well-Being

C. ROBERT CLONINGER

OXFORD
UNIVERSITY PRESS
2004

# OXFORD
UNIVERSITY PRESS

Oxford   New York
Auckland   Bangkok   Buenos Aires   Cape Town   Chennai
Dar es Salaam   Delhi   Hong Kong   Istanbul   Karachi   Kolkata
Kuala Lumpur   Madrid   Melbourne   Mexico City   Mumbai   Nairobi
São Paulo   Shanghai   Taipei   Tokyo   Toronto

Copyright © 2004 by Oxford University Press, Inc.

Published by Oxford University Press, Inc.
198 Madison Avenue, New York, New York, 10016
http://www.oup.com

Oxford is a registered trademark of Oxford University Press

Library of Congress Cataloging-in-Publication Data
Cloninger, C. Robert.
Feeling good: the science of well-being / C. Robert Cloninger.
p. cm.   Includes bibliographical references and index.
ISBN 0-19-505137-8
1. Health.   2. Psychiatry.   3. Psychophysiology.   4. Mind and body.
5. Consciousness.   6. Personality.   7. Philosophy of mind.
8. Happiness.   9. Love.
I. Title.
RA776.C625 2004   613—dc22   2003190053

9 8 7 6 5 4 3 2 1

Printed in the United States of America
on acid-free paper

# PREFACE

To be truly happy people must learn to live in radically new ways. Well-being only arises when a person learns how to let go of struggles, to work in the service of others, and to grow in awareness. Prior approaches to feeling good have small or brief benefits because they separate the biological, psychological, social, and spiritual processes of living that must be in harmony for a happy life. The introduction of modern drugs and psychotherapy techniques has not resulted in more people who are very happy with their lives than in the past. Psychologists know much about the psychosocial skills of people who are happy but know little about their biology or spirituality. Psychiatrists know much about the biomedical characteristics of people who are unhappy, but not those who are happy. No one has integrated the psychosocial and biomedical knowledge that is available about well-being in a coherent developmental perspective.

Fortunately, psychosocial and biomedical approaches to well-being can be fully integrated, as is done in this book for the first time. The path to well-being described here provides the foundation needed to transform human personality and cure mental disorders. This ambitious book is a holistic account of the principles and mechanisms underlying the path to the good life—that is, a life that is happy, harmonious, virtuous, and wise. "Feeling good" cannot be authentic or stable without "being good" because happiness is the effortless expression of coherent intuitions of the world. Authentic happiness requires a coherent way of living, including the human processes that regulate the sexual, material, emotional, intellectual, and spiritual aspects of experience. Sex, possessions, power, and friendships can be self-defeating or adaptive, depending on how aware people are of their goals and values. The degree of coherence of human thoughts and social relationships can be measured in terms of how well our thoughts and relationships lead to the harmony and happiness of the good life. This holistic approach quantifies the development of human self-awareness as a sequence of quantum-like steps, which has many implications for everyday life, neuroscience research, and the practice of mental health. Likewise, my own understanding of personality had to be expanded step by step in order to account for observed phenomena, such as self-awareness, free will, creativity, and quantum-like gifts of the mind and spirit that could not be explained otherwise. What eventually emerged is an integrated science of well-being that unifies all the traditional divisions of psychology, psychiatry, and neuroscience.

This book will interest a broad range of readers because of its wide scope. It is intended for all open-minded people who are interested in understanding as much as they can about basic human needs, consciousness, creativity, and well-being. It is written for the general reader as well as for students and practitioners in the fields of mental health.

The broad range of subject matter in the book required the writing to be accessible to any intelligent person because few people have expertise in all the fields into which it delves. Even experts in one field or another will find much that is new and provocative throughout the book. Each chapter contains all essential introductory material, as well as extensive references for further reading.

In addition to its broad scope, the book focuses in depth on the most fundamental questions about human life. What is good? Who am I really? How can I be happy and creative? These are questions for which there are no complete or simple answers. Those who think they already know the true answers will not want to read this book unless they are prepared to challenge their minds and reevaluate some cherished assumptions. On the other hand, those who recognize the inexhaustible nature of the mysteries embedded in these questions will enjoy the book. Useful general principles of living are described along with practical exercises for the mind to help in exploring the steps of the path to greater wisdom and well-being. Such exercises are essential to experience different levels of consciousness directly, rather than viewing them as abstract concepts. This book will also be of interest to theologians, philosophers, and social scientists because it provides contemporary scientific concepts and language for addressing the perennial human questions about being, knowledge, and conduct at the crux of civilized thought. It is designed to help each of us to reflect and ponder the basic questions that everyone has about healthy living. This book stimulates the reader to develop his or her own self-awareness without reliance on any external authority, including myself.

This is the first of several books I intend to write on the science of well-being. It is limited primarily to describing the foundations of normal development, especially the development of self-awareness. The assessment and treatment of mental disorders will be considered in more depth in a second book because the principles of well-being must be recognized before psychopathology can be effectively understood.

The path of development of self-aware consciousness is described here from several interdependent perspectives, including physics, genetics, physiology, psychology, sociology, and philosophy. However, my focus is on human psychobiology because no one can provide an adequate theory of everything. A broad range of biomedical and psychosocial sciences is synthesized here to provide a solid foundation from which to understand both normal and abnormal development. The principles derived from this foundation provide the clues that have long been needed for mental health to advance from a predominantly descriptive and empirical science to one that is founded solidly on a self-organizing theoretical understanding of the basic mechanisms of life.

Tentative intuitions about the mysteries of life are described and tested in rigorous scientific terms. Sometimes the metaphorical descriptions of transcendental writers provided inspiration when their terms could be translated into a scientific form that was measured, tested, and refined in a stepwise manner. It is wonderful to be living at a time when creative advances in science and culture allow a deep and inspiring understanding of what it means to be human. We now have the opportunity to examine old, universal, human questions within a current, quantitative, scientific framework.

*St. Louis, Missouri*                                                                C.R.C.

# ACKNOWLEDGMENTS

This book could not have been completed without the help of many others. Fiona Stevens and Jeff House at Oxford University Press provided lucid editorial advice and steadfast encouragement over many years. The Wallace Renard Professorship, the Sansone Family Center for Well-Being, and the U.S. National Institutes of Health gave stable support that allowed me to work in creative freedom. The collegial atmosphere characteristic of Washington University in St. Louis, particularly in the Departments of Psychiatry and Psychology, has been conducive to the integration of psychosocial and biomedical approaches. I have learned much from many colleagues all over the world, but especially the founding members of our local center, psychiatrist Dragan Svrakic, psychologist Richard Wetzel, anthropologist Tom Przybeck, physicist Nenad Svrakic, and administrator Gerri Wynne. Our commitment to open-minded inquiry into fundamental human issues in the Center for Well-Being continues the spirit I first experienced in Plan II at the University of Texas in Austin under the leadership of philosopher John Silber. Fortunately, the late psychiatrists Eli Robins and Samuel Guze wisely nurtured the same deep philosophical spirit in psychiatry at Washington University.

Writing this book has been a wonderful adventure shared with my family and friends. My parents Morris and Concetta taught me much about the principles of coherent living by the example of their own fully engaged lives. My wife, Sherry, and sons, Bryan and Kevin, are continual sources of inspiration and love as we all learn to follow the path of well-being together.

# CONTENTS

# INTRODUCTION

Within every person is a spontaneous need for happiness, understanding, and love, yet neither psychiatry nor psychology has been effective in understanding the steps that lead to such a happy life. In fact, these disciplines have almost exclusively studied the unhappy. Available treatments of mental problems are usually based on empirical discoveries that ignore the importance of growth in self-awareness for the development of well-being. Consequently, available treatments are palliative and incomplete, not curative. Most patients with common mental disorders remain ill with varying degrees of recurrent or chronic disability throughout their life despite conventional biomedical and psychosocial treatments. Available psychotropic drugs and psychosocial interventions are often effective for acute relief of some symptoms of mental disorder. Despite the use of modern therapies, however, there has been no overall increase in the proportion of people in the community who are happy and satisfied with their life.

The meager progress by psychiatry and psychology in understanding the science of well-being is in part related to a failure to integrate major advances in other fields of science. Some phenomena of human consciousness, such as creative gifts and free will, may be explainable only in terms of quantum physics. Nevertheless, most psychologists and psychiatrists assume people are essentially machines, like computers. The deterministic algorithms of computers cannot explain human creativity or freedom of will, which at least seem to be important to the happiness of self-aware individuals. The mental health field needs a general approach to describe and understand human consciousness that is compatible with the fundamental principles of quantum theory.

The mental health field also needs a way to describe and understand the regulation of human self-aware consciousness that is compatible with recent advances in psychobiology and neuroscience. Self-aware consciousness is the unique human ability to remember and reexperience the past in the immediacy of our own intuition. It is the basis for the awareness of one's self, the sense of subjective time, and recollection of personal events in the context of a particular place and time. Self-aware consciousness depends on the mature development of specific brain regions, such as the prefrontal cortex, that are well developed only in human beings. Quantitative methods of brain imaging have shown that the movement of thought in self-aware consciousness is synchronous with sudden transitions between discrete brain states. The transitions between discrete functional states of the brain depend on changing connections between distributed neural networks that span the whole brain. A human being is actually an integrated hierarchy of biological, psychological, and social systems that adapt to changes in context. The degree of adaptability of a person depends on his level of awareness of the context in which he lives. Awareness of context varies greatly between individual persons and within the same person at different times, frequently changing from moment to moment. Even at the level of individual cells in the brain, biologists have recently found that the regulation of gene expression is controlled by complex adaptive systems of learning and memory. The regulation of gene expression is described as "epigenetic" because it depends on information that is not translated into the proteins that make up the structure of the body and may be acquired through experience. In other words, the inheritance of acquired characteristics is essential to the adaptive development of cells in every organ system, especially the human brain. In contrast to the dynamic nature of human awareness and brain states, however, most psychologists and psychiatrists make the highly doubtful assumption that people can be diagnosed and treated as if they had fixed traits of psychological health or illness, such as a discrete diagnosis like major depressive disorder. The field of mental health is in great need of a fundamentally new system of assessment and classification that is dynamic and compatible with the fundamental findings of modern biology, genetics, and neuroscience. We need a new method for assessing self-aware consciousness that can explain personal growth and well-being as well as mental disorders.

Furthermore, the science of mental health must recognize that individuals operate within the context of the goals and values of society. In turn, self-aware human beings evaluate society within a spiritual context that is ultimately nondualistic. As people develop in maturity, they grow in the radius of their awareness of the many biological, psychological, and social influences on themselves and their relationships with others. The self-aware consciousness of a person progresses through a hierarchy of stages that leads to increasing levels of wisdom and well-being, as has been documented clearly in longitudinal psychosocial research. Consequently, the mental health field needs a method for describing self-awareness that recognizes its stage-like development.

In effect, the science of mental health has been stagnated by its division into two parts. The *biomedical* part studies the brain, whereas the *psychosocial* part studies the mind. Essentially these two approaches define two separate paradigms for understanding mental health and disease. The psychosocial approach is concerned with the *paradigm of the person* whose thoughts, feelings, and behaviors are understood mentally in terms of adaptive responses motivated by external and internal events. In contrast, the biomedical approach is concerned with the *paradigm of disease categories*, which are discrete entities described in terms of a set of causes, specific criteria for diagnosis, and predictable course of development. For example, in the first part of the twentieth century, psychoanalysis dominated the field of psychiatry based on its paradigm of the person. Later, the biomedical approach and categorical diagnosis began to dominate the field of psychiatry along with advances in basic neuroscience and psychopharmacology.

Unfortunately, each part of the science of mental health—that is, the paradigm of the person and the paradigm of disease categories—is an inadequate basis to understand the relations of the body and the mind. The psychosocial paradigm of the person has lacked a coherent model of the biomedical basis of mental processes. Likewise, the biomedical paradigm of discrete disease categories has been unable to identify any specific laboratory tests for any mental disorder or to develop any treatments that enhance self-awareness and well-being. Many psychoactive drugs are moderately effective for treating acute symptoms, and some reduce the risk of relapse as long as they are maintained on a long-term basis. However, no biomedical treatment cures a person of their vulnerability to future mental illness. Likewise, no biomedical treatments produce progressive improvement in character and satisfaction with the meaning of one's life.

Self-critical leaders of each approach have usually sought to integrate these two parts. For example, Emil Kraepelin studied with the experimental psychologist Wilhelm Wundt and wanted to integrate the understanding of emotional and intellectual processes using psychological, genetic, pharmacological, and anatomical techniques that were innovative for the time. Kraepelin originally thought that mental disorders could be explained as specific diseases that involved defects in specific brain regions, but toward the end of his career, he concluded that this was unlikely to be true. Likewise, Sigmund Freud originally wanted to establish the neurobiological basis for a scientific psychology but quickly recognized that the tools to do this were not available during his lifetime. Unfortunately, later followers of the disease category and personality paradigms have assumed that their approach provided an adequate explanation of the whole field.

Modern observers of the field have concluded that a science of well-being needs an approach that is neither mindless nor brainless. Studies of education suggest that psychologists and physicians can be trained in each approach. However, there are no required educational tasks that actually involve integration of biomedical and psychotherapeutic skills. As a result of such compartmentalized training, psychiatry and psychology are each divided into two parts, each inadequate alone and needing the other. These two parts have vacillated in dominance, while neglecting or deprecating the other part. I began my own training in the biomedical disease model but later began to study the psychology and biology of personality. My work on the psychology and biology of personality has allowed me to work on the development of a scientific synthesis that is designed to cut through the divisions that cripple the science of mental health. It was only later in my career that I was able to merge and integrate the paradigm of disease with the paradigm of the person.

My work on the integration of body and mind has required me to question my most basic assumptions about human nature. I found that there were two basic errors that have blocked the progress of a science of well-being; these basic errors are the fallacies of dualism and reductionism.

The first of these fallacies is the Cartesian error of separating the body and the mind. The Cartesian error can be corrected by recognizing what I call the path of the psyche. Human beings have a rich innate endowment that permits personality to develop preferentially along a common internally directed path, thereby facilitating communication among people despite great differences between individuals in their psychological experiences and biological background. I found that body–mind dualism could not be reconciled without recognition of this common path for the development of self-aware consciousness. Biomedical and psychosocial approaches to mental health are each merely steps in the path of development of self-awareness, which is ultimately nondualistic. Any expansion of self-aware consciousness involves an increase in intuitive understanding, which is at least in part free and creative. In other words, the human psyche follows a path made up of multiple steps, each of which is spontaneous to some degree. Psychological developments are spontaneous (i.e., "noncausal") when they are not fully determined by prior conditions or by algorithmic reasoning about prior knowledge. The path of the psyche cannot be adequately specified in dualistic terms like those that dominate contemporary psychiatry and psychology because of the importance of noncausal phenomena like creativity and free will.

The available fragments of the science of mental health have all lacked an integrative, comprehensive model of the path of the human psyche. Nevertheless, the path of the psyche has been repeatedly documented in descriptive terms for over a century in rigorous studies of emotional reactivity and detailed longitudinal studies of character development. Only recently have the scientific tools for studying the genetics of personality, functional brain imaging, and statistical dynamics been available to measure and understand the mechanisms underlying individual differences in the development of well-being.

The second error blocking the progress of the science of well-being is the Aristotelian fallacy of reducing thought to the algorithmic processing of physical sensations. The Aristotelian fallacy of reductive determinism can be corrected by recognition of the primary role of intuition in self-aware consciousness. Recent studies of learning in children, ordinary self-aware cognition in adults, and human creativity show that intuition is actually the initial step in thought, not the final product of prior reasoning and analysis. Even standard dictionaries define *intuition* as immediate awareness without reasoning. Intuition is characterized by the holistic preverbal recognition on which subsequent labeling, reasoning, and emotional responses are based. No reasoning or objective demonstrations can communicate the subjective qualities of intuitive recognition, such as the taste of honey or the joy of love. The empirical findings of modern cognitive neuroscience confirm the importance of rational intuition as the initial foundation for self-awareness of what is true, just as was recognized clearly by Plato, but not by his student Aristotle.

In fact, intellectual reasoning is actually an intermediate level of self-aware consciousness, which always depends on rational intuition. There is a hierarchy of stages in the development of self-aware consciousness, which involve distinct psychosomatic processes. As a result, human consciousness is not a homogeneous phenomenon. In the absence of self-aware consciousness, human thought is dominated by the algorithmic processing of physical sensations. In the higher stages of self-aware consciousness, however, human thought becomes increasingly creative and intuitive. Much discussion and research about human consciousness have been confused by failure to specify the stage of self-awareness under consideration. I planned this book to provide an orderly account of what is known and what we need to know about the psychology and biology of each of the distinct stages of development of human consciousness.

This book has a few interrelated goals. My fundamental goal is to describe a unified and nonreductive approach to understanding the path of development of human self-aware consciousness, which I call the path of the psyche. *Psyche* is the Greek word for "life, soul, or spirit," as distinguished from *soma*, which refers to the "body." In my opinion, recognition of the path of the psyche is essential for an adequate approach to psychology and psychiatry, which are the study and treatment of the psyche, and for an adequate understanding of human psychological health and illness.

To explore and investigate this new approach, I describe the steps in observation and thinking that led me along my own personal path of discovery. Because I progressed by identifiable steps in my prior publications, this will help readers who may be familiar with parts of my work along the way. It will also clarify what observations forced me to develop a change in perspective. Changing one's basic assumptions is never easy; there is always some inertia and resistance to change. It may be helpful for others to see what forced me to make changes to account for available facts, so that others will not need to persist in the mistakes I made. Of course, others may not agree with my solutions and will be able to weigh the adequacy of my solutions by seeing clearly my motives and the basis for my conclusions. I hope others can go along with me as I recollect my own journey because only personal or vicarious experience leads to insight. Because of the human gift of self-aware consciousness, vicarious experiences like reading a book can have a real impact on the reader's personal development.

I originally set out to write a book on personality in 1987 shortly after I developed a model of human temperament. I started over in 1993 when I realized that my model was inadequate without the addition of character dimensions. In 1997 I restarted for a third time when I realized that temperament and character were inadequate without consideration of how they are coherently integrated by intuition in self-aware consciousness. Finally, in the last few years I recognized that recent developments in the quantitative measurement of thought, brain imaging, genetics, and the statistical dynamics of complex adaptive systems provided an adequate way of describing and testing my intuitions about the science of well-being in rigorous scientific terms.

Each of the biopsychosocial foundations of the science of well-being is examined in this book. Individual chapters add a component to the foundation, beginning with a brief history of the philosophy of well-being to provide an overview of basic questions that need to be explored scientifically. I suggest that each chapter be read as a sequence of discourses or seminars for discussion and reflection. There is much to consider and to assimilate in each chapter. Such personal study should be done calmly and freely at one's own pace. I suggest that the most useful approach is a quest for a partial deepening of our understanding of questions about which we keep an open mind, rather than fixed judgment or unquestioning acceptance. If considered as a contemplative study, the reading of the book could be a stimulus for personal growth in self-awareness, which is the crux of any serious study of human consciousness. When discussing self-awareness, you must live what you are studying to be able to say anything with true understanding. Such growth in self-aware consciousness through reflection, meditation, and contemplation are the three stages of self-aware consciousness. Each of these stages is essential to prepare yourself to apply the principles of the science of well-being in clinical practice with efficacy and compassion.

I have found that the development of human consciousness involves movement in a nested hierarchy of complex adaptive systems. This hierarchy progresses from the quantum states of inanimate matter to epigenetic states of cellular life, brain states of the body, ego states of the self, moral states of members of society, and ultimately the creative states of human self-aware consciousness. Consequently, a rigorous understanding of the hierarchical development of human self-aware consciousness builds on many prior advances in physics, genetics, psychophysiology, psychology, sociology, and philosophy. Each successive step in this nested hierarchy is a dynamic system that provides the context for the prior step, providing a bridge from inanimate matter to nondualistic consciousness. Likewise, each chapter in this book is designed to provide a framework for reflection, meditation, and contemplation in a particular order that may help people to discover and understand their fundamental assumptions about the nature of reality, consciousness, and well-being.

It is noteworthy that both the beginning and the end of the hierarchy of life systems are enfolded within one another and have the quantum properties of spontaneity ("noncausality") and inseparability ("nonlocality"). In contrast, the intermediate steps involve dynamic systems with "small-world" properties, which are quantum like (but not quantum) in their dynamics. The basic idea of a small world is that apparently distant events can have widespread effects rapidly, as in the popular notion that there are only "six degrees of separation" between any two people. In fact, such small-world dynamics really are characteristic of most living systems, including both biomedical and psychosocial networks.

These biopsychosocial foundations provide a solid theoretical basis on which to base the principles of clinical practice that lead to well-being. Accordingly, I describe some techniques of clinical assessment and treatment that other mental health practitioners can learn to promote well-being in thought and in relationships. Some of these techniques are briefly described in this book on the biopsychosocial foundations of the science of well-being. The clinical methods of the science of well-being will be considered in more depth in a second book on psychopathology and its causes and treatment. These are the same methods I have found to be successful in my own active clinical practice, in my teaching about the science of well-being in our residency program at Washington University, and in lectures and workshops elsewhere for both professionals and nonprofessionals. However, what I have written allows a more thorough presentation of both the principles and the practice of the science of well-being than is practical in individual lectures or workshops. I hope that what I have written will allow more people to begin to study this scientific paradigm and clinical method on their own.

The methods of the science of well-being have greatly enhanced the reliability and depth of my clinical assessments. They have also resulted in much more rapid and effective treatment even with patients who were unresponsive to other approaches. In contrast to the dualistic concepts and techniques about mental health that are now often taught, the techniques I will describe in this book are fundamentally nondualistic and based on the primacy of intuition in the development of human relationships and self-aware consciousness. Soma and psyche exist in an irreducible correspondence with one another. *At every step in psychological development, there is synchronous correspondence between the development of our spiritual values, our social relationships, our thoughts, and our brain states as we move along the path of self-awareness to well-being.*

I hope that the skills that develop with growing self-awareness will allow mental health practitioners to understand and value the contributions of observations by investigators in the many diverse fields that contribute to the science of well-being. To understand human consciousness, we must understand that its foundations are embedded in physics, genetics, physiology, psychology, sociology, and philosophy. Together the findings of these many fields provide a wonderful foundation for ongoing discovery of the limitless mysteries of human development. I have tried to present the key findings of each field without assuming that the reader has previous training, experience, or knowledge. Nevertheless, to appreciate its amazing opportunities, psychology and psychiatry must undergo a paradigm shift as revolutionary as that made by quantum physicists nearly a century ago. My style of presentation is to be as clear and open as I can about my conclusions and their basis. I do this with the intention of stimulating others to reflect on their own assumptions, rather than to persuade others that I am right. In fact, I do not want you to agree with me. I would prefer that you disagree with me whenever your own intuitions differ from mine, so that you can recognize the questions about which you find that additional study is most needed by all of us.

We all know from repeated experience that even a carefully reasoned argument usually fails to elevate the level of another person's self-aware consciousness. Occasionally a reasoned argument will help someone recollect other facts they regard as certain or to reduce contradictions among various personal beliefs. However, insight is always intuitive. We can be led to new considerations by reasoning, but insight is always based on intuition and not on reasoning or experimental demonstrations. If reasoning or experimental results are inconsistent with our world view, we simply reject them with a statement like, "It must be wrong because (I think) it is impossible." Paradoxically, the resistance of a person to insights beyond their intuitive recognition is actually evidence of the hierarchical nature of self-awareness. Such resistance to reasoned arguments and empirical evidence is also strong evidence of the primacy of intuition in human self-aware consciousness.

Sadly, many people do not recognize this paradox and vehemently reject the reality of what they have not experienced intuitively. In contrast, let me say now that my world view is certainly incomplete and may contain errors of logic or fact of which I am currently unaware. I know I have frequently been wrong in the past and had to change my viewpoint and my conclusions repeatedly. I hope my ongoing process of discovery will continue as long as I am alive. Nevertheless, I have tried to state my observations and conclusions as clearly and emphatically as I felt to be justified, so that others may understand my thinking and disagree with me in developing their own self-awareness. What I find most valuable is the joy and well-being inherent in the unending process of discovery. If you experience that joy of discovery and insight in participating in this contemplative journey with me, then I will have communicated the spirit of the science of well-being. It is insight into the spirit of well-being that I hope to share, not fragmentary facts or opinions.

This work is a synthesis of what I have learned from many people in many fields throughout my life. Many, but not all, of these influences are co-authors of publications cited throughout the book. However, the basic ideas of the positive philosophers whose work I describe are a perennial heritage of all human beings. Whenever we seek to understand basic questions about life, consciousness, and human development, we find that others have repeatedly asked essentially the same questions. We are all on a common path in search of well-being. My only originality may be in beginning to communicate a contemporary idiom for expressing these perennial ideas so that they can be tested with scientific rigor and applied with clinical efficacy.

# Feeling Good

# 1

# A BRIEF PHILOSOPHY OF WELL-BEING

## THE BASIC TRIAD OF HUMAN NEEDS

People differ markedly from one another in the depth of their understanding of themselves and their relationships. Nevertheless, all human beings have a need for increasing coherence of personality, which can only come from growth in self-awareness. Consequently, people differ greatly in the degree to which they are wise and happy.

Even when people are currently happy, they want to understand how they can maintain and increase their satisfaction. Whether people are being treated for major mental disorders or are successful in their work and personal life, every-one ultimately seeks three inseparable goals in their life—greater well-being, self-understanding, and coherence. Concerning well-being, people ask, "How can I be happy?" or, more abstractly, "What is good?" or "How can I find God?" Concerning understanding, people may ask, "Who am I really?" or "What is life?" or "What is truth?" Concerning coherence, we may ask, "How can I have a healthier balance between work, play, and love in my life?" or "What do I really love?" or "What is beauty?" The words may vary but the essence of the questions about being, knowledge, or conduct remains the same. Human beings seek answers to these questions as their basis for the goals and values of life. Even the thera-pists, teachers, and philosophers who deal with these questions in their professions need help from others to cope with their personal fears, struggles, and lack of awareness.

The study of the individual differences in self-aware consciousness may be called the *science of well-being*, the *science of consciousness*, or the *science of personality*. The three names are synonymous because well-being, wisdom, and coherence of personality all depend on the level of a person's growth along the same path of development.

Because of the vast scope of human consciousness, the science of well-being rests on an orderly foundation made up of a hierarchy of information of increasing complexity—physics, genetics, physiology, psychology, sociology, and philosophy. Each of these layers of the foundation will be examined in subsequent individual chapters and then integrated in the final chapter.

Philosophy is unique in its systematic consideration of the whole of being, that is, all of what actually and potentially exists. A philosophy of life provides answers to the three fundamental human questions about being, knowledge, and conduct. Philosophy is literally the "love of wisdom," so its contributions to understanding consciousness and well-being are substantial. Wisdom is traditionally defined as the understanding of the truth, which leads to a life of virtue and well-being. Everyone wants to be happy, so it is natural for humans to seek wisdom. However, extensive empirical information shows that a radical transformation of self-aware consciousness is required to develop well-being, wisdom, and coherence.

Philosophy and science share a common focus on truth. Philosophy is the love of truth, and science is the knowledge of truth. Science literally means "knowledge," but knowledge that is not true is misunderstanding, not science. From this perspective, well-being requires the development of a scientific form of consciousness. Science is not mere empiricism, nor is it theoretical abstraction. In its full development, science goes beyond the loving search for truth to the immediate and effortless awareness of truth, as noted by Hegel in his *Phenomenology of Spirit* (1807). According to Hegel, true science leads to *wisdom*, which can be defined as the intuitive awareness of what is good, true, and beautiful. Scientific consciousness is a self-awareness that integrates facts about life with the spiritual good of virtue and the emotional good of happiness.

The search for self-understanding distinguishes human beings uniquely from all other animals. It is normal for people to search for an ever-more coherent understanding of themselves and of the world in which they live (Jung 1933; Jaspers 1951; Winnicott 1958; Frankl 1959; Kohut 1984). The human need for coherence has been called the "unitive sense" (Teilhard de Chardin 1978). People experience emptiness or the lack of coherence as strongly unpleasant and unsatisfying. In contrast, the freedom and love involved in coherent living are pleasant (Teilhard de Chardin 1978; Rogers 1980; Cervone and Shoda 1999).

Similarly, human beings have been described as "evolution conscious of itself"(Huxley 1959). Life seems to evolve along a path of ever-increasing awareness leading to recognition of cosmic coherence (Teilhard de Chardin 1959), which is also called the *universal unity of being*. We humans have an irresistible need to understand our nature, including our drive for boundless self-awareness. By recognizing what motives give rise to happiness and what motives give rise to unhappiness, we can learn how to live well.

Given the importance of self-awareness for human well-being, it is perhaps amazing that the nature of consciousness and self-awareness remains largely a mystery. It is useful to specify a few definitions for sake of clarity. First, *awareness* is a synonym for *consciousness*. According to standard dictionaries, consciousness is defined as awareness of one's existence, sensations, and thoughts. Furthermore, the words *aware* and *conscious* both refer to our sense of recognition of something in relation to our self. However, the word *conscious* emphasizes the state of inner realization, whereas the word *aware* emphasizes the intuitive feelings associated with inner recognition. A third word, *cognizant*, emphasizes outer recognition on the level of reason and intellectual knowledge rather than on the level of intuitive feelings.

Animals other than humans have some level of consciousness in the sense that they may be awake and responsive to sensory input in an adaptive manner. However, only human beings have self-awareness (Povinelli 2000; Tulving 2002). Some great apes can learn to recognize themselves in a mirror, but all normal human beings do this spontaneously without an external mirror.

Thus, a crucial feature of human consciousness is self-awareness, which by definition depends on intuition. According to standard dictionaries, *intuition* is defined as immediate apprehension, or direct perception and recognition, independent of any reasoning process. In other words, intuition is an inner sense or senses that act like an in-built mirror of our self and the world in which we live. Reasoning may be helpful in refining our understanding, but intuition provides the recognition of information about which we reason. Human cognition characteristically begins with information that is recognized by intuition. Infants have active intuitions about themselves and the world before the development of formal reasoning ability.

The controversies that surround the mystery of consciousness are expected because there are substantial differences among people in their level of self-awareness. Intuitions carry with them certainty of conviction, so people tend to believe what they think is true even when others disagree. Also, people often ignore or deny what is beyond their own capacity or experience, just as someone who is deaf may have difficulty understanding and accepting the concepts of sound and music except by analogies that are incomplete. Consequently, we need a way to systematize information about variability in levels of self-awareness. Such organization requires a general theory of the nature of self-awareness that is experimentally testable. Otherwise we remain enmeshed in endless controversies based on different intuitions about the nature of consciousness.

Although intuitions usually have a quality of certainty or truth, they can be fallible, much as reasoning or experimental observations can be false. Therefore, our intuition must be purified so that it is not biased by our fears and expectations, just as experimental observations need to be made under conditions that are unbiased. Intuition, reasoning, and experimentation are complementary processes by which we can arrive at reproducible scientific findings. A science of human consciousness and self-awareness must integrate an understanding of the ways that processes of intuition, reasoning, and observation are interrelated in both healthy and abnormal development. We need to know how we can develop pure rational intuition.

## HOW CAN WE BE HAPPY?

Everyone wants to be happy, but many people are dissatisfied with their life. In fact, most people are even confused about what can make them happy. Most people are unable to predict their future emotional responses accurately (Kahneman, Diener et al. 1999; Loewenstein and Schkade 1999). Our rationalistic disciplines of psychology, medicine, and religion teach that a civilized human being must learn to delay gratification of immediate desires for sake of future happiness. We are taught to postpone happiness, whereas what we really want is to be happy and to stay that way. People want to understand how to be happy and peaceful regardless of their external circumstances.

Most people prefer happiness rather than extrinsic achievements, such as fame, wealth, or social status (Myers 1992; Diener, Lucas et al. 2002). There is confusion over what constitutes happiness because of uncertainty about how to achieve intrinsic satisfaction and discrepancies between different measures of happiness (Larsen and Fredrickson 1999). For example, in a 2000 work on emotions, four concepts of happiness have been distinguished, as described in Table 1.1 (Averill and More). These differ in their level of arousal or their degree of objectivity. With regard to arousal, happiness can range from states of low activation (e.g., contentment or equanimity) to high activation (e.g., joy or eudaemonia). With regard to objectivity, happiness can range from subjective internal states (e.g., joy or contentment) to objective external activities (e.g., eudaemonia or equanimity). *Eudaemonia*, which means well-being or happiness, is derived from a Greek term meaning "to have a happy, good, or true spirit." It is what Aristotle called the "good life" and Augustine called the "happy life."

These modern ideas about happiness are rooted in early Greek philosophy of the mind, particularly the work of Aristotle. For Aristotle, happiness was the result of an active life governed by reason, as noted in Table 1.1. Such a good life was gratifying as a result of its being meaningful, achievable, and sustainable with effort and discipline. Aristotle's concept of happiness is dualistic and therefore incom-

**Table 1.1.** Four Concepts of Happiness

| | *Degree of Objectivity* | |
|---|---|---|
| *Level of Arousal* | *Subjective (Feeling Good)* | *Objective (Doing Well)* |
| | JOY | EUDAEMONIA |
| High | "Rejoice ye in that day and leap for joy." (Luke 6:23) | "If we are right in our view and happiness is assumed to be acting well, the active life will be the best." (Aristotle) |
| | CONTENTMENT | EQUANIMITY |
| Low | "What is the happy life? It is peace of mind, and lasting tranquility." (Seneca) | "Marvel at nothing—that is perhaps the only thing, Numicius, that can make a man happy and keep him so." (Horace) |

Luke is from New Testament
(Aristotle 1984) Politics, Book VII
(Seneca 1962) Ad Lucillium, Epis. XCII
(Horace 1966) Epistle VI
*Source*: Reprinted with permission from Averill, J. R. and T. A. More. (2000). Happiness. *Handbook of emotions*, 2nd ed. M. Lewis and J. M. Haviland-Jones, eds. New York, Guilford Press: 663–676. Copyright 2000.

plete, but more coherent than the desire for pleasure. Hedonism is an incoherent concept of happiness, because the insatiability of desire conflicts with the limitations of our physical capacities and mental powers.

Consequently, approaches to the science of happiness based on the rationalism of Aristotle seek to identify goals for people that are meaningful, productive, and restrained. For example, people may be taught to reframe their attitudes toward work, play, and love so that they are regarded as meaningful to oneself and beneficial to others (Frankl 1959; Rogers 1980; Seligman 2002). Aristotelian approaches to modern positive psychology teach that we should accept and idealize what is practical, even if this involves a positive illusion. Such a dualistic approach (Seligman 2002) unfortunately leads to the contradiction that the basis for "authentic" happiness is illusion and not the consciousness of reality.

Aristotle had a different understanding of how to be happy than did his teacher, Plato. According to Plato (Cornford 1941) and then Augustine (Augustine 400a), conduct is properly directed to the Good, which leads to living in virtue. The Good is the sole condition and guarantee of well-being. The Good is the ultimate end, or purpose, of living because it is desired for itself alone, whereas everything else is desired as a means to the Good. The only invariant source of happiness is awareness of the universal unity of being. In other words, virtue is its own reward, whereas honor, glory, money, and other extrinsic satisfactions are only indirect and inconsistent means to happiness, as has been confirmed in modern experimental research (Myers 1992; Myers and Diener 1996; Diener, Lucas et al. 2002).

Naturally, if a person has love of himself, he must wish for well-being. What makes well-being possible? According to Plato and Augustine, living in virtue was only possible for one who recognized the coherence of the universal unity of being and who sought to understand the truth of this unity through love. Love does not involve renunciation or rejection of any aspect of living. The coherence of the universal unity of being is what Plato called the Good and Augustine called God. Therefore, to be wise, to be a philosopher, to have well-being, and to love oneself was to love what was good and true and thereby to live in virtue and happiness.

According to Plato and Augustine (Augustine 386), only a life of virtue and boundless love gives permanent well-being in which there is increasing peace and joy as others grow in their well-being. Hence Plato and Augustine made clear that the growing boundlessness of love was the essential path to well-being. Augustine's pithy words in the *City of God* (Book 10, Chapter 4) are especially revealing for parents, for teachers, and for therapists in mental health: "To this Good we must be led by those who love us, and to it we must lead those whom we love" (400a).

According to Plato, the use of rational intuition is necessary to know the Good because God is the eternal and incorruptible essence of Goodness, Truth, and Beauty. God is immaterial and hence is beyond the grasp of the physical senses. Plato emphasized the role of prenatal awareness or innate recollection of the true essence of things as the basis of induction by intuition. According to Plato, people differ at birth in their intuitive ability to recollect the essence of things, such as their abilities in mathematics or music. The essence of something is the true reality underlying physical appearances. In modern psychology, excellence in recollection is called *giftedness*. We are aware of the essence of things by means of gifts of the intuitive senses, whereas we are aware of outward appearances using our physical senses. According to Plato, our response to education depends on our intuitive gifts as well as on our experiences.

## ARISTOTLE'S ERRORS

Later Aristotle suggested that well-being was the result of a life guided by reason. He emphasized the importance of practical demonstrations in experience as a source of induction of the axioms and principles that guide living (Barnes 1984). Aristotle recognized the need for both induction and deduction by the intellect, and he recognized that induction was an intuitive process. Like his teacher, he knew that individuals differ in their intuitive gifts, but, unlike Plato, he emphasized practical experience rather than purification of intuition as the basis for recognizing truth.

Aristotle did not recognize the importance of intuition in guiding behavior. Reason has a finite capacity to process the overabundance of information given in experience (Simon 1990). In addition, intuition is needed to discover and recognize the categories and schemas—that is, axioms and principles—from which reason draws its deductions. As a result, reliance on reason without the enlightenment of intuition leads to conflict and contradiction in life, rather than virtue, wisdom, and well-being. When we really see the truth, we know what to do and proceed happily without hesitation, choice, or conflict. However, the seeing of truth depends on insight, and not on fragmentary empirical demonstrations, observations, and analysis.

Aristotle's emphasis on reason and empirical demonstration is closely related to his assumption that nature is a composite of many independent substances, which are causally yet also contingently related. In Aristotle's world view, the universe has a more-or-less loosely knit order that is observable using the physical senses and understandable using reason. According to Aristotle, the universe is *not* fundamentally an inseparable whole. In contrast, Plato and other nondualistic philosophers, such as Augustine and Spinoza, assume that nature is fundamentally an inseparable whole and that this universal unity is intelligible by intuition.

The failure to recognize the universal unity of being has profound consequences for understanding human thought and behavior. The most universal idea in human thought is unity, which is also referred to as nonduality, inseparability, or nonlocality. Likewise, the idea of being is the most inclusive of terms, including all actual and potential forms of existence. Hence dualism rejects the unity of being as a fundamental characteristic of the universe, and this rejection has profound and pervasive consequences for philosophy and psychology.

A major consequence of Aristotle's dualism was his assumption of a mechanical model of causation, or what may be called *reductive determinism*. According to Aristotle, the world is fundamentally composed of many independent substances. Whatever degree of unity that occurs in the world is derived from the order and connections imposed on its components by their causal interactions with one another, and freedom is the result of contingency and chance. According to Aristotle, the world is like a machine, which is nothing but a number of individual substances arranged in a certain way. The universe as a whole has no intrinsic form.

In contrast, for Plato, following the Good gave rise to personal freedom, because freedom is an inherent property of the self-existing primal Unity, which has no constraining antecedent causes. Later, Spinoza (1955) clearly formulated the Platonic viewpoint that true freedom can be a property only of unitary self-existing substance, which is the universal source of all things. For Spinoza, the unity of being is the infinite substance from which all things originate and to which they return. In this way, everything is both free and necessary, one and many, nonlocal and dispersed without conflict or contradiction. The infinite source is free, whole, and indivisible, whereas the finite parts contained within it have a particular order, multiplicity, and dispersion in space-time. According to Plato and Spinoza, human beings are free and virtuous to the extent to which they live according to what is true, and what is true is intelligible by intuition and reason operating in concert.

Augustine later clarified Aristotle's account of information processing by reaffirming the importance of intuition guiding reason and the existence of differences between individuals in their intuitive gifts or recollection of the universal essences underlying particular experiences (Augustine 386, 400a, 400b, 400c) . During the Renaissance, Leonardo da Vinci (MacCurdy 1938), and later Bacon (Bacon 1620) and Pascal (Pascal 1662; O'Connell 1997) during the Enlightenment, clarified the complementary role of intuition and experimentation in developing certainty about the validity of our interpretations of experience. However, most of science from the Middle Ages through the present has perpetuated Aristotle's rationalistic tendency to emphasize observation and demonstration over intuition, as well as dualism over the unity of being.

Modern research on information processing has provided more support for Plato's theory of knowledge than for that of Aristotle. As in the theories of knowledge described by Plato, Augustine, da Vinci, and Spinoza, intuition is recognized as essential for discovering the gist of what is happening (Brainerd, Reyna et al. 1990; Bjorklund 1997; Miller and Bjorklund 1998; Reyna and Brainerd 1998). Such intuitive recognition is necessary before reasoning or experimentation. Intuition is essential for efficiency of living, which is not in practice based on exhaustive analysis of all logical possibilities in experience. Intuition is not always correct since our recollection is always finite and imperfect. The degree of imperfection in intuition varies among individuals according to their giftedness in particular domains. Experimentation and love of truth allow us to test and clarify our intuition. Hence, the proper use of our intellect requires the purification of rational intuition.

Nevertheless, the dualistic and rationalistic interpretation of Aristotle has usually been followed in modern versions of the psychology of happiness, as shown in Table 1.1 (Averill and More 2000). In modern positive psychology, eudaemonia has been described as full engagement and optimal performance of meaningful behavior, which is a dualistic concept of well-being. I will not use the term *eudaemonia* because its etymology suggests unnecessary metaphysical assumptions and its modern interpretation makes questionable dualistic assumptions. Instead, I will use the term *well-being* to refer to a stable condition of coherence of personality that leads to a full range of positive emotions and no negative emotions regardless of external circumstances. In my view, full well-being requires coherence, which transcends the dualistic distinction of the subjective and the objective.

My nondualistic approach is consistent with that of Plato because the aspects of coherence include virtue, wisdom, and well-being. My approach differs from dualistic approaches that try to base well-being on rationality without cultivating intuitive wisdom or that try to base happiness on the pursuit of extrinsic satisfactions like pleasure, honor, wealth, or other selfish desires. However, dualistic approaches still have much popularity in contemporary thought, so the differences between dualistic and nondualistic approaches are considered in more depth in what follows.

## THE WAY OF POSITIVE PHILOSOPHERS

The path to well-being described by Plato, Augustine, and Spinoza is not unique to a few philosophers. There has been a long succession of "lovers of wisdom" with similar basic assumptions. Lovers of wisdom will be called positive philosophers because they have had a positive view of human potential as well as a constructive role in the cultural advance of civilization. All positive philosophers have been drawn to the same core of beliefs about being, knowledge, and conduct. No one can fully state the inexhaustible mysteries of Truth, but some key assumptions can help to point us toward it. The basic assumptions about being, knowledge, and conduct that are shared by highly positive philosophers are summarized in Table 1.2.

Regarding being, positive philosophy recognizes a universal unity of all that actually or potentially exists. In other words, everything is interrelated and inseparable. This does not mean that there is no observable diversity in the various manifestations of being. Rather, there is great diversity in space and time, but all things are interrelated because they originate from a common source beyond space and time. In modern physics, this unity and inseparability is called "nonlocality." According to quantum field theory, all things are fundamentally inseparable because there is a universal field of energy and information from which all things originate and return (Bohm and Hiley 1993). In fact, there is strong experimental evidence for nonlocality, which is discussed in more depth in Chapters 3 and 5. The appearance of duality or independence of things is an approximation that breaks down when we consider the equivalence of mass and energy, quantum phenomena, or the uniformity of natural laws throughout the universe (Gamow 1966; Bouwmeester, Pan et al. 1997; Weihs, Jennewein et al. 1998; Walker 2000).

How, then, does the nondualist understand the incoherence that is observable in everyday life, such as the differences between good and evil, or the lack of unity

**Table 1.2.** Basic Assumptions of Positive Philosophy

1. *Being*: Monism (universal unity of being): All things that actually or potentially exist are indivisibly related through a common universal source.
2. *Knowledge*: Wisdom and rationality are the immediate and effortless consequences of self-awareness leading to coherence of rational intuition.
3. *Conduct*: Rational enjoyment of life and selfless love are the spontaneous expression of freedom of will by a self-aware being.

in function between the human body and mind? The positive philosophers Plato and Augustine were clear that all things are derived from the Good. Spinoza (1955) assumed that reality was synonymous with perfection. Then how can there be evil? According to the positive philosophers, what is evil is good in essence but has been perverted to oppose its natural function as a result of human pride and ignorance (Augustine 386). This perversion is ignorance because it leads to loss of well-being and ultimately is self-defeating because it does not involve love of the reality that all things are dependent on one infinite and perfect source.

Nevertheless, the perversion of nature is possible because of the human gift of free will, and the permissibility of such perversion is good to allow us to voluntarily grow in awareness from experience. The alternative absence of freedom is not good because we would be mechanically determined—robots without responsibility and the dignity that comes with responsibility. According to Hegel (1807), we need an exhaustive experience of all reality to purify our consciousness of any misunderstanding, such as recognition of the misleading appeal of selfish pleasure, wealth, and honor as a means to well-being. According to Ibn Al'Arabi (Bayrak 1997), the secret of the opposition of good and evil is that human beings need to realize that well-being only arises when we recognize that what is truly satisfying and what is good have one source. To stimulate the full realization of nondualistic consciousness, opposing stimuli must be very strong, as is the case for the human drives for pleasure, wealth, and honor. These strong desires are self-centered and provide immediate but transient satisfaction that only leads to more desire without growth in the stable sense of well-being. Evil often disguises itself as good. Nevertheless, experience with the insatiability of selfish desire can provoke awareness of the source of true satisfaction. That the only real and stable understanding must come from direct experience has long been recognized. In *Meccan Revelations*, Al'Arabi wrote,

> Knowledge of mystical states can only be had by actual experience, nor can the reason of man define it, nor arrive at any cognizance of it by deduction, as is also the case with knowledge of the taste of honey, the bitterness of patience, the bliss of sexual union, love, passion or desire, all of which cannot possibly be known unless one be properly qualified or experience them directly. (Al'Arabi 1980, page 25)

According to positive philosophers, the human body and the human mind are derived from the same source, so they should function in unity. The mind and the brain are neither independent nor the same; the mind and the brain are coordinated phenomena derived from one universal source. However, without conscious awareness of the potential mind–body coherence, there is resistance to the natural unity in function inherent in the universal unity of being. Spinoza (1955) made a clear effort to show that Descartes's (1650) assumption that the body and mind were independent substances involved errors in logic and understanding. According to Spinoza (1955), two infinite and independent substances cannot co-exist, so dualism is an inadequate view of the cosmic order.

Regarding knowledge, positive philosophy assumes that human intuition allows the immediate perception of truths, which are aspects of the universal unity. The stepwise increase in awareness of truth allows us to become increasingly wise or coherent in our understanding. This growth is based on the intuitive perception of truth, which is facilitated by reasoning but does not depend on it. When there is immediate awareness of what is true, there is no interest in what is untrue and hence maladaptive.

According to the coherence theory of truth, the coherence of the relationships within a totality assures that our pure intuition is rational (Lehrer 1990). Such rationality excludes any interest in the pursuit of immediate gratification that is harmful for self or others. Such rationality is spontaneous and effortless. For example, Gandhi stated that he always made decisions coherently, integrating intuition and reason; he said, "It is true that I do not depend upon my intellect to decide upon any action. For me the reasoned course of action is held in check subject to the sanction of the inner voice" (Iyer 1999, page 231). In other words, pure rational intuition is another way of describing integrated intelligence in which there is "harmonious growth of body, mind, and soul" (Iyer 1999, page 392).

Regarding conduct, positive philosophy assumes that growing self-awareness leads to freedom of one's will from past conditioning. As we grow in wisdom, we grow in adaptive flexibility and in serenity. Our will is less and less influenced by the past and increasingly influenced by what is true and adaptive in the present. As our awareness of the cosmic order increases, our freedom is naturally expressed as rational enjoyment of life, which includes heightened awareness of all our senses (physical and intuitive) as well as selfless love and service to others rather than self-centered motives. Consequently, the free person is also selflessly impartial and satisfied.

These basic assumptions about being, knowledge, and conduct point us toward the essence of the thought of positive philosophers throughout the ages, regardless of culture or religion. The positive philosophers find firm support from modern studies of physics, neurobiology, cognition, and well-being, which we examine throughout this book. At the present, I only want to make the basic assumptions clear and point out that positive philosophers have played an instrumental role in the advance of human civilization.

A partial listing of the most influential positive philosophers is given in Table 1.3. For example, we find the descriptions of human life as a journey of discovery and a quest for wisdom and well-being in the writings of Homer and the Jewish prophets during antiquity. A little later we find the positive philosophy described by Plato in Greece during its Classical Age (Cornford 1941) and by Al-Ghazali in Arabia during its Golden Age (Al-Ghazali 1978, 1979, 2000). We observe the positive philosophy again in the work of Petrarch and Leonardo during the Renaissance (MacCurdy 1938; Petrarch 1995). We find it embodied by Montaigne, Spinoza, and Voltaire during the Enlightenment (Voltaire 1927; Spinoza 1955; Montaigne

**Table 1.3.** A Chronology of Some of the Highly Positive Philosophers Who Have Made Outstanding Contributions to Civilization since Antiquity (1000 BC)

| Philosopher | Location | Time Period |
|---|---|---|
| ANTIQUITY | | |
| David | Israel | 1035–962 BC |
| Elijah | Israel | 927–840 BC |
| Homer | Greece | 8th C. BC |
| Isaiah | Israel | 777–680 BC |
| Jeremiah | Israel | 649–570 BC |
| | | |
| GREEK CLASSICAL AGE | | |
| Pythagoras | Greece | 575–500 BC |
| Phidias | Greece | 493–430 BC |
| Plato | Greece | 428–348 BC |
| Diogenes | Greece | 400–320 BC |
| Archimedes | Greece | 287–212 BC |
| | | |
| NEOPLATONISM AND CHRISTIANITY IN THE ROMAN EMPIRE | | |
| Cicero | Italy | 106–43 BC |
| Plutarch | Greece/Rome | 46–119 AD |
| Clement | Egypt | 150–215 AD |
| Iamblichus | Syria | 250–330 AD |
| Augustine | Africa | 354–430 AD |
| Benedict | Italy | 480–547 AD |
| | | |
| ARABIC GOLDEN AGE | | |
| Ali | Arabia | 600–661 AD |
| Al-Farabi | Turkistan | 878–950 AD |
| Al-Biruni | Afghanistan | 973–1048 AD |
| Al-Ghazali | Iran | 1059–1111 |
| Ibn Al-Arabi | Spain | 1169–1240 |
| | | |
| WESTERN SCHOLASTIC PERIOD | | |
| Peter Abelard | France | 1079–1144 |
| Albertus Magnus | Germany | 1200–1280 |
| Duns Scotus | Scotland | 1266–1308 |
| | | |
| WESTERN RENAISSANCE | | |
| Petrarch | Italy | 1304–1374 |
| Boccaccio | Italy | 1313–1375 |
| Brunelleschi | Italy | 1377–1446 |
| Leonardo | Italy | 1452–1519 |

*(Continued)*

**Table 1.3.** (*Continued*)

ENLIGHTENMENT

| | | |
|---|---|---|
| Montaigne | France | 1533–1592 |
| Pascal | France | 1623–1662 |
| Spinoza | The Netherlands | 1632–1677 |
| Voltaire | France | 1694–1778 |

TRANSCENDENTALISM

| | | |
|---|---|---|
| Hegel | Germany | 1770–1831 |
| Lamartine | France | 1790–1869 |
| Gandhi | India | 1869–1948 |
| Krishnamurti | India/United States | 1895–1986 |

1998). The positive philosophy recurs in Hegel and Gandhi during the Industrial Revolution (Gandhi 1957; Hegel 1996; Gandhi 2000). Krishnamurti wrote and lectured about the positive philosophy during the emergence of the modern quantum age (Krishnamurti 1975; Krishnamurti and Bohm 1985, 1999). Positive philosophy has been called the "perennial philosophy" (Huxley 1946) because it is a perennial and constructive aspect of human culture. It is the perspective of many of our wisest philosophers, scientists, and artists.

Yet such authority is not a criterion by which we will evaluate it because truth cannot be judged on the basis of tradition or authority. According to Leonardo da Vinci, "Anyone who conducts an argument by appealing to Authority is not using his intelligence, he is just using his memory" (MacCurdy 1938). Likewise, during The Enlightenment, Voltaire and other positive philosophers divorced themselves from all religious authority so that human intelligence would be free of all authority in the search for a science of well-being.

## THE WAY OF NEGATIVE PHILOSOPHERS

We can evaluate the validity of the assumptions of the positive philosophers by comparison to the consequences of following alternative assumptions. The antithesis of positive philosophy will be called "negative" philosophy because these types of philosophy are directly opposed in their assumptions. More properly, the "negative" philosophy can be regarded as the *absence of coherence*, that is, the absence of unity in being, knowledge, and conduct. A few distinguished philosophers have made assumptions opposite from those of the positive philosophers. Protagoras (485–410 BC), William James (1842–1910), David Hume (1711–1776), and Niccolo Macchiavelli (1469–1527) are outstanding examples. Ayn Rand (1905–1982) described a modern variant of the negative philosophy called objectivism (Rand 1957, 1962, 1964). Her writings are enjoying a resurgence of interest among business executives seeking to justify self-interested conduct as moral in the wake of exposures of widespread greed and corruption in major American corporations. In fact, the negative philosophy has been present alongside the positive philosophy throughout recorded history but has only sporadically found a spokesman willing or able to defend it seriously.

Plato wrote extensively about his criticisms of Protagoras and other sophists, who are early examples of what I am calling negative philosophers (Plato 1956). The term *sophist* is derived from a Greek word that refers to someone who considers himself wise in knowledge. Philosophers are lovers and seekers of wisdom, whereas sophists think they already have wisdom. The basic assumptions of the negative philosophers are summarized in Table 1.4. Regarding being, Protagoras and later negative philosophers are dualists or radical individualists. They assume that the universe is heterogeneous, fragmentary, and made up of transient things. In other words, individual people and things are separate and have fundamentally independent causes and powers. Therefore, the function of each thing is contingent on other things, leading to a wide variety of contrasts and conflicts, such as nature versus nurture, body versus mind, and good versus evil.

Protagoras claimed that values were relative so there could be no absolute distinction between good and evil; thus, all distinctions were matters of individual opinion. Consequently, Plato and Aristotle both charged Protagoras and the sophists with being concerned with opinions about transient or accidental occurrences, rather than about truth. According to Plato, the sophists dealt with what is not, whereas "lovers of truth" dealt with what is. Hence, not all dualists are negative philosophers. For example, Descartes and Kant are dualists but not negative because they make positive assumptions about knowledge and conduct. For them, the cosmic coherence is intelligible with the certainty of conviction of personal intuition, rather than a matter of questionable opinion and belief about appearances.

Regarding knowledge, the negative philosophers are probabilistic and relativistic pragmatists. For them, all knowledge is fragmentary and contingent on particular conditions. For them, there is no absolute truth or the possibility of immediate or certain knowledge of the truth. For the negative philosopher, immediate aware-

**Table 1.4.** Basic Assumptions of Negative Philosophy

1. *Being*: Dualism (The universe is fragmentary and composed of essentially separate individuals and things with independent causes.)
2. *Knowledge*: Probabilistic and relativistic pragmatism (Human beings are immediately aware only of fragmentary information from their physical senses. There is no absolute or universal truth, only differences judged by the individual according to practical consequences.)
3. *Conduct*: Freedom is the opportunity for individuals to strive to maximize their self-interests and desires for wish fulfillment.

ness is restricted to physical sensations that are fragmentary and incomplete in their grasp of what is given in experience. For example, the skeptic David Hume (1748) cast doubt on the rational basis of opinions about causal relationships. For Hume, causal relationships were not intelligible either by rational intuition or by observation. According to Hume (1748, page 46), "When we reason *a priori* . . . independent of all observation, it never could suggest to us the notion of the inseparable and inviolable connection between a cause and its effect." Hume did acknowledge that he realized that belief in causation was needed in practice for living. Consequently, Hume (1752) suggested that life must be guided by whatever is most expedient and practical. Following the pragmatic theory, the relative truth of a statement must be judged by its practical consequences for the individual, especially by agreement with subsequent experience (Haack 1992).

Not all pragmatists are negative. In fact, the pragmatic criterion of consequences can (and should) be combined with an appreciation of the need for coherence in the whole of knowledge to test and verify the correspondence between concepts and reality. For example, Francis Bacon said, "The fruits and effects are the sureties and vouchers, as it were, for the truth of philosophy" (Bacon 1992). Although Bacon had a pragmatic approach to the validation of ideas, he also had faith in absolute truth and the unity of being and knowledge. He disparaged the extremes of both empiricism and dogmatism:

> Those who have handled sciences have been either men of experiment or men of dogmas. The men of experiment are like the ant; they only collect and use; the reasoners resemble spiders, who make cobwebs out of their own substance. But the bee takes the middle course; it gathers its material from the flowers of the garden and of the field, but transforms and digests by a power of its own. Not unlike this is the true business of philosophy. (Bacon 1992)

Bacon emphasized the potential for the unification of knowledge to improve the quality of life for all people.

Unlike Bacon's bee, which works in service to the whole community, the negative philosophers take a self-centered perspective on conduct. Given that they see no fundamental unity among individuals, they view freedom as the opportunity for wish fulfillment. That is, negative philosophers wish to maximize extrinsic sources of satisfaction, such as pleasure, wealth, and power. Their preoccupation with extrinsic gratification in conduct derives from the negative theory of knowledge, which assumes that human beings are only immediately aware of information through their physical senses. According to the negative philosophers, human beings are strongly attracted to immediate gratification and make an effort to delay such gratification only to maximize it ultimately.

The maximization of personal gratification does not necessarily mean that people cannot act in a benevolent way when it is expedient or convenient. For example, Hume (1752) suggested that people might be happy to act benevolently on some occasions because, he suggested, such sympathy was a natural emotional predisposition or moral sentiment that we share with other animals, such as dogs. In other words, Hume claimed that kindness was an emotion like aggression, rather than a virtue that transcended conflict-based emotions. In contrast, Voltaire (1754) claimed that human morality and free will were divine gifts unlike anything observed in other animals. Unfortunately, if Hume was correct that love and hate are on the same level, then love cannot overcome hate, which would be contrary to the claims of positive philosophers. In any case, what negative philosophers admit is that the effort to maximize extrinsic gratification should not exclude the expedience of behavior involving aggression, which is caused by self-interest in response to threats or frustration of wish fulfillment. This negative concept of individual freedom as a right to struggle and fight may or may not be extended to the idea of reducing conflict by mutually satisfactory ("win–win") contracts, but the motivation for this is still utilitarian and ultimately self-centered.

When these negative assumptions about being, knowledge, and conduct are combined, the consequences are dramatic and often disastrous. Consider the problems inherent in the definitions of pornography or terrorism under such assumptions. Each individual is separate and motivated by wish fulfillment and is judged on the basis of practical consequences. Consequently, pornography and terrorism lie only in the eye of the beholder. For example, no international consensus on a definition of terrorism has been possible despite much effort during the past five decades because one person's "terrorist" is another person's "freedom fighter" (http://www.US-Israel.org 2002).

The philosopher Macchiavelli gives a lucid and candid account of the application of negative philosophy to political governance.

> Thus, it is well to seem merciful, faithful, humane, sincere, religious, and also to be so; but you must have the mind so disposed that when it is needful to be otherwise you may be able to change to the opposite qualities. And it must be understood that a prince, and especially a new prince, cannot observe all those things which are considered good in men, being often obliged, in order to maintain the state, to act against faith, against charity, against humanity, and against religion. (Machiavelli 1513)

To a remarkable degree, Machiavelli's assumptions about political governance are currently prevalent in politics throughout the world. National sovereignty, cultivation of nationalistic patriotism and xenophobia, pragmatic logic, and the acquisition and retention of power and money regardless of collateral damage to other people and the environment are the concepts and motives that dominate contemporary politics throughout the world. Power, wealth, and politics seem to have mutual affinities for one another. As a result of this affinity, tyrannies or plutocracies emerge in which people dominate government for their own self-interest, leading to an increasing inequality between the powerful and rich and the weak and poor. Such disparity of opportunity and resources between the rich and the poor has consistently lead to social instability and declines in the education, health, commercial productivity, and moral values of countries throughout history (Augustine 400a; Gandhi 1957; Phillips 2002). In other words, the negative philosophy is not only self-centered but also is self-limiting and brings about its own destruction.

Unfortunately, the tendency to try to achieve happiness by maximizing personal satisfaction without pity, fraternity, or love for others can be extremely destructive when the resulting problems are erroneously blamed on others. Furthermore, the assumption of dualistic pragmatism in the negative philosophy does lead to a tendency to blame one's problems on others. As a result, negative philosophy is not only self-defeating for its advocates but also can lead to extensive harm to others. This is illustrated by Adolf Hitler's autobiography *Mein Kampf* [*My Struggles*] (1927). It is revealing to compare Hitler's autobiography with those of the positive philosophers Augustine (400b) and Gandhi (1957). Recalling the biblical account of Cain's murder of his brother Abel, Hitler is like a latter-day Cain, filled with vanity, fear, hatred, and greed. In contrast, Augustine and Gandhi are like latter-day Abels, searching for truth and growing in well-being, wisdom, and love.

Some negative philosophers have cultivated broader social acceptance than Machiavelli. William James (1907) presented the negative philosophy in a genteel manner that attracted much approval. Nevertheless, he explicitly stated his agreement with the view of the "world which the antique skeptics conceived of— in which individual minds are the measures of all things, and in which no one 'objective' truth, but only a multitude of 'subjective' opinions, can be found." Furthermore, he claimed that personality traits are the cause of the differences between positive and negative philosophers, as summarized in Table 1.5. According to James, in his first lecture on *Pragmatism* (James 1907), "The history of philosophy is to a great extent that of a certain clash of human temperaments . . . you will practically recognize the two types of mental make-up . . . by the titles

**Table 1.5.** William James's Description of the Differences in the Philosophical Approaches of People Who Are "Tender-Minded" or "Tough-Minded" in Temperament

| *The Tender-Minded* | *The Tough-Minded* |
| --- | --- |
| Rationalistic (going by "principles") | Empiricist (going by "facts") |
| Intellectualistic | Sensationalistic |
| Idealistic | Materialistic |
| Optimistic | Pessimistic |
| Religious | Irreligious |
| Free-willist | Fatalistic |
| Monistic | Pluralistic |
| Dogmatical | Skeptical |

'tender-minded' and 'tough-minded.'" According to James, positive philosophers such as Plato and Hegel are simply "tender-minded" rationalists, in contrast to his own more pragmatic ("tough-minded") perspective. However, it is also revealing that in *The Varieties of Religious Experience*, he described tough-minded individuals like himself as having "sick souls" whereas those who were naturally tender-minded were "healthy-minded" (James 1999).

James was well regarded as both a philosopher and a psychologist. His studies of the varieties of religious experience have even made him influential in the philosophy of religion. His admission of having a "sick soul" in need of spiritual rebirth had a broad appeal. James described recovery from a major depression and suicide attempt to later academic success and greater self-confidence. However, despite his success and self-confidence, William James remained a "sick soul" who took pride in his "tough-mindedness." It is unwise to ask a person who is still not healthy minded to tell others how to achieve well-being. Hence, it is not surprising that James's basic assumptions about the path to spiritual rebirth are quite inconsistent with the message of healthy-minded positive philosophers whom James acknowledged to have shed the most light on the path to happiness.

Specifically, James claimed that the individual ego is the ultimate criterion of being or reality. In his *Principles of Psychology*, he wrote

> The world of living realities as contrasted with unrealities is thus anchored in the Ego. . . . Whatever things have intimate and continuous connection with my life are things of whose reality I cannot doubt. Whatever things fail to establish this connection are things which are practically no better for me than if they existed not at all. (James 1890, page 645)

Thus, James is only concerned with "practical" reality, not with impartial knowledge of the truth of what exists in general. For James, what we can verify and believe depends on an idea's consequences, which he called "truth's cash-value in experiential terms" (James 1911, preface, page ix). Furthermore, according to James, the pragmatic test of truth depends on an idea's appeal "to our aesthetic, emotional, and active needs" (James 1890, page 655). Regarding ethics, he concluded that "we have learned what the words, "good", "bad", and "obligation" severally mean. They mean no absolute natures, independent of personal support. They are objects of feeling and desire, which have no foothold or anchorage in Being, apart from the existence of actually living minds" (Castell 1948, page 74).

To account for emotion, James described what he called a "sensationalistic" theory in which the physical body is dominant in its influence, rather than emotion depending largely on mental or "intellectualistic" processing. In *Principles of Psychology*, he assumed that emotions are the consequence, not the cause of physiological events in the body (James 1890). For example, consider the situation in which a person meets a bear, becomes frightened and runs away. According to James, meeting the bear causes the person to run instinctively without mediation by conscious thought, and the sensations associated with the meeting and the running is interpreted as fear. In this sensation-based view, there is no role for intuition, no role for free will, and therefore no possibility of coherence in thought or action from awareness of the context of the events. According to James, human thought and action are dominated by physiological reactions to separate and extrinsic sensible objects. For this reason, James recognized that his "tough-minded" pragmatism was pessimistic and fatalistic, as shown in Table 1.5. The attempt by James to reduce human emotion to somatic reactions and human thought to a passive role was quickly and thoroughly discredited by evidence that differences between individuals in the active processing of information in the brain was the major cause, rather than the consequence, of emotions (Cannon 1927). Nevertheless, contrary to the assumptions of negative philosophy, it is well established that personal and social behavior depends on differences between individuals in their personality as well as on awareness of the meaning of events in their life (Cervone and Shoda 1999; Lewis and Haviland-Jones 2000; Snyder and Lopez 2002). Furthermore, our behavior involves the integration of psychobiological processes (Eisenberg 2000). Consequently, we need to avoid the fallacies involved in dualistic rhetoric about body versus mind, which pervade the writing of negative philosophers.

In summary, the negative philosophy is based on assumptions of separateness, self-determination, and self-interest. Throughout history the negative philosophy has sanctioned and encouraged pride, greed, and violence, although sometimes disguised in genteel or self-deceptive terms such as pragmatism or protection of national security. Nevertheless, negative philosophy is useful because it shows us what is not compatible with well-being. One approach to the path to wisdom and well-being is the progressively complete negation of the assumptions of negative philosophers. This is an explicit way of interpreting Plato's allegory of the cave (Cornford 1941) if we represent the positive philosophy by light and the negative philosophy by shadow or the absence of light. We move from ignorance to wisdom, or from the shadows to increasingly pure and intense light, as we increase our understanding of the positive philosophy and let go of the elements of the negative philosophy. According to Plato, we must become positive philosophers to eliminate conflict and contradiction. Unfortunately, wisdom is rare, so the positive philosophy may seem to be utopian. Can we have well-being by means of a less demanding transformation of our consciousness?

## THE WAY OF HUMANISTS

Perhaps the negative personal and social consequences of the negative philosophy depend mainly on the assumption that freedom is expressed as self-concern. There have been many rationalistic dualists who tried to base wisdom and well-being on reason alone using various concepts of human dignity. For example, Rene Descartes (1596–1650) sought to establish a coherent theory of the world and man's place within it on the basis of science, which he defined as systematic and reliable knowledge based on certain foundations. He regarded evidence from the physical senses as unreliable, but that skepticism reaches its logical limit in self-awareness (Descartes 1650). As Augustine had previously observed, we cannot doubt our own self-awareness without contradiction because the act of doubting is certain evidence of existence. In his *Discourse* (Part IV), Descartes's own famous conclusion was, "I think, therefore I am" (Descartes 1650). On the basis of this rational intuition, Descartes sought to deduce knowledge of the external world. However, as a dualist who assumed that the mind and body were essentially separate, Descartes concluded that he was unable to say anything with certainty about the external world unless he also accepted that his idea of a perfect creator was true. Subsequent philosophers and scientists were left to struggle with the task of finding a basis for human dignity that did not appeal to a divine guarantor of universal coherence.

In the search for coherence despite dualism, there have been three concepts of the basis of human dignity. These concepts of human dignity in philosophy correspond to concepts of human character in psychology that have been called self-directedness, cooperativeness, and self-transcendence (Cloninger, Svrakic et al. 1993). These concepts are hierarchical or complementary, rather than mutually exclusive. The simplest is the claim of John Locke (1632–1704), and later of Friedrich Nietzsche (1844–1900), that human dignity comes from human self-determination. Locke (1690) argued that all knowledge comes from experience acquired through the physical senses or from reflection about such sensations. Some pervasive ideas, such as unity, are derived from both experience and reflection. According to Locke, human beings have self-awareness and reasoning ability, which gives them freedom and responsibility for their conduct (Locke 1689). This concept has been developed in psychology as "autonomy," "internal locus of control," "agency," "self-efficacy," or "self-directedness," an aspect of human character involving responsibility, hopeful purpose, and resourcefulness (Cloninger, Svrakic et al. 1993). Nietzsche's psychology of power (1891) also formed the basis in psychiatry for Alfred Adler's work on overcoming feelings of inferiority (Ansbacher and Ansbacher 1956). A human being has dignity because of his ability to set his own goals with hope and to realize them with power.

Immanuel Kant (1724–1804) expanded the concept of human dignity by indicating that reason provided the basis for what Kant called the "dignity of a rational being" in *Metaphysics of Morals* (1996). Kant revolutionized the understanding of human cognition by his emphasis on the presence of innate ideas from intuition, which were active in giving form to our thoughts. Human knowledge was the result of sensation for Locke, but Kant emphasized that intuitive processes were responsible for forming thought. In *Critique of Practical Reason* (Chapter 3), a human being had a "personality by which alone they are ends in themselves" because human responsibility for their thoughts also implied freedom of will from mechanical determinism (Kant 1996). According to Kant, man has the dignity of a rational being who is endowed with at least some innate memories (e.g., recollectable ideas of space and time), understanding, and freedom of will.

Kant's focus on the functions of reason was stimulated by his dissatisfaction with David Hume's philosophy. Kant sought to show how reason alone could provide a basis for valid scientific knowledge, as well as healthy character development and morality (Kant 1996). According to Kant (1996), "We are indeed legislative members of a moral kingdom rendered possible by freedom, and presented to us by reason as an object of respect." The legislative function of reason endows man with great dignity and humanistic potential. Kant (1996) said, "It can be nothing less than a power which elevates man above himself (as a part of the world of sense), a power which connects him with an order of things that only the understanding can conceive. . . ." Kant further described the intelligible world as "a world which at the same time commands the whole sensible world, and with it the empirically determinable existence of man in time, as well as the sum total of all ends (which totality alone suits such unconditional practical laws as the moral)." According to Kant's influential formulation of the categorical imperative in *The Critique of Pure Reason* (1996), we should act with an awareness of the dignity of every rational being. In *Metaphysics of Morals* (1996), Kant said, "Act so that you use the humanity either in your own person, or in that of any one else always as an end, and never merely as a means." Only a rational being exists as an end in itself because of the freedom of self-determination, so a rational being must also recognize and tolerate the dignity of others in a consistent manner. According to Kant, fraternity and dignity are based on rationality and freedom of will; therefore, human conduct should be tolerant, empathic, and cooperative.

However, the effectiveness of this imperative in practice is weakened by Kant's dualistic theory of knowledge. Kant thought that the observer was separate from what was observed, so that a thing could not be known in itself. That is, we only know what we perceive, not what is given in experience. Nevertheless, Kant is conscious of the certainty of his rational intuition of the "intelligible" world of things in themselves, which he can conceive but not observe. In contrast, for positive philosophers, there is a possibility of purifying intuition so that there is direct intuition of what is. For example, Hegel was conscious with certainty from his own intuition of the evolving potential of human intuition being able to sense the essential aspects of things in themselves (Hegel 1807). To use the terminology of quantum physics (Krishnamurti and Bohm 1985; Bohm 1995; Krishnamurti and Bohm 1999), the observer is the observed when there is coherent awareness and understanding. Hegel spoke of the phenomenology of spirit, which is consciousness of what is immaterial but sensible by intuition in a state of loving union. For a dualist like Kant, such coherence of understanding by rational intuition is assumed to be impossible. Things in themselves are supersensible, even though they are intelligible in the sense of being conceived by our understanding.

Kant's thoughts about the limitations of knowledge and understanding had a substantial impact on the development of Sigmund Freud's approach to cognition and personality development. Kant's legislative function of reason corresponds to what is called "cooperativeness" in psychological studies of personality (Cloninger, Svrakic et al. 1993). For Kant, cooperative and moral behavior is ideal, but it is not ensured unless reason is purified. Unfortunately, when people think they are right, they are likely to forcefully impose their thinking on others, justifying such behavior as being for the good of others. Consequently, dualistic reason often fails to guarantee moral behavior because any appeal to its purity, universality, or coherence is uncertain.

According to positive philosophers, reason can only be purified by coherent intuition. Such pure reason is spontaneous and effortless wisdom. Only recognition of the totality of actual relationships guarantees coherence without conflict and contradiction. For example, Hegel (1770–1831) was initially a disciple of Kant but later rejected Kant's assumption of the dualistic limitations on rational intuition. He was deeply impressed by Kant's idealism but regarded it as "immature" and not fully coherent as a result of its dualism. Hegel said,

> In every dualistic system, and especially in that of Kant, the fundamental defect makes itself visible in the inconsistency of unifying at one moment what a moment before had been explained to be independent and therefore incapable of unification. . . . It argues an utter want of consistency to say, on the one hand, that the understanding only knows phenomena, and, on the other, assert the absolute character of this knowledge, by such statements as "Cognition can go no further"; "Here is the *natural* and absolute limit of human knowledge." But . . . No one knows, or even feels, that anything is a limit or defect, until he is at the same time above and beyond it. . . . A very little consideration might show that to call a thing finite or limited proves by implication the very presence of the infinite and unlimited, and that the awareness of limit can only be in so far as the unlimited is *on this side* in consciousness. (Hegel 1992)

In the preface to *Phenomenology of Spirit*, Hegel explained that Kant had rediscovered the three aspects of consciousness (rational agency, freedom of will, and intuition) but had not been able to transform his thinking from abstract reasoning, which is dualistic and lifeless, to rational intuition, which is nondualistic and living (Hegel 1807). Kant was trapped in the dualism that separates the subject and its object when the subject is not aware that the object of its consciousness has the same essence as itself. In such a dualistic state of consciousness, sometimes determinations of sense, such as awareness of beauty, truth, or goodness, are picked up by intuition. However, these intuitions are not recognized as spiritual essences, notions of truth, or things-in-themselves. Rather, Kant and other dualists treat such nondualistic intuitions as dualistic abstractions by analogy to external objects. As a result, Kant had not been able to move from a philosophy of rational idealism to the science of well-being.

Furthermore, Hegel could not reconcile Kant's idealism with the reality of irrational violence occurring throughout human history or with his faith in the human potential to evolve a greater consciousness of the spiritual foundation of nature. Hegel developed a positive philosophy in which human beings were evolving toward direct spiritual awareness of the universal unity of being (Hegel 1996). Hegel recognized that there were differences between individuals at any particular time in the level of the maturity and coherence of their awareness. That is, people may reach nondualistic consciousness at different rates. Some people may currently be materialistic skeptics, others may be dualistic in their consciousness, and still others may already be nondualistic in their consciousness. Dualistic consciousness, as in the reflections of Kant, was not the limit of human consciousness in Hegel's own experience. For Hegel, it was possible to transcend the artificial dichotomies of dualistic thinking in a process of evolution to pure rational intuition, which Hegel called variously "pure consciousness," "intuition," and "reason." Hegel said the evolutionary movement of knowledge as a phenomenon was the "path of natural consciousness" or the "path of the soul" (Hegel 1807, 1981):

> Knowledge as a phenomenon . . . can . . . be taken to be the path of the natural consciousness, which presses forward to true knowledge; or it could be taken as the path of the soul, which ranges through the succession of its configurations, as if through the stations naturally foreordained for it, so that, by attaining the knowledge of what it is in itself through an exhaustive experience of itself, it may purify itself into spirit. (Hegel 1981)

In contrast, skeptical ("eliminative") materialists like Hume and some contemporary philosophers like Dennett and the Churchlands have tried to deny the reality of phenomenal consciousness and related concepts such as spirituality, freedom of will, and the soul (Rey 1997; Seager 1999). Dualistic philosophers have accepted the ordinary concept of the reality of the phenomenon of consciousness but insisted that its qualitative aspects must be private. Dualists assume the consciousness of individuals is fundamentally separate so that there is no potential for transpersonal unity in being and knowledge. For materialists and dualists, Hegel's claims for the potential unity of being and knowledge must be illusory or idealized because they have never experienced such awareness themselves. The dualistic assumption that the consciousness of one individual is separate and private from other individuals is commonplace in contemporary society. For Hegel and other positive philosophers, the assumptions of both materialists and dualists are characteristic of the limited awareness of particular stages along the path of consciousness. For positive philosophers, the path of consciousness is ever widening until there is awareness of the universal unity of being and knowledge. Hegel also reaffirms what we have previously discussed in prior sections: history provides abundant evidence for the increasing coherence and practical advantages of growth along the path of consciousness.

With this impressive phenomenological statement of the positive philosophy, Hegel renewed interest in classical Greek thought by his insightful description of the writings of Plato and Aristotle. He also inspired the American transcendentalists, such as Emerson and Thoreau, who took as their central axiom that the human soul was substantive and had intuitive senses independent of the physical senses of the body (Miller 1957). Hegel's work integrated Kant's idealistic humanism about the potential of rational conduct with the reality of conflict throughout human history.

Nevertheless, Hegel remained optimistic because he observed that love, conceived as a union of opposites, was a form of consciousness in which contradictions (such as the finite individual and the infinite universal spirit) were intuitively synthesized. We only transcend dualism in a state of loving unity. Hence, pure consciousness is love, and love leads by its free movement to awareness of what is true, good, and universal. In other words, Hegel was conscious of his certainty that human intuition could sense the essence of a thing in itself in a state of loving awareness.

Therefore, paradoxically, it appears that pure reason must be nondualistic and can operate only by means of the coherence of intuition. If so, then the only fully coherent rationalists are nondualistic positive philosophers like Spinoza. Dualistic forms of rationality, which are effortful, are also essentially incomplete because they are based on a finite set of fragmented individual experiences, not on the relevant totality of actual and potential relationships.

The incompleteness of effortful reasoning was made clear by the work of phenomenologists in philosophy and psychology. In contrast to rationalism that focuses on conceptual reasoning, phenomenology is concerned with the intuitive foundation and verification of concepts, focusing on the flow of consciousness prior to reflection. Husserl (1859–1938) described phenomenology as "an analysis of essences and an investigation of the general states of affairs which are to be built up in immediate intuition. . . . Phenomenology proceeds by 'seeing,' clarifying, and determining meaning, and by distinguishing meanings" (Husserl 1992). Martin Heidegger (1889–1976), a student of Husserl, extended the work of Hegel and others about being and nothingness, setting the stage for the existential movement (Heidegger 1996). Heidegger emphasized the unique potential of human intuition. In *What Is Metaphysics?*, he said, "Readiness for dread is to say 'Yes!' to the inwardness of things, to fulfill the highest demand which alone touches man to the quick. Man alone of all beings, when addressed by the voice of Being, experiences the marvel of all marvels: that what-is is."

According to Karl Jaspers (1883–1969), a prominent existential philosopher and psychiatrist, by reason we can recognize that we are finite and derived from what is infinite (Jaspers 1951). However, to be wise, which is the only rational choice, requires transcendence. According to Jaspers, we are transcendent when we allow ourselves to be spontaneously aware of the universal unity and freedom inherent in being in the world, thereby giving rise to love and faith in what transcends our transient material existence. More generally, some existentialists, such as Sartre and de Beauvoir, have described transcendence as a state of being that is not fully identified with or instantiated in oneself, which allows freedom from empirical determinism and freedom for self-determination, morality, creativity, art, and wisdom. Similarly, the American transcendentalists led by Emerson had previously emphasized that such transpersonal consciousness of what is true, beautiful, and good was evidence of the function of the intuitive senses of the soul, which are not dependent on the physical senses of the body (Miller 1957).

The transcendental concept of human dignity corresponds to the trait of "self-transcendence" as measured in contemporary personality psychology (Cloninger, Svrakic et al. 1993). Dualistic reasoning is an incomplete basis for the dignity and wisdom that emerges in self-transcendent consciousness. The incompleteness of reason is also clearly demonstrated by Kurt Godel's theorem and his later work (1981). Godel proved that there must be truths that are neither provable nor disprovable within any logical or mathematical system. Consequently, logic and mathematics are essentially incomplete because no logical system can be proved within itself. The limit of reason is to recognize its own incompleteness. Likewise, in *Pensees*, Pascal (1662) observed, "Reason's last step is the recognition that there are an infinite number of things which are beyond it." This recognition of the incompleteness of reason does not mean that personal development is bounded in a predictable manner. Rather, the recognition of the incompleteness of reason merely opens the door for intuition and faith in search of understanding.

For example, Godel divided philosophies into two groups like those of William James: skepticism, materialism, and positivism on the left side and spiritualism, idealism, and theology on the right side. He compared these with the development of a child, which he suggested proceeds in two directions: one involving experimentation with material objects in the external world, and the other involving the development of consciousness in terms of ever-newer intuitions that transcend what we formerly took as the limits of truth. He suggested that the first (left or materialistic) direction corresponded to the development of empirical science and technology. On the other hand, the other (right or dialectical) direction corresponded to the development of mathematics. Godel has shown that new axioms, which do not follow by formal logic from those established earlier, repeatedly become evident in the course of the development of the understanding of any mathematical system. The incompleteness of any system of logic or mathematics suggests that the development of human understanding requires the intuitive grasping of ever-newer axioms that are unpredictable and logically independent from earlier ones (Godel 1961). Intuition is needed for an ever-deeper grasp of the meanings implicit in our experience, which go beyond the predictable reach of formal logic and other dualistic forms of rationality.

The complementary roles of dialectical and empirical thinking that Godel documented in mathematics was also recognized in the philosophy of science underlying personality theory (Rychlak 1968). Nevertheless, rationalistic dualism has remained a commonplace perspective in philosophy (Rey 1997; Seager 1999) and psychology (Seligman 2002). Hence, it is important to examine carefully why the lack of direct awareness of universal unity in being and knowledge makes it impossible for rationalistic dualists, like Kant and Freud, to achieve wisdom and unconditional well-being. We need only ask why this is the case, not whether it is so, because such dualists have been frank enough to admit that life is stressful for them.

## WHAT MAKES LIFE STRESSFUL?

The persistent conflict between happiness and sadness in dualistic consciousness was well recognized by the founder of psychoanalysis, Sigmund Freud (1856–1939), whose views remain highly influential in our modern thinking about civilization and its discontents (Freud 1929). Why can't we be permanently happy? Why do people suffer so frequently? Freud developed a theory of conscious and unconscious processes in human motivation that was consistent with the classic world views of Newton in physics, Darwin in biology, and Kant in the philosophy of mind (Freud 1974). Freud observed that the rational desires and beliefs of which we are conscious were shaped by other prerational drives concerned with basic bodily processes of which we are often unconscious (Freud 1938). Thus psychoanalysis is an extension of the Kantian tradition of dualistic rationality concerned with the description of how human mental processes limit the knowledge of reality (Hopkins 1992).

Freud's classic foundations defined a mechanical, dualistic, and rationalistic view of the world. Freud observed that living in a society required human beings to curtail their personal desires to some extent, thereby reducing their immediate happiness and bringing some distress, because to satisfy them would bring even greater distress. However, curtailing desires brings conflict, so happiness always remains in opposition to misery. Suppressed or repressed fears and desires continue to have an influence on our human relationships and emotional state, even if they are unconscious. According to Freud, the best human beings can do is to be persistent and conscientious in living according to their rational goals and values. This means that we must live in a constant tension between the forces of unconscious fears and irrational desires (Id), rational aspects of character (ego, or self-directedness), and other ideal and conscientious aspects of character (superego, or cooperativeness and self-transcendence). As a consequence in Freud's view, which is implicit to a large extent in most contemporary perspectives, human behavior inevitably results either in conflict (when character overrides emotion) or in character deficits (when emotion overrides character).

In his book *Civilization and Its Discontents* (1929), Freud concluded that it was impossible for human beings to love their neighbors as themselves and to be permanently happy. This conclusion followed from his rejection of the reality of human intuitions of the universal unity of being, which he called "oceanic feelings." Following Goethe, Freud recognized what distinguished human beings from other animals are science, art, and religion, which are the fruits of intuition and the basis of civilization. However, he was unable to accept human intuitions about the immortality of the soul, the providence and mercy of God, or other spiritual intuitions as anything but illusions arising from a need to console ourselves when dealing with fear, helplessness, and grief over the death of those we love. At the very beginning of *Civilization and Its Discontents*, he aptly described such intuitions of the universal unity of being as "a feeling of indissoluble connection to belonging inseparably to the external world as a whole." The sense that an individual is an inseparable part of the whole is described as an "oceanic feeling" because waves in a universal field are inseparable parts of the whole, just as an individual ocean wave is a part of the ocean. Freud considered such feelings to be natural residuals of the infant's innate and primary experience of the world in the fluid-filled amnionic sac of the mother. He recognized that ego boundaries were artificially constructed as a means of protection to avoid painful external influences (such as the withdrawal of the nurturing maternal breast). Furthermore, like Hegel, Freud also recognized that such artificially constructed boundaries between subject and object could be relaxed in a natural and healthy way in response to attraction and love of others. Nevertheless, he doubted and rejected the unity and inseparability of all life in the world. Freud recognized that "oceanic feelings" were the experiential basis of faith. However, Freud's own fears kept him in an endless ego-based struggle against both the external world and his innermost urges for perfection and pleasure. In his own words at the conclusion of *Civilization and Its Discontents*, Freud saw the basis for his own failing to point out the path to well-being to others. "My courage fails me, therefore, at the thought of rising up as a prophet before my fellow-men, and I bow to their reproach that I have no consolation to offer them; for at bottom this is what they all demand—the frenzied revolutionary as passionate as the most pious believer."

Despite Freud's many profound insights and widespread influence, his dualistic and rationalistic perspective is profoundly confused and obviously inadequate as an approach to well-being. Many people enjoy their life with an abiding sense of coherence, including intuitions of hope, love, and faith that cannot be explained dualistically. The occurrence of such coherent attitudes is common and well documented in large-scale surveys and through clinical examinations (Myers and Diener 1996).

For example, in the United States, the National Opinion Research Center at the University of Chicago surveyed a representative sample of about 1500 people each year since 1957. In these surveys, three in ten people say they are "very happy," and the majority describe themselves as "pretty happy." Only one in ten chooses the most negative description, "not too happy." Furthermore, such self-reports are moderately consistent over years of retesting and confirmed by interviews with their close friends, family members, and professional raters. Those who are happy and satisfied with their life are distinguished by the coherence of their personality rather than by demographic variables, such as age, race, and socioeconomic status, or extrinsic variables, such as increases in income. Americans now earn twice as much in current dollars as they did in 1957, but the proportion who report that they are "very happy" has declined from 35% to 29%.

In terms of personality, individuals who report that they are very happy are described as optimistic and sociable in temperament and creative in character. Very happy people have high self-esteem and describe themselves as more ethical, more intelligent, less prejudiced, better able to get along with others, and healthier than the average person (Myers and Diener 1996). Other studies show that these self-reports are valid. Those who are happy are more likely than those who are depressed to be married, to have several close friends, to have active religious affiliations, and to have good physical health. This suggests that happy people are more likely than depressed people to be physically healthy and to manifest the virtues of hope, love, and faith. These virtues and social characteristics are what distinguish coherence of personality from the simple absence of mental disease.

In brief, subjective reports of happiness are strongly associated with many indicators of physical and mental well-being in roughly one in every three individuals. What is remarkable about the observations that abiding states of well-being are a frequent experience of many people is that our theories and methods of clinical practice do not correspond to this well-documented reality. Such a striking error and gap between belief and reality is an important clue to understanding the nature of the resistance to coherent living associated with dualistic world views. Essentially, dualistic world views conceptualize well-being in conditional terms that always involve enduring struggle or conflict, whereas nondualistic views begin with hope in unconditional well-being.

The positive philosophy has had a perennial and constructive role in the cultural development of human civilization. The positive philosophy has always had an influential exponent at the times when cultures were at their peak, as in ancient Greece, the Golden Age of Arabia, the Renaissance, and the Enlightenment. In contrast, the negative philosophy has had only sporadic appeal and at times has been clearly destructive. Rationalistic and dualistic approaches to psychology are commonplace but seem to provide an inadequate account of human cognition. In particular, rationalistic dualism does not provide an adequate foundation for the development of wisdom and well-being.

Positive philosophers have made an inspiring contribution to society with their writings and their examples of how to live well. However, outstanding exponents of positive philosophy have often had limited success in helping their followers to develop coherence, as was recognized by Gandhi and Krisnamurti in recent times (Gandhi 1957; Jayakar 1986; Blau 1995). I have no doubt that Spinoza is an outstanding example of wisdom and well-being, and his exposition of his deductions from his intuitions are impeccable. However, many people are unable to experience the same certainty and clarity that Spinoza had about his definitions and axioms. Neither the problem nor the solution to well-being lies in reasoning. Rationality is the effortless consequence of intuitive coherence. Rather, we must ask, "Is it possible to learn to share the intuitions of a wise person?" "Can we develop the creative happiness that is well-being?" "Can we learn to see the world as did Leonardo da Vinci?" "How can we purify our own intuition so that we see clearly in a way that is unbiased by our fears and desires?" Before we can begin to answer such questions, we need a coherent model of human consciousness and personality.

It is interesting to consider the history of developments in the positive philosophy as a possible model of the path of consciousness. The basic elements of the positive philosophy have been consistent from the classical Greek period to the present. Alfred North Whitehead once remarked that "the safest general characterization of the European philosophical tradition is that it consists of a series of footnotes to Plato" (1929). More specifically, it appears that there have been five major steps in the development of these footnotes. The five steps correspond to the particular ways the positive philosophy was adapted to respond to the predominant concerns of society at different times. These five steps that can be discerned in Table 1.3 are (*1*) purification of superstition and magical thinking, (*2*) teaching of correct beliefs and practices for everyday living, (*3*) cultivation of aesthetics and harmonious emotional expression, (*4*) establishment of the scope of intellectual and scientific methods, and (*5*) nondualistic spirituality.

For example, in Table 1.3 the positive philosophers during the Neoplatonic period, such as Iamblichus (1999), dealt extensively with the superstitious concerns and magical practices of people at the time. Later, during the Arabic Golden Age and Western Scholastic Period, positive philosophers put more emphasis on conformity to beliefs and practices that were correct according to tradition and authority. Next, during the Renaissance, there was a reawakening of interest in art and beauty. During the Enlightenment (Montaigne through Voltaire), there was a special focus on understanding the abilities and limits of the intellect in general. Then, during the transcendental period (Hegel through Krishnamurti), there was special emphasis on listening to one's own soul without outside authority. This is a partial illustration of growth in the general level of society along the path of consciousness described by Hegel and Teilhard de Chardin. However, much remains to be done before we have a detailed scientific account of the path of self-aware consciousness.

## REFERENCES

Al'Arabi, I. (1980). *The bezels of wisdom*. Mahwah, New Jersey, Paulist Press.

Al-Ghazali (1978). *The just balance*. Lahore, Pakistan, Sh. Muhammad Ashraf.

Al-Ghazali (1979). *The alchemy of happiness*. Lahore, Pakistan, Sh. Muhammad Ashraf.

Al-Ghazali (2000). *The incoherence of the philosophers*. Provo, Utah, Brigham Young University Press.

Ansbacher, H. L. and R. R. Ansbacher, eds. (1956). *Individual psychology of Alfred Adler: A systematic presentation in selections from his writings*. New York, Basic Books.

Aristotle (1984). *The complete works of Aristotle*. Princeton, New Jersey, Princeton University Press.

Augustine (386). *The happy life; Answer to skeptics; Divine providence & the problem of evil, soliloques*. New York, Cima Publishing Co., 1948.

Augustine (400a). *City of God*. New York, Doubleday, 1958.

Augustine (400b). *Confessions*. Chicago, Illinois, Brittanica, 1996.

Augustine (400c). *The Trinity*. Brooklyn, New York, New City Press, 1991.

Averill, J. R. and T. A. More. (2000). Happiness. *Handbook of emotions*. M. Lewis and J. M. Haviland-Jones, eds. New York, Guilford Press: 663–676.

Bacon, F. (1620). Novum Organum. *Great books of the Western World*. M. J. Adler, ed. Chicago, Illinois, Britannica: 28: 105–198.

Bacon, F. (1992). The philosophical works of Francis Bacon. *A dictionary of philosophical quotations*. J. O'Grady, ed. Oxford, England, Blackwell: 33.

Barnes, J., ed. (1984). *The complete works of Aristotle*. Princeton, New Jersey, Princeton University Press.

Bayrak, T., ed. (1997). *Ibn 'Arabi's divine governance of the human kingdom*. Louisville, Kentucky, Fons Vitae.

Bjorklund, D. F. (1997). "In search of a metatheory for cognitive development (or, Piaget is dead and I don't feel so good myself)." *Child Development* 68: 144–148.

Blau, E. (1995). *Krishnamurti: 100 Years*. New York, Stewart Tabori & Chang.

Bohm, D. (1995). Interview about Krishnamurti. *Krishnamurti: 100 Years*. E. Blau, ed. New York, Stewart, Tabori & Chang.

Bohm, D. and B. J. Hiley (1993). *The undivided universe: An ontological interpretation of quantum theory*. London, Routledge.

Bouwmeester, D., J. W. Pan, et al. (1997). "Experimental quantum teleportation." *Nature* 390: 575–579.

Brainerd, C. J., V. F. Reyna, et al. (1990). "The development of forgetting and reminiscence." *Monographs of the Society for Research in Child Development* 5: 1–93.

Cannon, W. B. (1927). "The James-Lange theory of emotions: A critical examination and an alternative theory." *American Journal of Psychology* 39: 106–129.

Castell, A., ed. (1948). *Essays in pragmatism by William James*. New York, Hafner Publishing Co.

Cervone, D. and Y. Shoda (1999). *The coherence of personality: Social-cognitive bases of consistency, variability, and organization*. New York, Guilford Press.

Cloninger, C. R., D. M. Svrakic, et al. (1993). "A psychobiological model of temperament and character." *Archives of General Psychiatry* 50: 975–990.

Cornford, F. M., ed. (1941). *Plato's The Republic*. New York, Oxford University Press.

Descartes, R. (1650). Collected works. *Great books of the Western World*. M. J. Adler, ed. Chicago, Illinois, Brittanica: 28: 223–588.

Diener, E., R. E. Lucas, et al. (2002). Subjective well-being: The science of happiness and life satisfaction. *Handbook of positive psychology.* C. R. Snyder and S. J. Lopez, eds. New York, Oxford University Press: 63–73.

Eisenberg, L. (2000). "Is psychiatry more mindful or brainier than it was a decade ago?" *British Journal of Psychiatry* 176: 1–5.

Frankl, V. E. (1959). *Man's search for meaning: An introduction to logotherapy.* New York, Simon & Schuster.

Freud, S. (1929). *Civilization and its discontents.* New York, Jonathan Cape & Harrison Smith.

Freud, S. (1938). *A general introduction to psychoanalysis.* Garden City, New York, Garden City Publishing Company.

Freud, S. (1974). *Complete psychological works of Sigmund Freud.* London, Hogarth Press.

Gamow, G. (1966). *Thirty years that shook physics: The story of quantum theory.* New York, Dover Publications.

Gandhi, M. K. (1957). *An autobiography: The story of my experiments with truth.* Boston, Beacon Press.

Gandhi, M. K. (2000). *The Bhagavad Gita according to Gandhi.* Berkeley, California, Berkeley Hills Books.

Godel, K. (1961). The modern development of the foundations of mathematics in the light of philosophy. *Collected works.* New York, Oxford University Press: 3.

Godel, K. (1981). *Collected works.* New York, Oxford University Press.

Haack, S. (1992). Pragmatism. *A companion to epistemology.* J. Dancy and E. Sosa, eds. Oxford, England, Blackwell: 351–357.

Hegel, G. F. W. (1807). *Phenomenology of spirit.* Oxford, England, Oxford University Press.

Hegel, G. F. W. (1981). *The Berlin phenomenology.* London, Reidel Publishing Company.

Hegel, G. F. W. (1992). Encyclopedia. *A dictionary of philosophical quotations.* A. J. Ayer and J. O'Grady, eds. Oxford, England, Blackwell: 168.

Hegel, G. F. W. (1996). *Collected works.* Chicago, Illinois, Brittanica.

Heidegger, M. (1996). What is metaphysics? *Great books of the Western World.* M. J. Adler, ed. Chicago, Illinois, Brittanica: 55: 299–310.

Hitler, A. (1927). *Mein Kampf.* Boston, Houghton Mifflin.

Hopkins, J. (1992). Epistemology of Sigmund Freud. *A companion to epistemology.* J. Dancy and E. Sosa, eds. Oxford, England, Blackwell: 149–150.

Horace (1966). *Satires, epistles, and poetry.* Cambridge, Massachusetts, Harvard University Press.

Hume, D. (1748). *An inquiry concerning human understanding.* New York, Liberal Arts Press.

Hume, D. (1752). *An inquiry concerning the principles of morals.* New York, Liberal Arts Press.

Husserl, E. (1992). The idea of phenomenology. *A dictionary of philosophical quotations.* A. J. Ayer and J. O'Grady, eds. Oxford, England, Blackwell: 204–207.

Huxley, A. (1946). *The perennial philosophy.* London, Chatto and Windus.

Huxley, J. (1959). Foreword. *The phenomenon of man.* P. Teilhard de Chardin, ed. New York, Harper & Row: 11–28.

Iamblichus (1999). *On the mysteries and the life of Pythagoras.* Somerset, England, The Prometheus Trust.

Iyer, R., Ed. (1999). *The essential writings of Mahatma Gandhi.* New Delhi, Oxford University Press.

James, W. (1890). The principles of psychology. *Great books of the Western World*. M. J. Adler, ed. Chicago, Illinois, Brittanica: 53: 1–897.

James, W. (1907). *Pragmatism: A new name for some old ways of thinking*. New York, Longmans Green & Company.

James, W. (1911). *The meaning of truth*. New York, Longmans Green & Company.

James, W. (1999). *The varieties of religious experience: A study in human nature*. New York, Modern Library.

Jaspers, K. (1951). *Way to wisdom*. New Haven, Connecticut, Yale University Press.

Jayakar, P. (1986). *J. Krishnamurti: A biography*. London, Penguin Books.

Jung, C. G. (1933). *Modern man in search of a soul*. London, Routledge.

Kahneman, D., E. Diener, et al., Eds. (1999). *Well-being: The foundations of hedonic psychology*. New York, Russell Sage Foundation.

Kant, I. (1996). Collected works. *Great books of the Western World*. M. J. Adler, ed. Chicago, Illinois, Brittanica: 39: 1–613.

Kohut, H. (1984). *How does analysis cure?* Chicago, Illinois, University of Chicago Press.

Krishnamurti, J. (1975). *The first and last freedom*. San Francisco, California, HarperCollins.

Krishnamurti, J. and D. Bohm (1985). *The ending of time*. San Francisco, California, HarperCollins.

Krishnamurti, J. and D. Bohm (1999). *The limits of thought: Discussions*. London, Routledge.

Larsen, R. J. and B. L. Fredrickson (1999). Measurement issues in emotion research. *Well-Being: The foundations of hedonic psychology*. D. Kahneman, E. Diener and N. Schwarz. New York, Russell Sage Foundation: 40–60.

Lehrer, K. (1990). *Theory of knowledge*. Boulder, Colorado, Westview.

Lewis, M. and J. M. Haviland-Jones, eds. (2000). *Handbook of emotions*. New York, Guilford Press.

Locke, J. (1689). An essay concerning toleration. *Great books of the Western World*. M. J. Adler, ed. Chicago, Illinois, Brittanica: 33: 1–24.

Locke, J. (1690). An essay concerning human understanding. *Great books of the Western World*. M. J. Adler, ed. Chicago, Illinois, Brittanica: 33: 85–402.

Loewenstein, G. and D. Schkade (1999). Wouldn't it be nice? Predicting future feelings. *Well-Being: The foundations of hedonic psychology*. D. Kahneman, E. Diener and N. Schwarz. New York, Russell Sage Foundation: 85–108.

MacCurdy, E. (1938). *The notebooks of Leonardo da Vinci*. New York, Reynal & Hitchcock.

Machiavelli, N. (1513). The prince. *Great books of the Western World*. M. J. Adler, ed. Chicago, Illinois, Brittanica: 21: 1–37.

Miller, P., ed. (1957). *The American transcendentalists: Their prose and poetry*. Garden City, New York, Doubleday & Company.

Miller, P. H. and D. F. Bjorklund (1998). "Contemplating fuzzy-trace theory: The gist of it." *Journal of Experimental Child Psychology* 71: 184–193.

Montaigne, M. (1998). *The complete essays of Montaigne*. Stanford, California, Stanford University Press.

Myers, D. G. (1992). *The pursuit of happiness: Who is happy and why*. New York, William Morrow.

Myers, D. G. and E. Diener (1996). "The pursuit of happiness." *Scientific American* 273: 70–72.

Nietzsche, F. (1891). *Thus spoke Zarathustra*. Buffalo, New York, Prometheus Books.

O'Connell, M. J. (1997). *Blaise Pascal*. Cambridge, England, W. B. Eedmanns Publishing.

Pascal, B. (1662). Collected works. *Great books of the Western World*. M. J. Adler, ed. Chicago, Illinois, Brittanica: 30: 1–487.

Petrarch (1995). *Petrarch's secret: Three dialogues between himself and Augustine.* Westport, Connecticut, Hyperion Press.

Phillips, K. (2002). *Wealth and democracy.* New York, Broadway Books.

Plato (1956). *Protagoras.* Indianapolis, Indiana, Bobbs-Merrill Company, Inc.

Povinelli, D. J. (2000). *Folk physics for apes: The chimpanzee's theory of how the world works.* New York, Oxford University Press.

Rand, A. (1957). *Atlas shrugged.* New York, Random House.

Rand, A. (1962). Introducing objectivism. *The Objectivist Newsletter.* 1: 35.

Rand, A. (1964). *The virtue of selfishness: A new concept of egoism.* New York, New American Library.

Rey, G. (1997). *Contemporary philosophy of mind.* Oxford, England, Blackwell Publishers.

Reyna, V. F. and C. J. Brainerd (1998). "Fuzzy-trace theory and false memory: New frontiers." *Journal of Experimental Child Psychology* 71: 194–209.

Rogers, C. R. (1980). *A way of being.* Boston, Houghton Mifflin.

Rychlak, J. F. (1968). *A philosophy of science for personality theory.* Boston, Houghton Mifflin Company.

Seager, W. (1999). *Theories of consciousness: An introduction and assessment.* London, Routledge.

Seligman, M. (2002). *Authentic happiness: Using the new positive psychology to realize your potential for lasting fulfillment.* New York, Free Press.

Seneca, L. A. (1962). *Ad Lucilium epistulae morales.* Cambridge, Massachusetts, Harvard University Press.

Simon, H. A. (1990). "Invariants of human behavior." *Annual Review of Psychology* 41: 1–19.

Snyder, C. R. and S. J. Lopez, eds. (2002). *Handbook of positive psychology.* New York, Oxford University Press.

Spinoza, B. (1955). *Works of Spinoza.* New York, Dover Publications.

Teilhard de Chardin, P. (1959). *The phenomenon of man.* New York, Harper & Row.

Teilhard de Chardin, P. (1978). *The heart of matter.* New York, Harcourt-Brace-Jovanovich.

Tulving, E. (2002). "Episodic memory: From mind to brain." *Annual Review of Psychology* 53: 1–25.

Voltaire (1754). *Philosophical dictionary.* London, Penguin Classics.

Voltaire (1927). *The complete romances of Voltaire.* New York, Walter J. Black, Inc.

Walker, E. H. (2000). *The physics of consciousness: Quantum minds and the meaning of life.* Cambridge, Massachusetts, Perseus Books.

Weihs, G., T. Jennewein, et al. (1998). "Violation of Bell's inequality under strict Einstein locality conditions." *Physical Review Letters* 81: 5039–5043.

Whitehead, A. N. (1929). *Process and reality: An essay in cosmology.* New York, The MacMillan Company.

Winnicott, D. (1958). *Collected papers: Through pediatrics to psychoanalysis.* New York, Basic Books.

# 2

# THE SEARCH FOR
# AN ADEQUATE PSYCHOLOGY

## THE ESSENTIAL QUESTIONS OF PSYCHOLOGY

Like philosophers, psychologists disagree about the importance of the body, the mind, and the spirit in the development of well-being. Skeptics and materialists, such as Hume and James, recognize the body and its physical sensations and emphasize the body's role in determining human desires and fears. In contrast, rational idealists and humanists, such as Kant and Freud, recognize the dualism of body and mind and emphasize the role of rationality in shaping character development and thereby defining human dignity. Transcendentalists, such as Hegel and Krishnamurti, recognize the whole of being and emphasize the role of intuition in integrating experience.

Hegel refers to the intuitive aspects of consciousness that give form to our awareness before reflection or reasoning as "spirit." The word *spirit* is derived from Latin word *spiritus*, meaning "breath." According to *Webster's New International Dictionary*, *spirit* has several interrelated meanings. The fundamental meaning of spirit is the "breath of life," which animates material things by giving them consciousness. More precisely, the spirit, or breath of life, refers to self-aware consciousness. In other words, the spirit refers to the psyche or soul or, more specifically, to the characteristic attitude or disposition of the psyche or soul. The spirit of something is its essential quality, pervading tone, disposition, or intent as opposed to the literal or material form of something. As a verb, *spirit* means to infuse with energy, life, or a characteristic intention.

In reference to individual human beings, the term *spirit* refers to the immaterial intelligent part of a person that provides personality with its inward structure, dynamic drive, and creative response to the demands it encounters during development. Hence, the spirit, or *psyche*, of a person is distinguished from the body, or *soma*, which refers to the material outer form. The soma and psyche of a person are analogous to the dual character of light as both particle and wave.

Contemporary philosophers have sometimes distinguished dualistic concepts of mind as "mind 1" and nondualistic concepts of spirit as "mind 2." Essentially, the mind is that which is conscious. When our consciousness is focused on material things, a dichotomy can be distinguished between the subject (i.e., the mind, which is conscious) and the object (i.e., that which is other than the mind). Likewise, when we regard another conscious being as a material object, we are aware only of what is finite and transient. In this objective perspective, we assume there is an essential separation of subject and object, which implies the privacy of consciousness. This dualistic state of consciousness is called "mind 1." For example, Kant was a dualist who recognized innate ideas about space and time from the intuitive senses of the mind. According to such a dualistic view, we may have an intuitive awareness of our being (i.e., we know we are in space) and of our responsibility and freedom (i.e., we know we are able to change in time).

Even though Kant recognized a role for intuition, Hegel and other transcendentalists regard such dualistic views as those of Kant as incomplete. According to Hegel (1807), consciousness is purified as the mind increases in the fullness of its awareness of itself. The transcendental mind fully aware of itself is pure self-aware consciousness, which is nondual. According to transcendentalists, a mind fully aware of itself is unbounded spirit, nonlocal, and aware of participation in the universal unity of being. In concrete terms, transcendentalists believe that it is possible to intuit what another person is feeling or thinking, but they admit that the degree to which nonlocal awareness is achieved in practice varies greatly between individuals and depends on psychological conditions. For example, appropriate psychological conditions for nonlocal consciousness have been described as loving union with goodness (Plato 1986) or loving union in nature (Thoreau 1848; Krishnamurti 1999; Krishnamurti and Bohm 1999).

Materialists regard all claims of nonlocal consciousness as illusory. Transcendentalists, on the other hand, say the individual mind is like a node in a universal Internet of consciousness and that these individual nodes vary in the speed and depth of their access to the whole web. The different views of materialists and transcendentalists are based on their assumptions about the composition of a human being. Materialists assume a human being is only matter. In contrast, transcendentalists assume a human being is composed of both soma (i.e., the body, which is the material aspect of our being) and psyche (i.e., consciousness, which is the intelligent immaterial aspect of our being). The psyche can be focused on material things (in which case we call it mind or mind 1). The psyche can also be focused on itself (in which case we call it spirit or mind 2). When focused on itself, self-aware consciousness can expand in a stepwise fashion to access the universal Internet of consciousness of which it is an inseparable part.

These distinctions help to clarify the scientific questions about which materialists and transcendentalists disagree, which psychology must reconcile in its study of consciousness. Materialists claim that nothing but matter exists. Eliminative materialists regard consciousness as nothing but an illusion, and less extreme materialists claim that consciousness is an attribute of matter or the product of antecedent physical causes (i.e., Newtonian mechanical determinism). If consciousness is an attribute or product of matter, it is necessarily finite, determined by antecedent causes, and local.

In contrast, transcendentalists claim that consciousness has unique properties that cannot be produced or explained by antecedent physical causes, such as being nonlocal and noncausal (i.e., spontaneously free or underdetermined by antecedent causes). Fortunately, we can recognize from this difference between materialists and transcendentalists that there is finally consensus about the phenomena that are denoted by the spirit, regardless of uncertainty about terminology and the reality of putative explanatory mechanisms (Chalmers 1996; Rey 1997). Materialists attack even the possibility of the same phenomena that transcendentalists celebrate as the essence of life. Specifically, the phenomena of the spirit include the nonlocality of consciousness, freedom of will, and specific forms of noncausality called gifts. Examples of gifts or giftedness are special forms of creativity, such as musical or mathematical genius, and other aspects of coherence, such as well-being, wisdom, and virtues. Examples of nonlocal consciousness include pantheistic experiences of union in nature, as reported by transcendentalists like Emerson and Thoreau (Miller 1957) and others (Krishnamurti and Bohm 1985), and transpersonal communion, as reported by some therapists in close therapeutic alliances (Spiegelman 1996) or by individuals in love (Lamartine 1851, 1887).

Materialists regard the reports of the transcendental phenomena of consciousness as illusory. Transcendentalists suggest that materialists have little or no consciousness of transcendental phenomena because of their low level of self-awareness. Logically, it is always true that the absence of proof is not the proof of absence of phenomena under other conditions. However, logic is never compelling to people who do not have personal experience with a phenomenon. We really only have conviction about what we directly recognize by intuition.

As a result of this divergence of viewpoints, progress in understanding consciousness must measure and explain these spiritual phenomena in a rigorous manner that characterizes the conditions under which they can or cannot be experienced. These transcendental phenomena are designated as "spirit" specifically because they cannot be explained by Newtonian concepts of mechanical determinism. However, the transcendental phenomena of consciousness may be explained by more fundamental mechanisms, such as the quantum properties of noncausality and nonlocality, as we examine in Chapter 5. However, before that is scientifically feasible, we must know more about the psychological measurement of personality in general.

To move from philosophical discussion to scientific measurement about consciousness and well-being, I began by trying to understand how to measure personality and its various aspects such as temperament, character, and coherence. Personality has been defined as "the dynamic organization within the individual of those psychophysical systems that determine his unique adjustments to his environment" (Allport 1937; Cloninger, Svrakic et al. 1993). Each part of this definition is important. Personality is *dynamic*, not static, so personality is not a set of permanently fixed traits. Personality development is *psychophysical*; that is, personality is influenced by both psychological and physical variables. Finally, an adequate personality description must be *idiographic*; that is, changes are adaptive in a unique way for each individual.

Learning has been likewise defined as "the organization of behavior as a result of individual experience" (Thorpe 1956; Cloninger, Svrakic et al. 1993). In other words, personality is a description of the way we learn or grow in self-aware consciousness. The measurement of personality allows us to describe differences between people in their style of living and their level of self-aware consciousness.

My own research on the understanding of personality development has gone through three major phases. I refer to these three phases in terms of models of personality as temperament, self, and coherence. First, *temperament* corresponds to a materialist approach to personality as determined by individual differences in the perception of physical sensations. Second, the *self* includes both temperament and character, and so corresponds to a mind–body dualism in which higher cognitive processes regulate basic emotional drives. Third, *coherence of being* involves the integration of body, mind, and spirit; that is, coherence is defined as unity of function in all aspects of a human being.

These three phases of my search for an adequate psychology of well-being illustrate a hierarchy of models of consciousness and personality. They are truly a hierarchy of nested hypotheses about personality in which the model of coherence includes that of self as a special case and the model of self includes temperament as a special case. I have personally developed and tested each of these paradigms to see what each can do and cannot do as an account of human nature. I have been forced to develop more comprehensive models by experimental observations that could not be satisfied by the more restricted cases.

My study of a succession of three paradigms for personality illustrates what is meant when a theory is said to be incomplete. An incomplete theory is not completely wrong—it is only correct to a certain degree of approximation under particular conditions. For example, Newton's principles of physics can only approximate the predictions of the more general theory of quantum physics under particular conditions. Nevertheless, Newtonian physics is sufficiently correct under ordinary conditions to build bridges. However, the mechanical world view of Newtonian physics may mislead us if applied to human consciousness. Progress in science requires that we give serious attention to the exceptions that cannot be explained by currently fashionable models. As a corollary of this principle, once a more complete model is found, it is unwise to assume it is universally complete. The mysteries to be discovered and explained are inexhaustible.

In this chapter, I only sketch my own succession of scientific paradigms in sufficient detail to reveal the major conceptual and experimental mysteries that I have confronted, to spare the reader from adopting or retaining inadequate paradigms, which are unfortunately all too commonplace. The development of the third phase of my work on coherence and well-being is the major purpose of this whole book; here, I first describe the experimental findings that could not be explained by temperament and character alone. Then I introduce key concepts about transcendental phenomena that influence the development of coherence of personality, which is examined in more detail in later chapters.

## HUMAN PERSONALITY AS TEMPERAMENT

### Individual differences in temperament

My initial approach to describing human personality was to provide a description of individual differences in temperament. Temperament is described in terms of habits and skills that are elicited by simple stimuli perceived by the physical senses. Temperament is the model of human personality described by materialists, such as William James, and materialistic rationalists, like Locke, who believe that all thought is a consequence of sensory experience or reflection on sensory experience. Temperament has usually been defined as those components of personality that are heritable, developmentally stable, emotion based, or uninfluenced by sociocultural learning (Goldsmith, Buss et al. 1987; Cloninger 1994). According to materialism, once temperament is properly measured, other aspects of personality can be predicted as developments from these basic predispositions. Accordingly, I sought to describe the underlying neurogenetic basis of human personality in terms of multiple dimensions of temperament, which I defined as the automatic associative responses to simple emotional stimuli that determine differences in habits and emotional responses, such as fear, anger, and disgust.

At the time that I set out to develop my model of temperament, I thought it would be adequate because the consensus in the fields of behavior genetics and biological psychiatry was that there were only two or three heritable dimensions of personality. Following the materialist viewpoint of the developmental scientist Piaget, I also assumed that personality followed a predictable linear pattern of development that was an epigenetic construction using the building blocks of accumulated sensory experience guided by the emotional drives of temperament. The vast majority of scientists at the time viewed personality development with the same materialistic assumptions.

The same belief in materialism (or a materialist form of rationalism like that of Locke or Piaget) is prevalent today. In modern biological psychiatry and psychology, there is little or no awareness of the limitations of materialism that have been long recognized in physics and philosophy. For example, I was aware of humanistic criticism of materialism from my university studies, but this information was so dissonant from the prevailing views of my medical education that I did not even try to reconcile and synthesize my knowledge of philosophy and biological psychology. Consistent with the prevailing materialistic views, I thought human personality could be reduced to a small number of physical biases in reaction to specific sensations. As a result, this model was appropriately described by a Freudian commentator as "a humanist's nightmare" (Kramer 1993). Nevertheless, the approach was innovative for biological psychiatry because it provided a description of a few quantifiable traits that could explain the confusing overlap that occurs when personality disorders are diagnosed as if they were discrete categories of illness (Cloninger 1986, 1987).

When I began my empirical research on personality, I initially distinguished three quantitative dimensions of temperament based on prior research on the genetic structure of personality in humans, neurobiological studies in humans and other animals, phylogenetic analyses, and behavioral conditioning (Cloninger 1986, 1987). These temperament traits were defined in terms of variability in behavioral conditioning to specific types of stimuli perceived by the physical senses, thereby excluding any role for intuition. Any mental or spiritual phenomena were assumed to be epigenetic developments or generalizations from accumulated sensory experience motivated by temperament. The three dimensions of temperament that I described were called Harm Avoidance (anxiety-proneness versus outgoing vigor and risk taking), Novelty Seeking (exploratory impulsiveness versus stoic frugality), and Reward Dependence (social attachment versus aloofness).

I then developed reliable clinical measures of these dimensions, including a self-report questionnaire called the Tridimensional Personality Questionnaire (TPQ) and related rating procedures for clinicians and observers. Factor analytic studies confirmed that these three dimensions were nearly noncorrelated with one another and highly internally consistent except that Persistence (industry versus underachievement) emerged as an independent fourth temperament dimension. Persistence had originally been a subscale of Reward Dependence, but it proved empirically to be independently heritable in large-scale twin studies in the United States and Australia (Heath, Cloninger et al. 1994; Stallings, Hewitt et al. 1996).

The descriptors of high and low scorers on each of these four dimensions are summarized in Table 2.1.

These dimensions have been extensively studied in clinical, neurobiological, and genetic research, as reviewed in detail elsewhere (Cloninger 1998, 2000; Cloninger and Svrakic 2000). These four temperament dimensions are each about 50% heritable according to twin studies, and each is influenced by multiple specific genes according to linkage and association studies (Comings, Gade-Andavolu et al. 2000; Gillespie, Cloninger et al. 2003).

Clinical studies have confirmed my original hypothesis (Cloninger 1987) that these temperament dimensions distinguish subtypes of personality disorders. Specific subtypes of personality disorder are associated with a specific configuration of temperament features, as depicted in Figure 2.1. For example, antisocial personality disorder is associated with high scores in Novelty Seeking and low scores in Harm Avoidance and Reward Dependence. More generally, individuals with anxious personality disorders (called Cluster C in *DSM-IV*) are high in Harm Avoidance; those with impulsive personality disorders (Cluster B in *DSM-IV*) are high in Novelty Seeking, and those with aloof personality disorders (Cluster A in *DSM-IV*) are low in Reward Dependence (APA 1994). If a four-cluster system is used, obsessional patients are higher in Persistence. These results have been confirmed by independent investigators in many countries throughout the world,

**Table 2.1.** Descriptors of Individuals Who Score High and Low on the Four Temperament Dimensions

|  | *Descriptors of Extreme Variants* | |
| *Temperament Dimension* | *High* | *Low* |
| --- | --- | --- |
| Harm Avoidance | Pessimistic | Optimistic |
|  | Fearful | Daring |
|  | Shy | Outgoing |
|  | Fatigable | Vigorous |
| Novelty Seeking | Exploratory | Reserved |
|  | Impulsive | Rigid |
|  | Extravagant | Frugal |
|  | Irritable | Stoic |
| Reward Dependence | Sentimental | Critical |
|  | Sociable | Aloof |
|  | Warm | Detached |
|  | Sympathetic | Independent |
| Persistence | Eager | Apathetic |
|  | Determined | Spoiled |
|  | Ambitious | Underachiever |
|  | Perfectionist | Pragmatist |

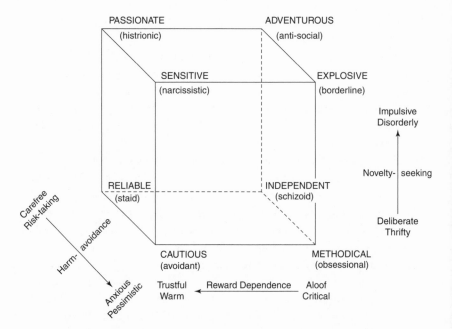

Figure 2.1. The temperament cube. (Reproduced by permission of the Center for Psychobiology of Personality, Washington University, St. Louis, Missouri)

showing the cross-cultural generality of this temperament model (Cloninger and Svrakic 2000). The major article describing the temperament model (Cloninger 1987) is one of the most frequently cited papers in the field according to the Science Citation Index.

However, I was shocked to observe that I could not distinguish my healthy friends from my patients based on temperament alone! As will be discussed in more detail later, systematic clinical studies showed that there are other aspects of personality besides these temperament dimensions. Furthermore, these additional dimensions of personality are needed to determine whether someone has a personality disorder, or to specify the degree of maturity of particular individuals (Cloninger, Svrakic et al. 1993; Svrakic, Whitehead et al. 1993).

In brief, temperament has been shown to describe differences between individuals in what they consciously experience and report to be emotionally salient. In other words, temperament describes what grabs our attention and how intensely we respond. Furthermore, the self-report measures agree strongly with clinical ratings by expert observers and also correlate with objective laboratory tests, such as individual differences in startle and regional brain activity (Cloninger 1998; Cloninger 2000; Sugiura, Kawashima et al. 2000; Paulus, Rogalsky et al. 2003). This indicates strong correspondence between subjective experience, objective performance, and self-reported knowledge of temperament.

The role of temperament in personality development

I had begun my work on temperament expecting that interactions among multiple temperament dimensions would predict patterns of personality development. In fact, we found that temperament dimensions were developmentally stable—they change little with increasing age, with psychotherapy, or with pharmacotherapy! We can measure the same temperament dimensions in children and adults regardless of age with age-appropriate questions that correspond to consistent psychological concepts (Constantino, Cloninger et al. 2000). Among a large sample of adults varying in age, we find little correlation between temperament scores and age (Cloninger 2003). Novelty Seeking does decrease with age but the other dimensions show no consistent pattern of change.

We found that temperament configuration did vary in the probability with which they were associated with immaturity. The relationship is moderately strong, as summarized in Table 2.2. Thus, individuals with an explosive configuration (high Harm Avoidance and Novelty Seeking, low Reward Dependence) have a high probability of being immature in character. However, the probability is not a certainty; temperament alone does not determine whether a person is mature or immature. In more clinical terms, temperament does not determine whether an individual has a personality disorder, is average in maturity, or is unusually well integrated.

**Table 2.2.** Relative Risk of Immaturity (i.e., Mild and Severe Personality Disorder) as a Function of Temperament Type in a Sample from the General Community

| Temperament Type | Configuration* | n | Immature (%) |
|---|---|---|---|
| HIGH RISK | | | |
| Explosive | NHr | 39 | 72 |
| Methodical | nHr | 44 | 59 |
| Adventurous | Nhr | 25 | 48 |
| Sensitive | NHR | 30 | 40 |
| AVERAGE | — | 15 | 33 |
| LOW RISK | | | |
| Cautious | nHR | 30 | 17 |
| Independent | nhr | 31 | 16 |
| Passionate | NhR | 50 | 12 |
| Reliable | nhR | 36 | 6 |
| TOTAL | | 300 | 33 |

*Novelty Seeking maybe high (N) or low (m), Harm Avoidance high (H) or low(h), Reward Dependence high (R) or low (r).

Source: From Cloninger et al., 1994.

Both the high and the low extremes of each temperament dimension have advantages and disadvantages depending on the context (Cloninger 1987). Accordingly, no genetic engineering or other manipulation can devise the optimal temperament for all circumstances. Adaptability lies in diversity within the whole population, which is based on conflicting drives within individuals. Consequently, temperament can never provide a complete solution to individual integration.

## Critique of personality as temperament

Temperament can be reliably measured and studied by self-report and by observations at many levels of organization from genetic, chemical, anatomical, and physiological to behavioral. Temperament provides a useful account of individual differences in processes of selective attention and emotional salience (Hansenne, Pinto et al. 2003), but does not stand alone as a description of human personality or consciousness. It provides no account of the self-organizing property of human personality, which gives it properties of executive control or empathic cooperation as observed in primates generally. It also provides no account of intuition or subjective awareness that underlies uniquely human characteristics, such as creativity, symbolic invention, or the drive for coherence and integration itself.

In addition, others have shown that behavioral conditioning in general is unable to explain human learning abilities, such as the way children acquire propositional logic or language (Chomsky 1980). Artificial intelligence programs can function well as expert systems but do not have the flexibility to make intuitive adaptations in the way that is characteristic of human consciousness. These findings by others and my empirical finding that temperament could not account for personality development led me to question materialism as an adequate account of human personality and consciousness. At the same time, awareness of the incompleteness of temperament as a model of personality opened the door for me to explore the role of rational processes in personality development.

## HUMAN PERSONALITY AS SELF

## Individual differences in character

When I observed that variation in temperament alone did not account for individual differences in degree of maturity or whether an individual had a personality disorder, I examined what aspects of personality were omitted in my model of personality. I compared the traits measured by the TPQ with other personality measurement systems, as well as the descriptions of human character in humanistic and transpersonal psychology and psychodynamic psychiatry. Character is what people make of themselves intentionally (Kant 1796). In other words, character is the reflection of personal goals and values. Accordingly, character traits can be specified in terms of subject–object relations. The subject–object dichotomy gives rise to three possible relations: namely, our concept of our self (subject–subject relations), our concept of our relations with others (i.e., subject-object relations), and our concept of our participation in the world as a whole (i.e., object–object relations). These three possible relations correspond to the three concepts of human dignity developed by dualistic rationalists, as discussed in Chapter 1.

To measure these three concepts of subject–object relations and human dignity, I extended the TPQ by developing reliable measures of three traits called Self-Directedness (self-concept), Cooperativeness (concept of relations with others), and Self-Transcendence (concept of our participation in the world as a whole) (Cloninger, Svrakic et al. 1993). The descriptors of high and low scores on these three character traits are presented in Table 2.3. The Temperament and Character Inventory (TCI) measures the four temperament dimensions (same as in the TPQ) and the three character traits of Self-Directedness, Cooperativeness, and Self-Transcendence. Thus, the TCI provides a dual-aspect description of self as the marriage of temperament and character.

The TCI is applicable in samples from the general population as well as in patients with psychiatric disorders. The factor structure is the same, but mean values are generally lower for the character traits in psychiatric patients (Svrakic, Whitehead et al. 1993; Bayon, Hill et al. 1996). Most important, the TCI character traits distinguish individuals with no personality disorder from those with per-

**Table 2.3.** Descriptors of Individuals Who Score High and Low on the Three Character Dimensions

|  | Descriptors of Extreme Variants | |
|---|---|---|
| *Character Dimension* | *High* | *Low* |
| Self-Directedness | Responsible | Blaming |
|  | Purposeful | Aimless |
|  | Resourceful | Inept |
|  | Self-Accepting | Vain |
|  | Hopeful | Deliberating |
| Cooperative | Reasonable | Prejudiced |
|  | Empathic | Insensitive |
|  | Helpful | Hostile |
|  | Compassionate | Revengeful |
|  | Principled | Opportunistic |
| Self-Transcendent | Judicious | Repressive |
|  | Idealistic | Practical |
|  | Transpersonal | Dualistic |
|  | Faithful | Skeptical |
|  | Spiritual | Materialistic |

sonality disorders diagnosed by expert clinicians using structured interviews (Svrakic, Whitehead et al. 1993). In fact, personality disorders are not discrete diseases but differ only quantitatively in degree of maturity from others. There is more information about maturity preserved by quantifying the character configuration of people using the TCI than by assigning discrete diagnoses.

A useful indicator of maturity overall is simply the sum of scores in TCI Self-Directedness and Cooperativeness. However, the three-dimensional character configuration provides additional information. Descriptors of traits associated with the possible configurations of the TCI character dimensions are shown in Figure 2.2.

The psychobiology of these character dimensions is being actively investigated. Initially, character was expected to be less heritable than temperament and more influenced by sociocultural learning and environmental influences shared by siblings who are reared together. However, twin studies and genetic association studies now contradict this. Each of the character dimensions shows moderate heritability and associations with multiple candidate genes (Comings, Gade-Andavolu et al. 2000) and little or no effects of environmental influences shared by siblings reared together (Gillespie, Cloninger et al. 2003).

In brain imaging studies, individual differences in TCI Self-Directedness has been found to correlate strongly with activity of the medial prefrontal cortex during executive tasks (Gusnard, Ollinger et al. 2003), as described in depth in Chapter 3. In addition, TCI Self-Transcendence is strongly correlated (–0.8) with serotonin$_{1a}$

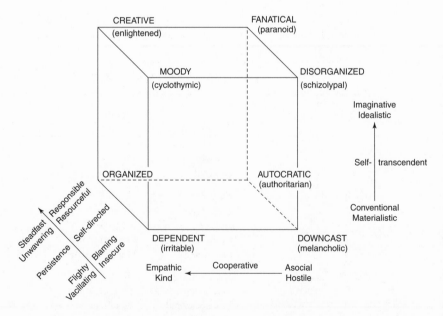

Figure 2.2. The character cube. (Reproduced by permission of the Center for Psychobiology of Personality, Washington University, St. Louis, Missouri)

(5-HT$_{1a}$) receptor density in the neocortex, hippocampus, and raphe nuclei (Borg, Andree et al. 2003). In psychophysiological studies, individual differences in TCI Self-Directedness have moderately strong correlations with the evoked potential P300, which is an indicator of individual differences in emotional relief from updating of expectancies. Furthermore, only Self-Directedness, and no other temperament or character trait, is correlated with P300 (Vedeniapin, Anokhin et al. 2001). Cooperativeness and Self-Transcendence are related to measures of Contingent Negative Variation (Cloninger 1998). These results are especially important because they show that human emotional conditioning is supervised and modulated by higher-order cognitive processes that are described as rational.

Furthermore, individual differences in rational cognitive processes (i.e., character) are largely unexplained by individual differences in the conditioning of behavioral response to stimuli perceived by the physical senses (i.e., temperament). In other words, the psychological assumptions of materialists (i.e., behaviorism in any of its forms) are excessively reductive. Materialism and behaviorism often erroneously diminish the importance of higher cognitive processing. As a result, most contemporary psychological research is based on cognitive-behavioral theories.

## Character development

Initially, my colleagues and I observed that character traits increased with age, particularly during the transition from adolescence to early adulthood (Cloninger, Svrakic et al. 1993), as summarized in Table 2.4. There are some increases with age, particularly for Cooperativeness from adolescence into early adulthood. However, the amounts of increase in character with age are small on average, and negligible after middle age.

The different possible configurations of character are described in Figure 2.2. For example, individuals high in all three traits of character are labeled as creative,

**Table 2.4.** Character and Age: Proportions of Items Endorsed on TCI Scales of Temperament by Age in a Cross-Sectional Sample of 1800 Individuals Older than Seventeen Years from the General Population

| Age (yr) | Self-Directed | Cooperative | Self-Transcendent |
|---|---|---|---|
| <21 | 0.64 | 0.80 | 0.50 |
| 21–30 | 0.71 | 0.79 | 0.51 |
| 31–40 | 0.74 | 0.83 | 0.51 |
| 41–50 | 0.74 | 0.84 | 0.50 |
| 51–60 | 0.76 | 0.86 | 0.53 |
| 61–70 | 0.77 | 0.86 | 0.52 |
| 71+ | 0.77 | 0.84 | 0.53 |

*Source*: Adapted from Cloninger, 2003.

and those who are low in Self-Directedness but high in the other two are labeled as cyclothymic. We observed that there are nonlinear relations among temperament and character configurations (Cloninger, Svrakic et al. 1997). Specifically, different temperament configurations are associated with the same character configuration (i.e., show equifinality). In addition, the same temperament configuration can lead to different character configurations (i.e., show multifinality). Using the labels for temperament configurations given in Figure 2.1, we can describe the correspondences between temperament and character configurations. For example, individuals with histrionic and reliable temperaments account for 29% and 20% of individuals with a creative character configuration (that is, high in all three character dimensions); this is an example of equifinality, or different temperaments leading to the same character. However, these same temperament configurations can result in character configurations other than the creative character; the histrionic temperament also often leads to a cyclothymic character, whereas the reliable temperament also often leads to an organized character. Such multifinality is another indication of the nonlinearity of relations between temperament and character. If the relations were linear, there would be one-to-one relations among temperament and character. Furthermore, predictions about the nonlinear dynamics of personality development were confirmed in longitudinal data about 593 individuals followed over a period of 1 year (Cloninger, Svrakic et al. 1997).

Next, we examined the pattern of character development in more depth by studying the sequence of changes in subscales of the three characters. Each character dimension has multiple subscales, which may each represent a distinct step in development. In fact, we observed that increases in subscale scores tended to follow a characteristic temporal sequence. This typical or canonical sequence is summarized and compared with the sequences described by Piaget, Freud, and Erikson (Table 2.5). The pattern of development is actually not linear, as is described in detail in Chapter 3, but there is sufficient correspondence to suggest that what I have called character development was what others have observed as cognitive maturation, psychosexual development, or ego development. This is also supported by findings that character traits are strongly related to maturity of ego defenses assessed with the Defense Style Questionnaire (Mulder, Joyce et al. 1996). Further studies of character development are examined in Chapters 3 through 6.

Another crucial aspect of character development is the possibility of improvement in response to treatment. The hope of therapy is that treatment leads to fundamental improvement in personality, particularly in character. Empirically, what is often found in therapeutic interventions is that the level of Self-Directedness at the beginning of therapy predicts the degree of improvement. This has been observed with cognitive-behavioral therapy for bulimia and depression, as well as in the treatment of depression with antidepressants (Joyce, Mulder et al. 1994; Tome, Cloninger et al. 1997; Bulik, Sullivan et al. 1998; Cloninger and Svrakic

**Table 2.5.** Comparison of Different Descriptions of Personality Development

| TCI Developmental Step | Piaget | Freud | Erikson |
|---|---|---|---|
| [1] sd1—responsible | Sensorimotor (reflexive) | | |
| [2] co1—tolerant | Sensorimotor (enactive) | Oral | Trust |
| [3] st1—sensible | Self-object differentiation | | |
| [4] sd2—purposeful | Intuitive | Anal | Autonomy |
| [5] co4—forgiving | | Phallic | Initiative |
| [6] st4—idealistic | Operational (concrete) | Latency | Industry |
| [7] sd4—self-accepting | | | |
| [8] co2—empathic | | Early genital | |
| [9] st2—transpersonal | | | |
| [10] sd3—resourceful | Operational (abstract) | | Identity |
| [11] co3—helpful | | Later genital | Intimacy |
| [12] st5—faithful | | | Generative |
| [13] sd5—hopeful | | | Integrity |
| [14] co5—charitable | | | |
| [15] st3—spiritual | | | |

2000). There are often some benefits from cognitive-behavioral therapy, but most patients treated for personality disorders have not made fundamental changes in their character with conventional treatments. That is, stable change in cognitive schemas, or what can be called their initial perspective, has been infrequent (Sperry 1999). Patients are most likely to return to their usual or best level of adjustment before the crisis that brought them to therapy. What is accepted as a good outcome of therapy is for a patient with personality disorder to become their own self-directed therapist for their persistent cognitive distortions (Beck 1996). Such limited benefits underscore the need for better understanding of the fundamental mechanisms of character development, as described in Chapter 5.

Critique of personality as self

In the model of personality as self, individual differences in human personality are described in terms of temperament and character. This description provides a useful account of behavioral conditioning in terms of temperament and of higher cognitive functions in terms of character, such as executive functions (Self-Directedness), legislative functions (Cooperativeness), and judicial functions (Self-

Transcendence). These traits together provide a rich account of normal personality and its disorders. As a result the major article describing the dimensions of temperament and character (Cloninger, Svrakic et al. 1993) is extensively used in the assessment of both normal and abnormal personality. Subsequently, it has also become one of the most highly cited articles in the field as measured by the Science Citation Index. Rather than characterizing only pathology, we can begin to understand how disorders can arise and be maintained despite association with much suffering.

## HUMAN PERSONALITY AS COHERENCE OF BEING

### What is self-aware consciousness?

After I developed my model of temperament (Cloninger 1986, 1987), I observed that temperament did not fully predict individual differences in degree of the maturity of character (Cloninger, Svrakic et al. 1993; Svrakic, Whitehead et al. 1993). Likewise, after I developed the model of temperament and character, I observed that these variables did not fully predict individual differences in level of awareness of reality or the unity of being (Cloninger and Svrakic 1997; Cloninger 1999, 2002). To be precise, I observed that people with both high and low levels of character development still varied substantially in their awareness of the world. For example, mature materialists are aware primarily of knowing facts, whereas mature transcendentalists are concerned with self-awareness (i.e., awareness of one's own intentions).

Detailed studies of human learning and memory have also shown that memories based on single observations include more than one type of memory (Tulving 1987, 2002). Tulving has distinguished procedural memory (i.e., incremental learning based on repetition of stimulus-response sequences) from two types of conceptual recognition and recall that occur after a single observation (Table 2.6). Procedural memory underlies associative learning and involves presemantic perceptual processing of information from the physical senses that can operate independently of abstract conceptual and/or volitional processes. In contrast, intuitive learning based on immediate recognition from a single episode of observation involves higher cognitive functions of abstraction and symbolization.

One type of memory based on immediate recognition is knowledge of general facts that are impersonal and timeless, which has been called "semantic memory" or "Mind 1." The second type of recognition memory is awareness of one's own intentions, which has been called "episodic memory" or "Mind 2." In other words, episodic memory involves self-awareness and recall of events in a personal context in time and space. Episodic memories describe the personal meaning of "when" and "where" events occur in the path of our life.

**Table 2.6.** Description of Tulving's Ternary Memory Classification

| Characteristic | Level I | Level II | Level III |
|---|---|---|---|
| Memory type | Procedural | Semantic | Episodic |
| Acquisition | Overt Behavioral conditioning (incremental exposure) | Observation (one-trial) + covert cognitive restructuring | Observation (one-trial) + covert cognitive accretion |
| Representation | Prescriptive Stimulus-response (sensory modality specific) | Descriptive abstract model (modality general) | Descriptive event in personal spatiotemporal context |
| Expression | Automatic Overt act | Factual reference Knowledge | Intentional recall |
| Level of consciousness | Anoetic (unaware) | Noetic (knowing) | Autonoetic (self-aware) |

*Source*: From Tulving (1987).

Episodic memory is what philosophers have called "recollection" or "rational intuition." Likewise, contemporary psychologists refer to episodic memory as recollection because it is what enables human beings to remember past experiences. In contrast, semantic memory is knowledge of general facts, which involves abstracting what is general from what is unique to each individual in a variety of life situations. Self-aware consciousness involves awareness of many volitional possibilities in life, but semantic memories reduce this flexibility to a single choice, much like the collapse of a quantum wave function by the measurements of an external observer.

It was shocking to me when I realized that memory does not necessarily involve "recollection," that is, an intuitive reexperiencing of the past in the immediacy of our self-aware consciousness. We also acquire intellectual "knowledge" of our personal past by semantic learning without having the ability to travel through time in self-aware consciousness. *Recollection* involves the immediate experience of personally travelling through time, whereas intellectual *knowledge* does not require any awareness of (or relationship to) time. It is normal for modern human beings to be able to do both (i.e., know the facts and recollect the context in which we learned the facts). Consequently, we often falsely assume that these two forms of memory necessarily go together. However, some people have deficits in episodic memory and are unable to recollect their past consciously, although they are also able to learn lessons in school and acquire the intellectual knowledge ("just the facts") needed to adapt in the activities of daily living at a practical and objective level. However, they do not have the normal human self-awareness that is the basis for development of art, science, or spirituality.

Self-aware consciousness is alive and free, whereas intellectual knowledge (i.e., semantic memories of concepts and general facts) is "dead" or "frozen" abstraction. For example, character traits like Self-Directedness are general concepts abstracted from a variety of situations that have unique meanings to each individual. They are not alive in the way that an autobiographical recollection communicates information in a personal and social context that is unique for every individual. In other words, self-awareness is "idiographic" (i.e., unique to every individual), whereas character traits are "nomothetic" (i.e., general facts about one's self-concept and object relations).

Initially, episodic memory was defined in terms of materials and tasks, such as intentions (i.e., one's self in a spatiotemporal context) (Tulving 1987). Subsequently, the concept of episodic memory has been refined and elaborated in terms of awareness of one's self, the sense of subjective time, and a state of consciousness in which there is recollection of personal events in space and time. Tulving (2001, 2002) now describes episodic memory as autobiographical, self-aware or "auto-noetic" consciousness, which is consistent with other descriptions of ordinary human self-awareness as based on immediate recognition by the intuitive senses. Tulving (2001) and others have found no evidence that such intuitive self-awareness is present in any animal species except human beings. Self-aware consciousness is lacking even in chimpanzees (Povinelli 2000; Povinelli and Giambrone 2001).

Procedural, semantic, and episodic memory can be functionally dissociated from one another. For example, individuals with Parkinson's disorder, characterized by striatal lesions, exhibit deficits in procedural learning but not in semantic or episodic memory. Individuals with an amnestic syndrome, characterized by lesions in the medial temporal lobe, have deficits in semantic learning of new facts but not in procedural learning or episodic consciousness. Individuals with amnestic syndrome have an anterograde amnesia for new facts but may have no deficit in their immediate sense of self-awareness. Bilateral lesions in the human hippocampus can lead to deficits in self-awareness (i.e., episodic consciousness or the intuitive recognition of one's self in a spatiotemporal context) without deficits in procedural or semantic memory. Episodic memory is served by a widely distributed network of cortical and subcortical brain regions that overlaps with, but also extends beyond, the networks serving other memory systems. Key regions in this network include the hippocampus and closely connected regions of the prefrontal cortex.

Essentially, the human episodic memory system acts like a mirror that provides spontaneous self-awareness to humans, whereas other primates require provision of an external mirror to recognize themselves. This mirroring function depends on hemispheric specialization in the encoding and retrieval of information. Left prefrontal cortex is more involved in encoding episodic memories and retrieval of semantic memories, whereas right prefrontal cortex is more involved in the retrieval of episodic memories. The episodic retrieval mode is a state of consciousness (in which a person is actively recollecting or remembering their past) that involves the strong activation of sites in the right prefrontal cortex and weaker activation of sites in the left prefrontal cortex and medial anterior cingulate.

The experimental evidence that human beings have an intuitive form of learning and memory as the basis for their unique capacity for self-awareness is now strong but its significance has yet to be widely appreciated (Brainerd, Reyna et al. 1999; Tulving 2002; Eichenbaum and Cohen 2001). Episodic memory is a recently evolved memory system that appears to be unique to human beings, just as components of the episodic network, such as prefrontal cortex, are recent evolutionary developments. As expected for a recently evolved function, episodic memory develops later than procedural or semantic learning. Children younger than four years of age do not yet have a mature episodic memory system (Tulving 2002), so people generally have no direct recollection of their past before four years of age. In contrast, basic emotions like fear and anger are present at birth, and self-object differentiation occurs between eighteen months and three years of age. Human children start to recognize themselves in mirrors once they develop self-object differentiation around eighteen months of age (Parker, Mitchell et al. 1994). The episodic memory ("mentalizing") system of the brain is mature enough at this point to allow implicit, but not explicit, attribution of intentions and other states. Self-recognition in photographs starts around two years of age, followed by signs of self-evaluative emotions (e.g., shame and pride). The sequence of these signs of implicit mentalizing ability is the same in apes as in humans, but it develops more slowly (Parker, Mitchell et al. 1994). In humans, but not in any other animals, explicit mentalizing becomes possible between the ages of four and six years, and from this age children can explain the misleading reasons that lead to false beliefs (Frith and Frith 2003). Only human beings develop beyond implicit signs of self-recognition to explicit self-aware consciousness (Parker, Mitchell et al. 1994; Povinelli 2000; Tulving 2002).

Current evidence suggests that the hippocampus is necessary for encoding of episodic memories but not for the acquisition of factual knowledge (Tulving and Markowitsch 1998; Tulving 2001; Tulving 2002). The hippocampus processes all sensory information available to a person about both one's external and one's internal milieu. Moreover, this pan-sensory information is constantly updated, allowing the registration and recall of ongoing life experiences in a personal context that is unique to each individual. The hippocampus is also known to maintain its plasticity throughout life, including the ongoing generation of new neurons as it adapts to ongoing experience.

The prefrontal cortex is involved in prospective autobiographical memory along with the hippocampus (Burgess, Quayle et al. 2001; Maguire, Henson et al. 2001; Burgess, Scott et al. 2003). There is also some evidence for the development of new neurons during adult life in regions to which the hippocampus has dense projections, such as the prefrontal cortex. In contrast, long-term declarative memories, such as factual knowledge and self-reported character traits, are stored in brain networks that show greater stability and less plasticity than the hippocampus. These findings about self-aware consciousness have accumulated gradually over the past three decades, with a more rapid increase recently as a result of improved methods of brain imaging. As the data accumulated, I began to consider with increasing seriousness the possibility that individual differences in self-aware consciousness were a crucial aspect of personality development. Self-aware consciousness seemed to offer a fundamental explanation for the importance of factors unique to the individual in personality development and of the substantial resistance to change of character and related cognitive schema. The plasticity of the hippocampus and its role in self-awareness also suggested a crucial role for growth in self-awareness as a means of experiential transformation of personality. However, I realized that much more work was needed to develop a clinical psychology of self-aware consciousness before it could provide a precise account of individual differences in personality development.

### Individual differences in self-aware consciousness

In particular, as I assessed the differences in self-awareness among individuals clinically, I observed that there were more than two levels of intuitive consciousness in human beings. More specifically, I observed a hierarchy of levels of awareness that I could measure by discussions of what are sometimes called the innate ideas or intuitions about being and human nature (Cloninger 2002).

In making these clinical observations, I developed an empathic understanding of the way another person was conscious of being, freedom of will, beauty, truth, and goodness, which provide markers of a hierarchy of levels of awareness (Cloninger 2002). These five aspects of our consciousness depend on our intuitive awareness of the world. The awareness of facts and intentions, as described by Tulving, are only two of the empirically observable levels of awareness. I initially observed five major levels of self-awareness, which are summarized in Table 2.7. Table 2.7 shows the levels of self-awareness in relation to the corresponding levels of character traits and types of mental problems that are most frequently (but not invariably) associated with the various deficiencies in self-awareness. Eventually I recognized that the five levels of self-awareness I recognized clinically in a qualitative manner could be quantitatively measured by individual differences in the five TCI subscales for Self-Directedness. TCI Self-Directedness is a global indicator of the degree of development along a hierarchical path of increasing self-awareness, and each of its five subscales measures the stepwise development of one of the levels of awareness.

For example, first I observed that some patients with severe personality disorders complain of "emptiness," which is a fearful feeling of isolation, separateness, annihilation, or lack of being. Such patients lack a stable awareness of their

**Table 2.7.** A Hierarchical Model of Mental Order and Disorder Based on Level of Self-Awareness

| Character Deficits | Associated Mental Health Features |
| --- | --- |
| LEVEL I (DEFICIENT SENSE OF BEING AND PERMANENCE) | |
| [ 1] sd1—victimized | Self-injurious behavior |
| [ 2] co1—mistrusting | Hypochondriasis |
| [ 3] st1—repressive | Emotionally unstable, hopeless |
| LEVEL II (DEFICIENT SENSE OF FREEDOM AND PURPOSEFULNESS) | |
| [ 4] sd2—aimless | Unemployment, criminality |
| [ 5] co4—revengeful | Polysubstance abuse |
| [ 6] st4—no moral ideals | Lack of charity and kindness |
| LEVEL III (DEFICIENT SENSE OF LOVE AND BEAUTY) | |
| [ 7] sd4—selfish | Social insecurity, jealousy |
| [ 8] co2—inconsiderate | Resentment, lack of intimacy |
| [ 9] st2—individualistic | Ungiving in attachments |
| LEVEL IV (DEFICIENT SENSE OF TRUTH AND FAITH) | |
| [10] sd3—inept | Inadequate, depressive |
| [11] co3—unhelpful | Hostility and tension |
| [12] st5—skeptical | Lack of faith and creativity |
| LEVEL V (DEFICIENT SENSE OF GOODNESS AND UNITY OF BEING) | |
| [13] sd5—compromising | Mastery-seeking perfectionism |
| [14] co5—self-serving | Lack of wisdom and well-being |
| [15] st3—materialistic | Lack of coherence and virtue |

Character subscales are designated by sd (Self-Directedness), co (Cooperativeness), st (Self-Transcendence) and the subscale (1–5) that is most frequently (but not invariably) characteristic of the corresponding level of intuitive self-awareness.

being and permanence, so they are sometimes described as having a borderline level of personality organization. The qualia of being can also be defined as the subjective awareness of the difference between self and other, which is needed for a sense of basic confidence in oneself and the sense of personal agency. Individual differences in personal agency are measured by the SD1 subscale of TCI Self-Directedness called "responsibility versus controlled and blaming." Individuals who lack a sense of agency feel controlled, victimized, or abused. Typical TCI items are "I usually am free to choose what I will do" (Yes if responsible) and "My actions are determined largely by influences outside my control" (No if responsible). Impaired self-object differentiation is characterized by difficulty in sublimation, intolerance of distress, distortions of reality testing, and poor self-acceptance. Without clear self-object differentiation there is a deficit in reasoning about misleading impressions that lead to false beliefs, so facts are frequently distorted (Frith and Frith 2003). Their unstable sense of being (i.e., lack of spiritual fullness, identity, permanence, and vitality) makes them so emotionally unstable and desperate that they often mutilate themselves or attempt suicide. About 1% of persons are chronically deficient in the intuitive sense of being and experience life with a borderline organization chronically. An additional 1% of persons experience such disorganization and emptiness intermittently under stress. In contrast, the vast majority of people have a well-developed awareness of being all the time. This level of awareness involves memory of existence with a stable sense of being, that is, without fear of annihilation.

Second, other people usually had a hopeful confidence in their being but felt that they were slaves to extrinsic influences. In other words, they had a lack of flexibility in their actions, or little freedom of will. The qualia of freedom or voluntariness can be defined experimentally as the subjective awareness of freedom in the purposeful choice of what is wanted (Spence, Brooks et al. 1997; Farrer and Frith 2002; Blakemore, Oakley et al. 2003). The intuition of free will is needed for the sense of power, voluntary intention, and purposefulness. The sense of power can be measured by the TCI Self-directedness subscale called purposefulness versus aimlessness (lack of goal-direction). Typical TCI items are "Each day I try to take another step toward my goals"(Yes if purposeful) and "Often I feel that my life has little purpose or meaning"(No if purposeful). In addition freedom of choice is indicated by strong development of the ability to delay gratification and to be charitable to others, as measured by TCI Cooperativeness, particularly by the subscale "compassionate and forgiving versus revengeful." The lack of awareness of freedom can be so complete that some people are fatalistic materialists and claim that freedom of will is an illusion or something in which they are lacking. Their own intuition contradicts that of humanists and dualists who believe that rational responsibility and freedom of will are what give human beings their dignity. About 10% of persons experience a lack of freedom chronically throughout their lives. This corresponds closely to traditional definitions of personality disorder, which involve lack of freedom or flexibility in adaptive behavior. Empirically, personality disorder is measured by low scores on TCI Self-Directedness and Cooperativeness (Svrakic, Whitehead et al. 1993). In contrast, most people have a stable intuitive sense of their freedom and responsibility for their intentions. More generally, this level of awareness involves a person's awareness of their voluntary intentions in a social context.

Third, some people have no intuitive sense of what is beautiful and lovable. The qualia of lovability and beauty can be defined as the subjective awareness of the choice to be kind, to give love, or to create beauty in art or personal relationships. We cannot demand love of others but we can be self-accepting and give love if our awareness is allocentric (that is, recognizing relationships with others that are not completely egocentric) (Farrer and Frith 2002). The intuition of beauty is needed for the sense of emotional contentment, which allows an acceptance of both oneself and others. The sense of acceptance of oneself and others is measured by the TCI subscale called Self-Acceptance versus succorance (approval and sympathy seeking), which is nearly equally correlated with the total Self-Directedness and Cooperativeness scales. A typical TCI item is "I want many things that I don't have" (No if self-accepting) and "I don't want to be more admired than everyone else" (Yes if self-contented). Those who had attained each level always had awareness of the lower levels, but not the higher levels of consciousness. For example, those with an awareness of beauty also had awareness of being, freedom, but not necessarily an awareness of truth or goodness. In other words, these indicators of consciousness define a hierarchy of levels of awareness. I was shocked and amazed that some patients with personality disorders have no recollection at any time in their lives of feeling a sense of wonder and admiration for the beauty of any poem, painting, or nature scenes! Imagine what it would mean if you had never experienced beauty and love. When such unaware individuals see a rainbow, they do not feel it is beautiful or wonderful! They just see physical colors and shapes with no conscious recognition of beauty. The complete absence of any sense of love and beauty is rarely acknowledged, occurring in only about 3% of individuals, but many more show little intensity in their appreciation of beauty in my clinical experience. Even though they know what opinions are fashionable, it has little or no impact on their ordinary awareness. Individuals with an unstable sense of beauty are consequently unstable in their capacity for love and emotional intimacy in relationships. On the other hand, aesthetic sensitivity is a highly developed intuitive sense in romantic poets and novelists, such as Lamartine and Emerson, and in romantic musicians, such as Schubert.

Fourth, other individuals had a sense of being, freedom, and beauty at least sometimes but never had any intuition of absolute truth. The qualia of truth can be measured experimentally as the subjective awareness of the ability to control intentions to be meaningful. The awareness of control of intentions can be distinguished experimentally from the awareness of choice about what is wanted (Frith, Blakemore et al. 2000). Some people, nevertheless, do not appreciate the distinction between the qualia of freedom and truth because they fail to be able to differentiate what is attractive and desirable from what is true and meaningful. The intuition of absolute truth is needed for a sense of faith, creativity, and resourcefulness. A person's resourcefulness can be measured by the TCI Self-Directedness scale resourcefulness (creativity) versus inadequacy (lack of self-sufficiency and identity). Typical items like "I usually look at a difficult situation as a challenge or opportunity"(Yes if resourceful) and "I often wait for someone else to provide a solution to my problems"(No if resourceful). The degree of development of faith is also measured directly by the supplementary TCI Self-Transcendence subscale called "faithful versus skeptical." Typical TCI items are "Faith provides my greatest sense of fulfillment and contentment" (Yes if faithful) and "I am grateful for supernatural guidance"(Yes if faithful). The failure to recognize absolute truth is typical of individuals who describe themselves as skeptics, pragmatists or objectivists. Such individuals also are usually agnostic or atheists because they have no intuition of their participation in a unity of consciousness, which gives rise to what Freud called "oceanic feelings" from the direct intuition of truth and hence to faith. About 10% of individuals in the United States are atheists or agnostics according to nationwide public opinion polls in the United States of America. According to a Gallup poll conducted in 2000, about nine of ten (86%) of Americans believe in God, but the majority do not believe that institutional religions are adequately inspiring and satisfying their spiritual needs. Eight percent of Americans do not believe in God but do believe in a universal spirit or higher power. Only 5% of people are atheists who also deny belief in a universal spirit or higher power. Similar results have been obtained in many surveys over the past fifty years (Popenoe 1983; Gallup and Jones 1989; Bishop 1999).

The intuitive sense of truth is prominent in many scientists, such as Teilhard de Chardin and Carl Rogers. It is even more fully developed in highly elevated positive philosophers, such as Hegel, Leonardo da Vinci, and Gandhi, who viewed their lives as experiments in truth.

Fifth, still other individuals had a sense of being, freedom, beauty, and truth at times in their lives but never had any intuition (i.e., direct awareness) of the intrinsic goodness of all things despite the perversions and corruptions that exist in the world. The sense of goodness is indicated by the TCI Self-Directedness subscale called "enlightened second nature" or hopefulness versus deliberation. Individuals who score high on the enlightened scale may be described as "light," whereas those who score low are "heavy." Typical items are "I think my natural responses are usually consistent with my principles and long-term goals" (Yes if light) and "I have so many faults that I don't like myself very much" (No if light, Yes if heavy). Unfortunately, the heavy group includes nearly all of us at times when we complain about the existence and nature of evil, compromise with what is good, or seek retribution and revenge against other human beings who threaten or attack us, or perhaps only frustrate us. Teilhard de Chardin (1978) related the human need for coherence to the intuitive sense of cosmic unity, which he called the "cosmic sense." The human cosmic sense has been well documented throughout history (Bucke 1951), as exemplified by the positive philosophers described in Chapter 1 and many other transcendentalists. However, the intuitive sense of goodness and unity is well developed only rarely. There is a partial awareness of it in individuals who are highly developed in all three character traits, including Self-Transcendence, such as the American transcendentalists like Emerson and Thoreau. A well-developed awareness of goodness and unity occurs only in highly developed positive philosophers, such as Plato, Augustine, and others listed in Table 1.3.

Finally, it became clear that there was only a crude relationship between a person's typical level of character development and the dynamic flow of their thoughts in self-aware consciousness. Character traits represent only abstract summaries of the way a person usually thinks, feels, and acts. Even the levels of development described in Table 2.7 represent only the maximum levels of thought a person has reached during their life; the levels represent the point in the flow of thought where a person is blocked or arrested in development. In psychotherapy, great flexibility is needed to follow along with the thoughts that are important for the patient at the moment. It is counterproductive to reduce thoughts to something frozen in a step in development, which only abstract thought from its freedom of flow in time. Descriptions of temperament and character are useful for diagnostic assessment and to help the patient begin to become more self-aware. Ultimately, progress in treatment requires a shift to attend directly to the movement of thought.

The description of temperament and character gave me only an incomplete account of these aspects of self-awareness in human consciousness. As a consequence, I was faced again with the need to extend my model of personality to provide a more adequate empirical psychology of human consciousness. The dualism of mind and body is an incomplete account of what it means to be a human being. To know our self fully, we must let the mind become conscious of itself.

When I discussed my observations about individual differences in the levels of self-aware consciousness with my fellow clinicians and scientists, many thought that further study was beyond the scope of psychiatry and psychology. Many of my colleagues believed that psychiatrists and clinical psychologists were primarily concerned with the treatment of disease and not with the development of optimal health and happiness. After carefully considering their hesitation, I came to the definite conclusion that I had to proceed in my studies because *health is more than the absence of disease.* Health involves coherence, which includes wisdom and well-being. We cannot provide well-being and cure of disease unless we have an adequate model of what makes us coherent. Even medical students learn about the normal function of healthy bodies before studying diseases, but psychology and psychological medicine has largely neglected the study of mental health. Just as a genuine scientist must persist in the search for truth, so must every person face reality to be well. The popular contemporary idea that authentic happiness can be based on illusions, mantras, and medication seemed to me to indicate serious flaws in current approaches to psychological medicine.

In addition, rigorous neuroscience research was demonstrating that self-aware consciousness is an important biological reality that is distinct from the semantic memories underlying character traits and the procedural memories underlying temperament traits. The different aspects of self-awareness can be experimentally defined and measured in ways that reveal the operation of distinct brain networks that are important in understanding both mental health and diseases like schizophrenia (Frith, Blakemore et al. 2000; Frith, Blakemore et al. 2000; Frith and Frith 2003). Furthermore, the biological reality of self-aware consciousness is what distinguishes human beings from all other animals. It seemed unsatisfactory to ignore what makes us uniquely human. Also, it seemed unwise to ignore the aspect of consciousness that retains the greatest plasticity during adult life. To be blunt, without an assessment of self-awareness, the description of personality is just a dead abstraction. So I ventured further along the path of the consciousness in my search for an adequate psychology of self-awareness and well-being.

## THE TRANSCENDENTAL PHENOMENA OF DEVELOPMENT

### Nonlinearity in complex dynamic systems

To characterize any phenomenon, you must experience it and then describe it in a way that is natural for that phenomenon. I have worked intensely since 1995 on the study of the spiritual aspects of consciousness (i.e., those involving self-awareness). Gradually, I have found ways and terminology to characterize the phenomena of self-awareness that are relevant to the development of well-being. When I began this phase of my studies, I looked for ways to observe and understand the processes of spiritual development in addition to my clinical work and research studies in the general population. I thought this was necessary because most contemporary clinical work, including my own up to 1995, has often neglected the self-aware aspects of consciousness. The first clinical question I had was whether it was possible to facilitate the development of the character trait of Self-Transcendence in people who had an organized character. That is, if someone is a mature dualistic rationalist (i.e., high in Self-Directedness and Cooperativeness but low in Self-Transcendence), under what conditions does he or she increase in Self-Transcendence? This is just another way of asking under what conditions does the mind begin to become aware of itself, reject rational materialism, question rational idealism, and explore and cultivate rational intuition.

Once I had observed that there was a hierarchy of differences between people in their consciousness of being, freedom, beauty, truth, and goodness, I worked to extend my model of character development to include these aspects of self-aware consciousness. The decision to do this did not require any assumption about the validity of spiritual phenomena, even though there was already solid evidence that self-aware consciousness is an important biological reality. Rather, I sought a way of systematically describing the observed differences between individuals in their life experiences. A model that cannot account for observed differences in perspective is simply incomplete. Therefore, I developed a tentative model of the stepwise development of personality that included the spiritual phenomena of consciousness (Cloninger and Svrakic 1997). This descriptive model integrated earlier work on temperament and character with other work on self-awareness and spiritual development. In addition, I sought to evaluate available techniques that have been suggested to expand self-awareness, using meditation techniques from different traditions. These traditions provided techniques from psychological medicine (Schultz and Luthe 1959; Benson 1975), integrative psychotherapy (Jung 1939; Assagioli 1965, 1991), mindfulness training (Cleary 1983; Nobu 1986; Goldstein and Kornfield 1987; Goleman 1989; Low 1989), and contemplative prayer (John of the Cross 1991; Burke 1992; Keating 1995). The techniques derived from these traditions were designed "to promote direct awareness of an intuitive consciousness more basic than categorization or the logical analysis of experience" (Cloninger and Svrakic 1997).

More specifically, I focused on the development of increasing awareness of being, freedom, beauty, truth, and goodness through a sequence of steps. These steps extended and elaborated the linear stepwise models of development of personality, such as those of Piaget, Freud, and Erikson and the twelve-step model of Alcoholics Anonymous (Cloninger and Svrakic 1997). Despite the widespread use of stepwise models to describe development in the past, I was surprised to find that psychological development is not really linear. In a one-year follow-up of 593 individuals in the general population, we tested my stepwise model and found that the dynamics of change were highly nonlinear (Cloninger, Svrakic et al. 1997). That is, development is poorly predicted by initial conditions and involved substantial unpredictability as to who would change. If a person did change, we could predict changes in character in terms of the nonlinear dynamics of a complex adaptive system defined by the initial configuration of temperament and character. Despite substantial differences between individuals, there is a recognizable path that is most frequent, which we called the "canonical sequence." This canonical sequence is what is usually described in linear stepwise models. The canonical sequence is an approximate description of overall group tendencies, but it does not say anything with precision about any particular individual. In fact, we could not tell who would or who would not change! In other words, the unpredictability of individuals—perhaps, that is, their freedom of will—is an intrinsic property of each individual that is unexplained by their initial temperament and character.

Likewise, in clinical therapeutic work, I began to face the reality that people simply do not think or change in a predictable linear sequence of developmental steps. When a person's thoughts are observed in their natural state of flow (i.e., in free association as described by Freud), they often range widely over many concerns, such as sexuality, aggression, attachments, intellectual questions, and spirituality—all in a rapid succession of complex patterns during one meeting. Furthermore, an individual's interest and motivation to change varies across this full range in a way that is proportional to his or her level of maturity.

Likewise, our interpersonal relationships, which substantially influence psychological development, are not predictable from information about the individuals in isolation from one another except at the extreme of inflexibility seen in severe personality disorder. Rather, relationships generally depend on factors that are unique to the particular relationship and its context. Furthermore, our interpersonal relationships with different individuals vary across many aspects of life, including sexuality, aggression, emotional attachments, intellectual issues, and spirituality.

As a result of these clinical and research findings, I concluded that the dynamic organization of thought and interpersonal relationships must involve a complex matrix of states of consciousness, which is not reducible to a linear sequence of development. Following this conclusion, in 1997 I looked for a better way to understand and describe human consciousness. This required a fundamental shift in my own way of thinking. I realized that psychological development simply could not be explained within the framework of mechanical determinism in which initial conditions or antecedent causes predict subsequent effects, as in Newtonian physics. Rather I became increasingly aware that well-being and certain phenomena of consciousness were better described in terms of nonlinear dynamic systems with properties analogous to the coherence phenomena of quantum physics (Cloninger, Svrakic et al. 1997; Cloninger 2002).

Also, I became increasingly aware that personality development could be facilitated but not controlled by a therapist. Personality development really involves an increase in self-awareness, which can only occur in a state of calmness, acceptance, and freedom. Personality development is not something that can be forced along a predetermined sequence of steps by another person whether they are therapist, parent, or spouse. In other words, a person cannot be trained to be free. Personality must unfold in its own unique and spontaneous way. Once I grasped this essential point, my clinical work started to become easier and more effective.

There are three basic phenomena that I have found most important to understand in the development of self-aware consciousness. I refer to these phenomena as *gifts*, *listening to the psyche*, and the *path of the psyche*. Each of these phenomena indicates a quantum-like characteristic of consciousness. First, gifts are discrete (i.e., dissociable like quanta, which are discrete packets of energy and information). Second, listening to the psyche is nondualistic and hence nonlocal (i.e., under appropriate conditions of self-awareness, consciousness transcends material sensation and becomes unbounded or unrestricted by proximity in space-time). Listening to the psyche is sometimes called listening to the inner voice, soul, or heart, but I think the most unassuming term in scientific psychology is simply psyche. Third, the path of the psyche is noncausal (i.e., free, not determined by initial conditions or private desires). The path of the psyche refers to the pattern and direction of movement in self-aware consciousness.

These developmental phenomena may be unfamiliar to many readers, as they were for me when I began to study them in 1995. Accordingly, I will illustrate them with quotations from the American transcendentalists, who are studied in more depth in Chapter 4. The American transcendentalists are at an intermediate stage of developing coherence so their writings will be supplemented with those of their great contemporary Alphonse de Lamartine, one of the positive philosophers described in Chapter 1.

Many of the terms and illustrative quotations express ideas that contradict popular assumptions about materialism and causality. To learn the new language of rational intuition, remember that it is essential to listen and understand what is being described before developing a more precise scientific model on which rigorous tests can be carried out. There is a huge gap between the romantic and metaphorical language of the transcendentalists and an explicit scientific theory of self-aware consciousness and well-being. Nevertheless, the ideas of the transcendentalists are what we must describe and understand if we are ever going to understand the source of their wisdom and well-being. A new language can never be learned if a person rejects the unfamiliar as absurd before considering it in the context of other ideas that have not yet been described. Consequently, we must first relax, let go of our critical resistance to the unfamiliar, and calmly immerse ourselves in a novel perspective with an open mind. A greater familiarity with the world view of the transcendentalists may help us to understand the basis of their wisdom and well-being, which is all too lacking in contemporary dualistic thought. Remember that the beginning of wisdom and well-being is humility, not pride or judgmental thinking.

## Gifts and the quantum-like nature of memory in the psyche

Gifts are innate intuitive abilities that occur spontaneously without training, reflection, or reasoning (Winner 1996). Gifted individuals are characterized by their immediate recognition and understanding, by rapid development of skill to an exceptional depth, and by love for exercising the gift. Gifted children with no personal or family experience for what they are doing, nevertheless, behave as if they already had the memory for doing it and are simply refreshing their recollection by a little practice. For example, the mathematical genius Ramanujan was untutored in mathematics, and his genius was recognized only when he wrote a professor at Cambridge University to seek comments on some of his intuitively derived mathematical formulas (Kanigel 1991). Likewise, gifts of the spirit often occur in uneducated people in situations that oppose rather than facilitate their expression. This is clearly demonstrated for example, in the wisdom of Catherine of Siena (Thorold 1907). Despite being an uneducated woman, she was widely acknowledged for her wisdom and sought out as an adviser to many people with extensive formal education.

Gifts, such as exceptional poetic or mathematical genius, have the quality of calling for their own use and further development. A gifted person feels calm and contented when using his or her gift but frustrated and anxious if unable to use it.

Everything else is gladly sublimated to use the gift. According to Emerson (1841, page 67), "The one condition coupled with the gift of truth is its use. . . . 'If knowledge,' said Ali the Caliph, 'calls into practice, well; if not, it goes away.'"

Similarly, Lamartine says in the *Stonecutter of St. Point* (1851, page 91), "God has given to each one his own taste, that every condition may be filled with contentment." Likewise, in *Christopher Columbus* (Lamartine 1887, page 4), the inspiration to use a gift of genius is compared with the pull of a magnet.

> Inspiration is truly a mystery of mankind, the source of which it is difficult to find in man himself. It seems to come from a higher and more distant origin, and, for this reason, we have also given to it a mysterious name, which is not well defined in any language: Genius. The birth of a man of Genius is the work of Providence. Genius is a gift. It is not acquired by work, it is not even attainable by virtue; it either is or is not, without it being possible for the very man who possesses it to give an account of its nature or of its possession. To this genius Providence sends inspiration. *Inspiration is to genius what the magnet is to metal.* She draws it, independently of all consciousness and will, to something fatal and unknown, like the pole. Genius follows the inspiration that leads it on. . . .

Gifts of the mind are most easily recognized when the gifted person has low general intelligence. In the case of such "idiot savants" or the "savant syndrome," the gift stands out like an island of light in an ocean of darkness (Treffert 2000). However, the discrete nature of gifts is also noticeable when one ability is remarkably greater than others, such as Mozart's gift for music, Ramanujan's gift for mathematics (Kanigel 1991), or Thoreau's gifts for language and naturalistic observation.

Examples of general genius do occur, as in the person of Leonardo da Vinci. However, genius is usually particular to a specific domain, like mathematics, language, singing, or music. More generally, the discrete nature of gifts is the basis for the theory of multiple intelligences (Gardner 1983, 1993, 1993). The variation between individuals is not an all-or-none phenomenon, so there are many grades of genius in a wide range of abilities. This semiquantitative variation does not undermine the essential discrete nature of gifts, but it does make it difficult to detect small gifts in people of average or higher general intelligence. We usually refer to the most frequent forms of exceptional ability as "talents." However, the transcendentalists distinguished between "genius" (which they regarded as gifts inspired by the soul because of their spontaneity) and "talents" (which they regarded as products of the body because of the effort and training required for their deliberate acquisition). According to the transcendentalists, as a result of the deliberate effort needed to acquire talent, talent is not a gift. In contrast, genius is a gift precisely because it cannot be acquired on demand or by training.

In addition to gifts of the mind, there are gifts of the spirit, such as wisdom, well-being, creativity, patience, counsel (compassion), piety (reverence), and awe of God (humility). Developmental studies show that these gifts of the spirit develop in a discrete stepwise manner, but their sequence of development is unique to each individual and only weakly predictable, as previously discussed (Cloninger, Svrakic et al. 1997).

The discreteness of gifts warrants their description as "quantum" or "quantum-like" phenomena, which simply means discrete. The term *quantum* was first applied to physics when it was discovered that light was emitted as discrete packets of energy (Gamow 1966). The analogy to quantum physics is remarkable because the standard model of particle formation in quantum physics requires the assumption of a universal field of energy and information, which is called the Higgs field. According to quantum field theory, quanta are constantly arising from, and returning to, a universal field that is filled with energy and information beyond the detection of the physical senses (Bohm 1980). Likewise, according to the intuition of Emerson (Emerson 1841, pages 54–55), long before the description of quantum field theory,

> One who conceives the true order of nature . . . *beholds the visible as proceeding from the invisible.* . . . The wholeness we admire in the order of the world is the result of infinite distribution. . . . Nature can only be conceived as existing to a universal and not to a particular end.

Likewise, gifts arise like discrete packets of light and are regarded by transcendentalists as the recollection of bits of information from a universal field or ocean of memory. In this way, gifts behave as quantum-like phenomena and not as expected if the memories of the psyche were determined mechanically or algorithmically by initial conditions. According to transcendentalists, gifts all have a common cause beyond space and time in the universal unity of being. The thought of gifted people involves intuitive leaps or quantum jumps, not deductive algorithms (Winner 1996).

Artistic creations were described poetically by Walt Whitman as "leaves of grass." Likewise, creations were described by Thoreau as "ripe fruits" that fall from a tree and can only be plucked by a "genius." According to Thoreau, someone who is blind to the spirit of truth cannot pick these fruits, even when they are available and ripe. For example, the spiritual genius Gandhi (Gardner 1993) plucked Thoreau's essay on *Civil Disobedience* and Tolstoy's essays on nonviolence and integrated them with his unique creative inspirations to advance his spiritual movement for Indian self-awareness and freedom from servitude to Great Britain. The fruits of Thoreau and Tolstoy had been there all along, but it took the genius of Gandhi to harvest them at the right place and time. Thoreau succinctly described the fundamental transcendental attitude about gifts and their creative role in the unfolding of the universal design of being. As quoted in Miller (1957, p. xi),

> There is no ripeness which is not, so to speak, something ultimate in itself, and not merely a perfected means to a higher end. In order to be ripe it must serve a transcendent use . . . and only the genius of the poet can pluck it.

More generally, the aspects of coherence of personality, such as wisdom, well-being, and creativity, involve the development of gifts of the spirit. Likewise, coherence is characteristic of quantum phenomena in general. The correspondences and differences in the meaning of coherence are further considered in other chapters in relation to physics (Chapter 5), physiology (Chapter 6), personality (Chapter 3), and theories of truth (Chapter 1).

Dualistic theories of mind have assumed that Newtonian physics provides an adequate description of mental phenomena (Rey 1997). This traditional assumption is being seriously questioned by many people in philosophy, physics, and psychology (Eccles 1989; Penrose 1994; Chalmers 1996; Stapp 1999; Walker 2000). Accordingly, in later chapters we examine the possibility that the noncausal and nonlocal phenomena of consciousness are better described by quantum physics and the quantum field theory than by the mechanical determinism of Newtonian physics. It is important here only to recognize that the discrete nature of gifts has profound implications for our fundamental concept of causality. The discreteness of gifts and their spontaneous demand for enthusiastic use provide psychological phenomena for investigation into the development of a testable science of well-being.

## Listening to the psyche

Another concept that is fundamental to spiritual movements like American transcendentalism is the need for the mind to become aware of itself. Growth in self-awareness involves a transformation of consciousness that depends on listening to one's own consciousness rather than depending on extrinsic authority, tradition, or written dogma. Gandhi called this "listening in" or "listening to one's inner voice." In more theological terms, Augustine referred to listening to the soul. In Hegel, listening to the soul is synonymous with consciousness becoming aware of itself. As a psychiatrist, I refer to the process of cultivating rational intuition as "listening to the psyche" because "psyche" means all these things (i.e., consciousness, spirit, soul, the inner voice, or conscience) and avoids premature assumptions about its own nature.

The concept of listening to the psyche is a way of describing the primacy of intuition in understanding and "insight." The process of growth in self-awareness requires the purification of rational intuition by the mind's becoming aware of itself. Emerson believed that it was possible to retain the direct quality of life within language so that others could experience the same life with their intuitive senses. "We hope to draw thoughts and feelings, which being alive can impart life" (Emerson and Fuller 1840, page 142). Words that are alive are those that stimulate self-awareness, that is, vivid imagery of personal life experiences in their natural spatial and temporal context. In contrast, semantic memories that reduce life to abstract concepts and general facts seem lifeless.

The feeling that nature and words are alive is often described as pantheistic. According to the transcendental worldview, all things in nature are imbued with living spiritual qualities that can be detected by our intuitive senses. Therefore, people can transform their consciousness by immersion in the spirit of the movement. According to the transcendentalists,

> You need not speak to me, I need not go where you are, that you should exert magnetism on me. Be you only whole and sufficient, and I shall feel you in every part of my life and fortune, and I can as easily dodge the gravitation of the globe as escape your influence. (Emerson and Fuller 1840)

Life is something divine and infinite to the transcendentalists. For example, the divine Word communicates to the humble stonecutter (Lamartine 1851, page 131) that "*I am All*, and nothing can escape Me but in annihilation, and annihilation is a word of finite man—there is no emptiness: I fill the universe; and My true name is *Life*."

The American transcendentalists all agree with Augustine and other Christian theologians that listening to the psyche is communication through the medium of love. For example, according to Emerson's Method of Nature, the transcendental atmosphere is simply love:

> What is Love? . . . Is it not certain admirable wisdom, preferable to all other advantages . . . in which the individual is no longer his own foolish master, but inhales an odorous and celestial air, is wrapped round with awe of the object, blending for the time that object with the real and only good, and consults every omen in nature with tremulous interest? (Emerson 1841, page 64)

Similarly, Lamartine described love as the means by which he came to know himself and thereby to know virtue and the universal unity of being. In the novel *Raphael* (Lamartine 1857, pages 53–55), he says,

> Love was the torch which, while it fired my heart, enlightened all nature, heaven, and earth, and showed me to myself. . . . I entered into the heaven of my soul, as my heart and eyes fathomed the *ocean of beauty, tenderness, and purity* which expanded hourly in the eyes, in the voice, and in the discourse, of the heavenly creature who had manifested herself to me. . . . In a word, I saw and felt, I worshiped God himself, through the medium of my love! If life were to last in such a condition of the soul, nature would stand still, the blood would cease to circulate, the heart forget to beat; or rather, there would be neither motion, precipitation, nor lassitude, neither life nor death in our senses. There would be only one endless and living absorption of our being in another's, such as must be the state of the soul at once annihilated and living in God!

Emerson called his predominant approach to listening to the psyche the "method of nature." If we will only listen to the urgings of our soul, Emerson thought we would learn how to live wisely, creatively, and happily. Listening to the psyche is a graphic way of describing contemplation. More specifically, Emerson regarded listening to the psyche to be piety or reverence, which is a gift of the spirit expressed as loving veneration of the primal cause of nature. In *The Method of Nature* (Emerson 1841, page 62), he wrote that "By piety alone, by conversing with the cause of nature, is man safe . . . because all knowledge is assimilation to the object of knowledge, as the power or genius of nature is ecstatic, so must its science or the description of it be."

The conscious experience of union in nature is so pleasant and enjoyable that Emerson described it as producing a state of ecstasy, which combines joy with faith in the cause of nature. The ecstatic states of union in nature described by the transcendentalists are what Freud called "oceanic feelings" in *Civilization and Its Discontents*. For example, in the passage from *Raphael* quoted earlier, Lamartine referred specifically to "the ocean of beauty, tenderness, and purity." Freud recognized such ecstatic experiences as the basis for religious faith, and this connection of ecstasy and faith is well illustrated by the transcendentalists.

According to the transcendentalists, such states of ecstasy are rational and even wise because of the coherence of superconsciousness. *Superconsciousness* refers to consciousness of the "superincumbent tendency" by which all life is supposed to be organized as part of the cosmic order (Emerson 1841, page 57). Emerson's disciple Bronson Alcott described the psyche as an oracle to which we should listen with enthusiasm.

> Believe, youth, that your heart is an oracle; trust her instinctive auguries, obey her divine leadings; nor listen too fondly to the uncertain echoes of your head. The heart is the prophet of your soul, and ever fulfils her prophecies; reason is her historian; but for the prophecy the history would not be. (Alcott 1840, page 87)

The functions of the soul as an oracle or inner voice are multifaceted according to transcendentalists. Initially, Homer distinguished the essence of understanding (i.e., sentient life or Greek *quh'c*) from the will (i.e., Greek *jum'ov*). According to the Orphic mysteries, recognition of the true path of spiritual knowledge also depended on inspiration from the Lake of Memory, which allowed people to recognize the divinity within themselves (Geldard 1989). The human drive for coherence requires the integration of these three functions. Growth in self-awareness increases understanding, but recognition is required before understanding. Recognition depends on memory, and the will of the psyche is to do spontaneously what is understood to lead to well-being. Therefore, to learn is to remember and to act.

By the time of Plato, the three functions of self-aware memory, understanding, and will were regarded as interdependent functions of the indivisible psyche, thereby permitting coherence to arise by growing awareness of what is divine within all things. According to the transcendentalists, the key to any radical transformation of consciousness (i.e., metanoia) is the contemplation of the unity of being, which requires the mind to be aware of itself. Hence, when we listen to the psyche, the appearance of a subject–object dichotomy is eliminated. When we pass beyond the narrow gate of dualism, which appears to separate physical matter from its surrounding immaterial atmosphere, we enter into awareness of oceanic feelings. According to the naturalist Thoreau (1848), such contemplative thinking is merely the awakening of the "common sense."

Materialists, of course, regard the "common sense" as simply a romantic illusion. Reliance on the physical senses alone leads toward the negative philosophy, whereas listening to the psyche leads toward the positive philosophy. Questions about the role of intuition in consciousness are at the crux of disputes about whether human beings can know the truth of reality directly by intuition or only through appearances from the physical senses. The understanding of materialists is that belief in the nonlocal consciousness and phenomena like spiritual healing are illusory. Materialists also doubted the possibility of nonlocality in quantum physics, but it is now experimentally proven in a rigorous manner for what are called "entangled" particles (Bell 1993; Bouwmeester, Pan et al. 1997; Tittel, Brendel et al. 1998; Zeilinger 2000). It is shocking to think that the same consciousness can be in more than one place at once! Jung's ideas about a collective unconscious have been resisted because they violate familiar assumptions of local realism. Yet the nonlocal communality of consciousness is exactly what transcendentalists claim when they speak of the "common sense," which produces the ecstasy and joy of communion in nature.

Such communality of consciousness would violate the conviction of the privacy of consciousness of every materialist and nearly all but the most transcendent of rational dualists. If listening to the psyche provides a means to both increased self-awareness and awareness of the joy of nonlocal consciousness, then psychology must prepare for a revolution in its notions of causality, knowledge, and well-being. As a result, this disagreement about the possible nonlocality of consciousness, as well as the role of the intuitive senses in awareness of what is pleasant, provides other phenomena for investigation in the empirical psychology of well-being.

## The path of the psyche

A third fundamental concept that is important for understanding the thought of transcendentalists is that the psyche is an indestructible entity that has a path with a direction in time. The notion of a path of consciousness cannot be understood without the corollary concept of freedom of will, which involves the capacity to be responsible for one's thoughts and actions rather than being controlled by prior conditioning. According to Emerson (1880, page 6), "the new race is stiff, heady and rebellious; they are fanatics in freedom; they hate tolls, taxes, turnpikes, banks, hierarchies, governors, yea, almost laws. . . . They rebel against theological as against political dogmas; against mediation, or saints, or any nobility in the unseen."

Similarly, free will is well accepted by humanists and rational idealists such as Kant, who was much admired by Emerson. However, freedom of will really implies more than is sometimes recognized by rational idealists. According to Spinoza and other positive philosophers, freedom is by definition unbounded, so full freedom requires an unending evolution of the path of the psyche. In other words, increasing freedom of will leads ultimately to the absolute (i.e., pure consciousness).

Hence, freedom of will implies a path of consciousness. There is a direction to the path of the psyche, just as there is an arrow of time in physics. Time can be described as the freedom accorded to movement along the path of the psyche. As a result, in psychology there are frequent references to the "stream" or "river" of consciousness, which is freely flowing unless it encounters a dam or obstacles, such as human desires and fears causing attachments and aversions to extrinsic objects. Without attachment or aversion to extrinsic objects, consciousness is inherently free in the unbounded flow of its development in time. Consequently, if we are in a state of free flow (i.e., when we love what we are doing), the passage of time is unnoticed subjectively, so subjective estimates of how much time has passed during a state of free flow are shorter than indicated by objective standards. In Lamartine's words (1851, page 92), when we are free and undistracted in work or play, "time passes away . . . as if it had never been." In contrast, when we are trying to control or resist the natural flow of events, time drags (i.e., subjective estimates of the passage of time are longer than indicated by objective standards). In Krishnamurti and Bohm's words (1985), when discursive thought is silent and our consciousness flows freely, there is an "ending of time."

Paradoxically, self-awareness leads to nondualistic consciousness, which is self-forgetful and ultimately selfless. Still people encounter obstacles to their growth in self-awareness. According to Lamartine in the *Stonecutter of St. Point,*

> Every man has an atmosphere which surrounds him, and spreads around either good or evil influences, heat or cold,—as his heart is more or less set on high, and reflects more or less of the divinity that shines on him. Repulsion and attraction are only the sensations awakened within us by these human atmospheres: some draw us toward them like a lover, others repel us like a serpent, without our knowing why; but nature knows, and these repulsions and attractions must be listened to and obeyed, as the instinctive warnings of the soul. Almost every attraction is a revelation of some hidden virtue; every repulsion, the spirit of some concealed vice. Souls, too, have their physiognomics: we do not scrutinize them it is true, we experience them. Who has not said, on approaching some men,—I feel myself a better being near these? (Lamartine 1851, pages 62–63)

In other words, our personal "atmosphere" is the energetic field of our consciousness, which is the function of our psyche (i.e., our soul with its various virtues and vices). We may have a harmonious atmosphere, which is helpful and pleasing to others, or we may be experiencing a destructive storm as a result of emotional conflicts. Furthermore, the consciousness of people may differ markedly in level of awareness. In other words, every psyche has a characteristic level of elevation that influences thought. Lamartine said,

> It requires a great concentration of mind, a rapt elevation of soul, not to be distracted in inward intercourse with the good God; not to be deafened by the tumults of the world; not to be chained down to the current of petty thoughts. *In a word, one must be endowed with a peculiar faculty, a sense which is common indeed to all men, but has not in all the same measure of development*; a sense more intellectual and divine than all our other senses . . . (Lamartine 1851, page 41)

In other words, all human beings have some degree of self-awareness, but each psyche varies in its measure or magnitude (i.e., level of development along the path of the psyche). According to the level of the psyche, each individual is more or less well attuned to divine inspiration, which transcendentalists describe as the collective atmosphere or ocean of light in which we live and breathe. The level of the psyche is a gift, however, so we cannot change it by demand or training. Lamartine (1851, page 134) says without complaint "I cannot see beyond the sight Thou give." The higher the level or magnitude of the psyche, the greater is our memory of what is good, true, and beautiful (Augustine 388).

Nevertheless, there is still freedom in the range of our thoughts regardless of the level of the psyche.

> God is like the architect of an iron dome, who leaves, as I have seen, space between the materials that form its timber-work, in order that the iron may expand or contract freely, according to the seasons. This provision of the Architect above, who gives effect to His immutable will in giving effect to the invocations of men, I recognize in prayer. (Lamartine 1851, page 132)

Consequently, human beings can advance step by step if they use their freedom of will (i.e., the space free for expansion and contraction with the seasons) to move along the ascending path of consciousness by keeping their thoughts elevated in search of what is beautiful, true, and good.

> This is then God's will, that the soul should labor like the body in search of nourishment . . . that our minds may be always thinkin.g of Him, advancing slowly step by step toward His perfect knowledge; for if we could reach that knowledge at a bound, we should walk on and search no more; but to be ever seeking after truth—this is to live. (Lamartine 1851, page 138)

Hence, there is freedom of will to grow in awareness along the path of the psyche. Such growth is an evolution of the degree to which we can see and recollect the interdependent influences on our life. As we grow in awareness (i.e., as we "awaken"), what was formerly part of the collective unconscious becomes conscious, according to Jung's terminology. Growth along the path of the psyche is the awakening of awareness of the cosmic order in the individual being. The finite cannot hold the infinite within itself, but it can participate in the infinite with ever-decreasing resistance. Such nonresistance must involve freedom of will because what is unbounded is necessarily free. The free and stepwise reduction of our resistance to the intelligibility of the cosmic order is the path of the psyche.

According to the transcendentalists, we differ in our capacity for selfless love in proportion to our awareness of the truth that all humanity participates in the universal unity of being. Our little individual self in space-time becomes one with the universal Self that transcends space and time. Lamartine illustrated the human capacity for nearly universal love and mercy by the selfless life of the stonecutter Claude. Lamartine has the stonecutter explain the source of his inspiration:

> I lie down at summer-time in the middle of the day, my back on the turf or the sand, my eyes half-closed, turned toward the rays that strike from heaven on my face. . . . They run through me—they illumine me—they kindle the depths of my heart. It is as if I was bathed in a lake of subtle light, which penetrated all my members, coursed in my veins, commingled with my very spirit. Then, I fancy that these rays of living light, these waves of dazzling luster, are the sea of God in which I swim; that I am transported beyond space,—light and transparent as air. (Lamartine 1851, pages 48–49)

Emerson describes the path of the psyche as resembling freedom of movement along a spiral staircase leading toward ever-deeper awareness of what is beautiful, true, and ultimately a divine Unity. The spiral path of our self-aware consciousness is like the spiral patterns common in all forms of life, even vegetation, as described later in Chapter 8. In his essay *Beauty*, he wrote,

> The spiral tendency of vegetation infects education also. Our books approach very slowly the things we most wish to know. . . . Wherever we begin, thither our steps tend: an ascent . . . up to the perception of Plato that globe and universe are rude and early experiences of an all-dissolving Unity—the first stair on the scale to the temple of the Mind. (Emerson 1860)

In addition, Emerson described the movement along the path of the psyche as fluid and free, like flowing water, action and reaction in the cycles of nature, or beautiful dancing:

> Beauty is the moment of transition, as if the form were just ready to flow into other forms. Any fixedness, heaping, or concentration on one feature . . . is the reverse of the flowing, and therefore deformed. Beautiful as is the symmetry of any form, if the form can move we seek a more excellent symmetry. The interruption of equilibrium stimulates the eye to desire the restoration of symmetry, and to watch the steps through which it is attained. This is the charm of running water. . . . This is the theory of dancing to recover continually in changes the lost equilibrium, not by abrupt and

angular but by gradual and curving movements. . . . To this streaming or flowing belongs the beauty that all circular movement has . . . the annual wave of vegetation, the action and reaction of Nature; and if we follow it out, this demand in our thought for an everonward action is the argument for the immortality. (Emerson 1860, pages 178–179)

In contrast, materialists deny the possibility of free will and think that everything is caused by something in the past, which may or not be measured. This leads materialists to regard people and the world as deterministic machines for which love is a dispensable convenience, rather than an intrinsic living spontaneity. For materialists, what is unpredictable is the result of not knowing what to measure or the action of chance in nature. Nevertheless, according to modern physics, freedom is a fundamental quantum phenomenon underlying all things. There is underdetermination of all events in space-time, such that only probabilistic statements can be made about material events. More exactly, there is a limit to the precision with which any material event can be predicted in space-time. The unpredictability of physical events is another way of talking about freedom.

In brief, the claim of rational materialism is that what is unexplained is due to chance. In contrast, the claim of rational intuition is that what is unexplained in human behavior involves the freedom of will, which gives rise to acts of spontaneous kindness. However, the demonstration of quantum uncertainty under particular conditions does not necessarily imply that such unpredictability is a characteristic of human consciousness. On the other hand, if unpredictability is due to chance, it is not clear why subjective feelings of freedom should predict systematic bias in estimating subjective time or the frequency of spontaneous acts of kindness.

The alternative explanations of unpredictability lead to different expectations about the path of the psyche. If unpredictability is an intelligible property of consciousness (i.e., freedom of will), then there should be a measurable dimension of movement in self-aware consciousness related to individual differences in free will and the expression of spontaneous kindness. Fortunately, then empirical examination of the concept of the path of the psyche by studies of human consciousness and personality development provide a way to test the alternative assumptions of materialists and transcendentalists about a possible dimension of freedom in human self-aware consciousness.

More generally, transcendentalists claim that the path of the psyche is influenced by all of the basic phenomena described here—gifts, listening to the psyche, and freedom of will. As previously described, gifts lead to individual differences in creativity of thought and degree of contentment experienced in sublimation of other needs for the sake of such creativity. Likewise, listening to the psyche leads to individual differences in anticipation and awareness of what is joyful and pleasant in life. Freedom of will is associated with individual differences in spontaneous kindness and in estimation of subjective time, so that a person in free flow is beyond all fear and conflict (i.e., is in "love") and beyond effortful control (i.e., experiences the "ending of time").

Up to now, the concepts of transcendentalists have been illustrated only so that we can become familiar with their distinct way of thinking. The empirical evidence for the path of the psyche, including its structure and function, is examined in detail in later chapters. For the sake of clarity and precision, however, it is first essential to develop a reliable scientific method for the measurement of human thought in self-aware consciousness, as described in Chapter 3.

## REFERENCES

Alcott, A. B. (1840). Orphic sayings. *The American transcendentalists: Their prose and poetry*. P. Miller, ed. Garden City, New York, Doubleday & Company: 86–91.

Allport, G. W. (1937). *Personality: A psychological interpretation*. New York, Holt Rinehart & Winston.

Assagioli, R. (1965). *Psychosynthesis: A manual of principles and techniques*. Wellingborough, England, Crucible.

Assagioli, R. (1991). *Transpersonal development: The dimension beyond psychosynthesis*. Wellingborough, England, Crucible.

Augustine (388). The magnitude of the soul. *Writings of Saint Augustine*. New York, Cima Publishing Co.: 51–59.

Bayon, C., K. Hill, et al. (1996). "Dimensional assessment of personality in an outpatient sample: Relations of the systems of Millon and Cloninger." *Journal of Psychiatric Research* 30: 341–352.

Beck, J. S. (1996). Cognitive therapy of personality disorders. *Frontiers of cognitive therapy*. P. M. Salkovskis, ed. New York, Guilford Press: 165–181.

Bell, J. S. (1993). *Speakable and unspeakable in quantum mechanics*. Cambridge, Cambridge University Press.

Benson, H. (1975). *The relaxation response*. New York, Avon.

Bishop, G. (1999). What Americans really believe. *Free Inquiry* 19: 38–42.

Blakemore, S. J., D. A. Oakley, et al. (2003). "Delusions of alien control in the normal brain." *Neuropsychologia* 41(8): 1058–1067.

Bohm, D. (1980). *Wholeness and the implicate order*. London, Routledge.

Borg, J., B. Andree, et al. (2003). "The serotonin system and spiritual experiences." *American Journal of Psychiatry* 160(11): 1965–1969.

Bouwmeester, D., J. W. Pan, et al. (1997). "Experimental quantum teleportation." *Nature* 390: 575–579.

Brainerd, C. J., V. F. Reyna, et al. (1999). "Conjoint recognition." *Psychological Review* 106: 160–179.

Bucke, R. M. (1951). *Cosmic consciousness: A study in the evolution of the human mind*. New York, Dutton.

Bulik, C. M., P. F. Sullivan, et al. (1998). "Predictors of 1-year treatment outcome in bulimia nervosa." *Comprehensive Psychiatry* 39: 206–214.

Burgess, P. W., A. Quayle, et al. (2001). "Brain regions involved in prospective memory as determined by positron emission tomography." *Neuropsychologia* 39: 545–555.

Burgess, P. W., S. K. Scott, Quayle, et al. (2003). "The role of the rostral frontal cortex (area 10) in prospective memory: a lateral versus medial dissociation." *Neuropsychologia* 41(8): 906–918.

Burke, G. (1992). *Lighting the lamp: Practical instruction in interior prayer according to the hesychastic tradition of the Christian East.* Essex, England, St. George Press.

Chalmers, D. J. (1996). *The conscious mind: In search of a fundamental theory.* New York, Oxford University Press.

Chomsky, N. (1980). "Rules and representations." *Behavior and Brain Sciences* 3: 1–61.

Cleary, T. (1983). *Entry into the inconceivable: An introduction to Hua-Yen Buddhism.* Honolulu, Hawaii, University of Hawaii Press.

Cloninger, C. R. (1986). "A unified biosocial theory of personality and its role in the development of anxiety states." *Psychiatric Developments* 3: 167–226.

Cloninger, C. R. (1987). "A systematic method for clinical description and classification of personality variants: A proposal." *Archives of General Psychiatry* 44: 573–587.

Cloninger, C. R. (1994). "Temperament and personality." *Current Opinion in Neurobiology* 4: 266–273.

Cloninger, C. R. (1998). The genetics and psychobiology of the seven factor model of personality. *The Biology of Personality Disorders.* K. R. Silk, ed.. Washington, D.C., American Psychiatric Press: 63–84.

Cloninger, C. R. (1999). "A new conceptual paradigm from genetics and psychobiologyu for the science of mental health." *Australian and New Zealand Journal of Psychiatry* 33: 174–186.

Cloninger, C. R. (2000). "Biology of personality dimensions." *Current Opinions in Psychiatry* 13: 611–616.

Cloninger, C. R. (2002). Implications of comorbidity for the classification of mental disorders: The need for a psychobiology of coherence. *Psychiatric Diagnosis and Classification.* M. Maj, W. Gaebel, et al., eds. Chichester, England, John Wiley & Sons, Ltd: 79–106.

Cloninger, C. R. (2003). Completing the psychobiological architecture of human personality development: Temperament, character, & coherence. *Understanding human development: Dialogues with lifespan psychology.* U. M. Staudinger and U. E. R. Lindenberger, eds. Boston, Kluwer Academic Publishers: 159–182.

Cloninger, C. R. and D. M. Svrakic (1997). "Integrative psychobiological approach to psychiatric assessment and treatment." *Psychiatry* 60: 120–141.

Cloninger, C. R. and D. M. Svrakic (2000). Personality disorders. *Comprehensive textbook of psychiatry.* B. J. Sadock and V. A. Sadock, eds. New York, Lippincott Williams & Wilkins: 1723–1764.

Cloninger, C. R., D. M. Svrakic, et al. (1993). "A psychobiological model of temperament and character." *Archives of General Psychiatry* 50: 975–990.

Cloninger, C. R., N. M. Svrakic, et al. (1997). "Role of personality self-organization in development of mental disorder and disorder." *Development and Psychopathology* 9: 881–906.

Comings, D. E., R. Gade-Andavolu, et al. (2000). "A multivariate analysis of 59 candidate genes in personality traits: The Temperament and Character Inventory." *Clinical Genetics* 58: 375–385.

Constantino, J. N., C. R. Cloninger, et al. (2002). "Application of the seven-factor model of personality to early childhood." *Psychiatry Research* 109: 229-243.

Eccles, J. (1989). *Evolution and the brain: Creation of the self.* London, Routledge.

Eichenbaum, H., N. J. Cohen (2001). *From conditioning to conscious recollection: Memory systems of the brain.* New York, Oxford University Press.

Emerson, R. W. (1841). The method of nature. *The American transcendentalists: Their prose and poetry.* P. Miller, ed.. Garden City, New York, Doubleday & Company: 49–68.

Emerson, R. W. (1860). Beauty. *The American transcendentalists: Their prose and poetry.* P. Miller, ed. Garden City, New York, Doubleday & Company: 172–186.

Emerson, R. W. (1880). Historic notes on life and letters in New England. *The American transcendentalists: Their prose and poetry.* P. Miller, ed. Garden City, New York, Doubleday & Company: 1–20.

Emerson, R. W. and M. Fuller (1840). The editors (of the Dial) to the readers. *The American transcendentalists: Their prose and poetry.* P. Miller, ed. Garden City, New York, Doubleday & Company: 139–142.

Farrer, C. and C. D. Frith (2002). "Experiencing oneself vs another person as being the cause of an action: the neural correlates of the experience of agency." *Neuroimage* 15(3): 596–603.

Frith, C. D., S. Blakemore, et al. (2000). "Explaining the symptoms of schizophrenia: abnromalities in the awareness of action." *Brain Research—Brain Research Reviews* 31(2–3): 357–363.

Frith, C. D., S. J. Blakemore, et al. (2000). "Abnormalities in the awareness and control of action." *Philosophical Transactions of the Royal Society of London-Series B: Biological Sciences* 355(1404): 1771–1788.

Frith, U. and C. D. Frith (2003). "Development and neurophysiology of mentalizing." *Philosophical Transactions of the Royal Society of London-Series B: Biological Sciences* 358(1431): 459–473.

Gallup, G. J. and S. Jones (1989). *Religion in America: One hundred questions and answers.* Princeton, New Jersey, Princeton Religion Research Center.

Gamow, G. (1966). *Thirty years that shook physics: The story of quantum theory.* New York, Dover Publications.

Gardner, H. (1983). *Frames of mind: The theory of multiple intelligences.* New York, Basic Books.

Gardner, H. (1993). *Creating minds: An anatomy of creativity seen through the lives of Freud, Einstein, Picasso, Stravinsky, Eliot, Graham, and Gandhi.* New York, Basic Books.

Gardner, H. (1993). *Multiple intelligences: The theory in practice.* New York, Basic Books.

Geldard, R. G. (1989). *The traveler's key to ancient Greece.* New York, Alfred A. Knopf.

Gillespie, N. A., C. R. Cloninger, et al. (2003). "The genetic and environmental relationship between Cloninger's dimensions of temperament and character." *Personality and Individual Differences* 35: 1931–1946.

Goldsmith, H. H., A. H. Buss, et al. (1987). "What is temperament? Four approaches." *Child Development* 58: 505–529.

Goldstein, J. and J. Kornfield (1987). *Seeking the heart of wisdom: The path of insight meditation.* Boston, Shambala.

Goleman, D. (1989). *The meditative mind: The varieties of meditative experience.* Wellingsborough, England, Crucible.

Gusnard, D. A., J. M. Ollinger, et al. (2003). "Persistence and brain circuitry." *Proceedings of the National Academy of Sciences USA* 100: 3479–3484.

Hansenne, M., E. Pinto, et al. (2003). "Harm Avoidance is related to mismatch negativity (MMN) amplitude in healthy subjects." *Personality and Individual Differences* 34: 1039–1048.

Heath, A. C., C. R. Cloninger, et al. (1994). "Testing a model for the genetic structure of personality: A comparison of the personality systems of Cloninger and Eysenck." *Journal of Personal and Social Psychology* 66: 762–775.

John of the Cross, S. (1991). *The collected works of St. John of the Cross.* Washington, D.C., Institute of Carmelite Studies.

Joyce, P. R., R. T. Mulder, et al. (1994). "Temperament predicts clomipramine and desipramine response in major depression." *Journal of Affective Disorders* 30: 35–46.

Jung, C. G. (1939). *The integration of personality.* New York, Farrar & Rinehart, Inc.

Kanigel, R. (1991). *The man who knew infinity: A life of the genius Ramanujan.* New York, Charles Scribner & Sons.

Kant, I. (1796). *Anthropology from a pragmatic point of view.* Carbondale, Illinois, Southern Illinois University Press.

Keating, T. (1995). *Open mind, open heart: The contemplative dimension of the gospel.* New York, Continuum.

Kramer, P. D. (1993). *Listening to Prozac: A psychiatrist explores antidepressant drugs and the remaking of the self.* New York, Viking.

Krishnamurti, J. (1999). *This light in oneself: True meditation.* San Francisco, Harper.

Krishnamurti, J. and D. Bohm (1985). *The ending of time.* San Francisco, HarperCollins.

Krishnamurti, J. and D. Bohm (1999). *The limits of thought: Discussions.* London, Routledge.

Lamartine, A. de (1851). *The stonecutter of Saint Point.* London, George Routledge & Co.

Lamartine, A. de (1857). *Raphael; or, pages of the Book of Life at twenty.* New York, Harper & Brothers.

Lamartine, A. de (1887). *Christopher Columbus.* Toronto, Sutherlands.

Low, A. (1989). *An invitation to practice Zen.* Rutland, Vermont, C. E. Tuttle Co.

Maguire, E. A., R. N. Henson, et al. (2001). "Activity in prefrontal cortex, not hippocampus, varies parametrically with the increasing remoteness of memories." *Neuroreport* 12(3): 441–444.

Miller, P., ed. (1957). *The American transcendentalists: Their prose and poetry.* Garden City, New York, Doubleday & Company.

Mulder, R. T., P. R. Joyce, et al. (1996). "Towards an understanding of defense style in terms of temperament and character." *Acta Psychiatrica Scandinavica* 99: 99–104.

Nobu, N. (1986). *The crystal and the way of light: Sutra, Tantra, Dzogchen.* London, Routledge and Kegan Paul.

Parker, S. T., R. W. Mitchell, et al., Eds. (1994). *Self-awareness in animals and humans: Developmental perspectives.* Cambridge, UK, Cambridge University Press.

Paulus, M. P., C. Rogalsky, et al. (2003). "Increased activation in the right insula during risk-taking decision making is related to harm avoidance and neuroticism." *NeuroImage* 19: 1439–1448.

Penrose, R. (1994). *Shadows of the mind: A search for the missing science of consciousness.* New York, Oxford University Press.

Plato (1986). *The dialogues of Plato.* New York, Bantam Books.

Popenoe, D. (1983). *Sociology.* Edgewood Cliffs, New Jersey, Prentice Hall Inc.

Povinelli, D. J. (2000). *Folk physics for apes: The chimpanzee's theory of how the world works.* New York, Oxford University Press.

Povinelli, D. J. and S. Giambrone (2001). "Reasoning about beliefs: a human specialization?" *Child Development* 72: 691–695.

Rey, G. (1997). *Contemporary philosophy of mind.* Oxford, Blackwell Publishers.

Schultz, J. H. and W. Luthe (1959). *Autogenic training: A psychophysiologic approach to psychotherapy.* New York, Grune & Stratton.

Spence, S. A., D. J. Brooks, et al. (1997). "A PET study of voluntary movement in schizophrenic patients experiencing passivity phenomena (delusions of alien control)." *Brain* 120(Pt 11): 1997–2011.

Sperry, L. (1999). *Cognitive behavior therapy of DSM-IV personality disorders: Highly effective interventions for the most common personality disorders.* Philadelphia, Pennsylvania, Brunner/Mazel.

Spiegelman, J. M. (1996). *Psychotherapy as a mutual process.* Tempe, Arizona, New Falcon Publications.

Stallings, M. C., J. K. Hewitt, et al. (1996). "Genetic and environmental structure of the Tridimensional Personality Questionnaire: Three or four temperament dimensions?" *Journal of Personal and Social Psychology* 70: 127–140.

Stapp, H. (1999). "Attention, intention, and will in quantum physics." *Journal of Conscious Studies: The Volitional Brain* 6: 143–164.

Sugiura, M., R. Kawashima, et al. (2000). "Correlation between human personality and neural activity in cerebral cortex." *NeuroImage* 11: 541–546.

Svrakic, D. M., C. Whitehead, et al. (1993). "Differential diagnosis of personality disorders by the seven factor model of temperament and character." *Archives of General Psychiatry* 50: 991–999.

Teilhard de Chardin, P. (1978). *The heart of matter.* New York, Harcourt-Brace-Jovanovich.

Thoreau, H. D. (1848). *The Maine woods.* Princeton, New Jersey, Princeton University Press.

Thorold, A. (1907). An introduction on the life and times of the Saint. *The dialogue of the Seraphic Virgin Catherine of Siena.* A. Thorold, ed. Rockford, Illinois, Tan Books.

Thorpe, W. H. (1956). *Learning and instinct in animals.* Cambridge, Massachusetts, Harvard University Press.

Tittel, W., J. Brendel, et al. (1998). "Violation of Bell inequalities by photons more than 10 km apart." *Physical Review Letters* 81: 3563–3566.

Tome, M. B., C. R. Cloninger, et al. (1997). "Serotonergic autoreceptor blockade in the reduction of antidepressant latency: personality and response to paroxetine and pindolol." *Journal of Affective Disorders* 44: 101–109.

Treffert, D. A. (2000). Extraordinary people: Understanding savant syndrome. New York, Ballantine Books.

Tulving, E. (1987). "Multiple memory systems and consciousness." *Human Neurobiology* 6: 67–80.

Tulving, E. (2001). "Episodic memory and common sense: how far apart?" *Philosophical Transactions of the Royal Society of London—Series B: Biological Sciences* 356: 1505–1515.

Tulving, E. (2002). "Episodic memory: From mind to brain." *Annual Review of Psychology* 53: 1–25.

Tulving, E. and H. J. Markowitsch (1998). "Episodic and declarative memory: Role of the hippocampus." *Hippocampus* 8: 198–204.

Vedeniapin, A. B., A. A. Anokhin, et al. (2001). "Visual P300 and the self-directedness scale of the temperament-character inventory." *Psychiatry Research* 101: 145–156.

Walker, E. H. (2000). *The physics of consciousness: Quantum minds and the meaning of life.* Cambridge, Massachusetts, Perseus Books.

Winner, E. (1996). *Gifted children: Myths and realities.* New York, Basic Books.

Zeilinger, A. (2000). "Quantum teleportation." *Scientific American* 282: 50–59.

# 3

# THE MEASUREMENT AND MOVEMENT
# OF HUMAN THOUGHT

## THE PATH OF THE PSYCHE

An adequate psychology of self-awareness requires a more precise description of the basic concepts of gifts, listening to the psyche, and the path of the psyche than has been given by transcendentalists. Furthermore, we need to develop the scientific psychology of well-being in more detail to be able to describe and analyze the American transcendentalist movement. All three concepts are interrelated, so I will focus on the path of the psyche and describe the other two concepts in relation to it. I began the development of a fuller description of the path of consciousness by extending the work of Hegel, who had given the most detailed previous description of the path of consciousness in psychological terms.

Hegel described three stages in the development of self-aware consciousness. He first described the science of the experience of consciousness in his *Phenomenology of the Spirit* (Hegel 1807), which he wrote in Jena. Later he clarified his insights in successive editions of *Encyclopedia of the Philosophical Sciences in Outline* (Hegel 1981). Fortunately, the notes of his final course on the phenomenology of consciousness that he gave as professor in Berlin were translated (Hegel 1981), based largely on the final edition of the encyclopedia. According to Hegel's *Berlin Phenomenology* (1981, pages 29–30), there are three stages in the development of self-aware consciousness. The first stage is "immediate sensuous consciousness," which is the determination of the physical and intuitive senses in the here-and-now, as is typical of ordinary states of self-centered thinking in people after the age of 4 years. The second stage is "consciousness of the reflected object," which is an abstraction from time and place, as is typical of meditation and some mature idealistic states of dualistic thinking. The third stage is "consciousness of the object as that which is within itself, as living being or spiritual essence," which is characteristic of contemplation and nondualistic thinking. Such spiritual consciousness includes time and place without being limited to what is immediately present. Hence, consciousness can be recognized as having three stages, and as evolving toward a "triadic form" in which immediate intuition, reasoning, and awareness of the living movement of being in time are recognized as coherent aspects of one living whole.

In doing clinical work on my patients' understanding of their fears and other problems, I recognized that Hegel's three phases of self-aware consciousness corresponded directly with Krishnamurti's three stages of awareness in the solution of any human problem (Krishnamurti 1992, Volume IV, pages 26–27). As described by Krishnamurti, the first stage of self-awareness is the increasing awareness and acceptance of the real causes and effects of the problem. The second stage is growing in awareness of its dual or contradictory process, that is, the conflict of opposites that is always present when the thinker and his thought are experienced as separate. The third stage is the enlargement of consciousness to choiceless self-awareness in which knowing is acting in freedom because the thinker and his thought are experienced as one. Fears and other problems always continue, perhaps in a more subtle form, until the third stage of radical transformation in choiceless awareness of the problem is reached. The descriptions of Hegel and Krishnamurti will be summarized for each of the stages of self-aware consciousness because their viewpoints are complementary. Hegel provides the philosophical foundation, whereas Krishnamurti describes a practical psychology of the same stages of consciousness.

It may be difficult to grasp what Hegel and Krishnamurti meant by their descriptions of the three stages of self-aware consciousness when they are stated in only general and abstract terms. Furthermore, such general descriptions do not have much use as a practical psychology for understanding the development of an individual person or the movement of groups of people. Fortunately, the meaning of Hegel and Krishnamurti becomes much clearer when both are considered in an integrative manner in relation to levels of consciousness similar to that of Freud's topographical model of consciousness. The first stage of self-awareness is cognition, that is, the ordinary human consciousness of normal children after age 4. The second stage of self-awareness is what follows cognition, that is, metacognition, or thinking about thinking. Nearly everyone experiences the second stage of self-awareness occasionally when they recollect and consider the meaning of their experiences, as in psychotherapy. Metacognition is also called *meditation*, which is derived from the Latin word meaning "to measure" by reflection in thought—to weigh the quantity, dimensions, and value of something in relation to an intuitive standard, such as wisdom, virtue, or well-being.

In the second stage, thoughts that are "preconscious" or "subconscious" may be brought into consciousness rather than suppressed. The conflicts and contradictions of thought and feeling are processed in the subconscious, often outside of conscious awareness. However, subconscious thoughts can be brought into conscious awareness by the thinker in observing the flow of his own inner thoughts or in expressing them to others when writing in a journal or speaking to a friend or therapist, as in the states of impartial self-observation that Freud called "free association." Hegel observed that there is no dependence on anything but thought itself when the thinker observes his own thought (Hegel 1981). Hence, self-observation leads to freedom of thought from external constraints.

Likewise, in *The Interpretation of Dreams*, Freud (1900) described the state of self-observation associated with free association in terms of being tranquil, not critical, and absolutely impartial so that nothing is suppressed from consciousness. In this state, Freud observed that attention became mobile, allowing unlimited thoughts to come to consciousness, so that pathological ideas and dreams could be interpreted. Freud recognized the critical importance of self-awareness and of not being resistant or self-critical in free association. He distinguished the nonresistance of impartial self-observation from intellectual reflection, which is associated with tension and self-criticism. Freud said,

> I have noticed in the course of my psychoanalytical work that the psychological state of a man in an attitude of reflection is entirely different from that of a man who is observing his psychic processes. In reflection there is a greater play of psychic activity than in the most attentive self-observation; this is shown even by the tense attitude and the wrinkled brow of the man in a state of reflection, as opposed to the mimic tranquillity of the man observing himself. In both cases there must be concentrated attention, but the reflective man makes use of his critical faculties, with the result that he rejects some of the thoughts which arise into consciousness after he has been aware of them, and abruptly interrupts others, so that he does not follow the lines of thought which they would otherwise open up for him; while in respect of yet other thoughts he is able to behave in such a manner that they not become conscious at all—that is to say, they are suppressed before they are perceived. In self-observation, on the other hand, he has but one task—that of suppressing criticism; if he succeeds in doing this, an unlimited number of thoughts enter his consciousness which would otherwise have eluded his grasp. With the aid of the material thus obtained—material that is new to the self-observer—it is possible to achieve the interpretation of pathological ideas, and also that of dream-formation. As will be seen, the point is to induce a state which is in some degree analogous, as regards the distribution of psychic energy (mobile attention), to the state of the mind before falling asleep—and also, of course, to the hypnotic state. (Freud 1900, pages 84–85)

Freud noted that most of his patients are able to enter this state of freely mobile awareness after his first instructions. He found he could do so completely if he assisted the process by writing down the ideas that flashed through his mind. However, Freud noted that some people do not find it easy to enter the state of free association. Freud said, "The 'undesired' ideas habitually evoke the most violent resistance, which seeks to prevent them from coming to the surface." He quoted Friedrich Schiller's advice to a friend that it is not difficult to adopt an attitude of uncritical self-observation if we simply withdraw "the watchers from the gates of the intellect." The poet and philosopher Schiller suggested that the essential condition of poetic creation involved a mental attitude similar to free association. In correspondence with a friend who complained of his lack of creative power, Schiller wrote,

> The reason for your complaint lies, it seems to me, in the constraint which your intellect imposes upon your imagination. Here I will make an observation, and illustrate it by an allegory. Apparently it is not good—and indeed it hinders the creative work of the mind—if the intellect examines too closely the ideas already pouring in, as it were, at the gates. Regarded in isolation, an idea may be quite insignificant, and venturesome in the extreme, but it may require importance from an idea that follows it; perhaps, in a certain collocation with other ideas, which may seem equally absurd, it may be capable of furnishing a very serviceable link. The intellect cannot judge all these ideas unless it can retain them until it has considered them in connection with these other ideas. In the case of a creative mind, it seems to me, the intellect has withdrawn its watchers from the gates, and the ideas rush in pell-mell, and only then does it review and inspect the multitude. You worthy critics, or whatever you may call yourselves, are ashamed or afraid of the momentary and passing madness which is found in all real creators, the longer or shorter duration of which distinguishes the thinking artist from the dreamer. Hence your complaints of unfruitfulness, for you reject too soon and discriminate too severely. (Schiller, letter to Koerner, December 1, 1788, quoted by Freud, 1990, pages 85–86)

Furthermore, the radical transformation of undesired ideas actually occurs only in the third stage, not in the second stage of self-aware consciousness. Consciousness is only enlarged by new understanding of what had been unconscious before the third stage of consciousness. The expansion of consciousness in the third or unitive stage of self-aware consciousness is also described as the "purification of rational intuition," because expanded consciousness involves a greater awareness of what is true. Consciousness is enlarged by contemplation, which is going still deeper and accessing material that is usually unconscious but can come into consciousness under particular conditions. On the one hand, when a person is tired or under stress, information from the unconscious is more likely to emerge as unintentional slips of the tongue or acts ("parapraxes") than would occur under usual conditions. On the other hand, intentional access to unconscious information may occur in states of contemplation, in which a person is deeply calm and dualistic judging is quiet.

According to transcendentalists, the domain of the unconscious is beyond time, space, and conflict, which agrees with the observations of Freud and later Csikszentmihalyi (1991) in descriptions of states of psychological flow or optimal states of consciousness. However, according to transcendentalists, the unconscious is not limited to unrealistic instinctive drives as assumed by Freud based on his studies of the mentally ill. In fact, the third stage of self-aware consciousness is regarded by Hegel, Krishnamurti, and Csikszentmihalyi as the only truly scientific level of consciousness and the only level of self-awareness in which well-being can be attained by a full understanding of emotional conflicts and intellectual contradictions. Only in the third stage of awareness do human beings directly experience pure intuitions without effortful reasoning.

Most people experience the third stage of self-aware consciousness from time to time and can recognize its characteristics. We enter this state when we are fully absorbed in something we love to do without hesitation or struggle. In a state of flow, people typically feel happy, alert, in effortless control, not self-conscious, and at the peak of their abilities. According to Csikszentmihalyi, too great a challenge or too little challenge may interfere with a state of flow. Both the sense of time and all worry about problems seem to disappear in a state of joy and serenity. There is a deepening of understanding, which leads to growth of consciousness, lightening the unconscious and enriching the subconscious. Our abilities and character improve in a way that is effortless (Csikszentmihalyi 1991, 1993).

There is a sense of freedom and joy of self-discovery in flow states. The necessary and sufficient condition for entering this stage of consciousness is non-resistance to self-discovery and creative change without tension or struggle. The conditions and the experience cannot be separated because in this stage, the action and the thought, the thought and the thinker, the thinker and the world, all are united in a state of coherent flow, which is knowing and acting simultaneously. Thus, the third stage of self-aware consciousness begins in contemplation and culminates in the constant awareness that is wisdom and well-being.

The third stage of self-aware consciousness is the stage of awareness that is most useful in clinical work, but this has seldom been done because of a lack of understanding of its nature, the way to facilitate its development, or its clinical importance. However, if it is true that well-being and wisdom depend on growing in awareness, then it is crucial for everyone to understand each of the stages of self-awareness.

These general descriptions of the stages of self-aware consciousness demonstrate their existence but do not provide a rigorous psychological description that can be readily used in individual assessments or other clinical work. Hegel did not have knowledge of the topographical structure of consciousness, which Freud later described. Similarly, Krishnamurti spent nearly all of his life in contemplative thought, so he had little appreciation of how much unconscious and subconscious processes influence other people. Consequently, I have found it essential in clinical work to integrate the work of Hegel and Krishnamurti with a model of the topography of consciousness similar to that described by Freud and later psychoanalysts.

## EXPERIENCING THE STAGES OF SELF-AWARE CONSCIOUSNESS

The most recently evolved region of the brain in vertebrates is the prefrontal cortex of humans (MacLean 1985; Nauta and Feirtag 1986; Eccles 1989). Modern human beings have a greater development of the prefrontal cortex than do other primates. In particular, modern humans have well developed frontal poles (Brodmann area 10), which is essential for coherent orchestration of multiple tasks and prospective autobiographical memory (Burgess, Veitch et al. 2000; Burgess, Scott et al. 2003). The prefrontal cortex of the modern human being has access to all the sensory windows through which a person apprehends the external world, as well as all the sensory gateways to the internal world of the person (MacLean 1985; Nauta and Feirtag 1986). Likewise, the immediate sensuous objects of the first stage of self-awareness include information from both the physical and intuitive senses. The information about the external environment is derived from the five physical senses of touch, taste, smell, hearing, and sight. The information about the internal environment is derived from the corresponding intuitive senses of being, freedom, beauty, truth, and goodness, as described in Chapter 2. In the first stage of self-aware consciousness, the intuitive senses are asleep to a substantial degree because of lack of awareness of unconscious information, leading to the development of a "false self" (Winnicott 1958). As the intuitive senses awaken in the second and third stages of self-awareness, people experience an awakening to their "true" or "authentic" being (Winnicott 1958; Kohut 1984; Thermos 2002). At this state, people also awaken to the intelligible wonders that fill the world in which they live, as is described well by transcendentalists in search of union in nature. This awakening of the intuitive senses by union in nature has been compared to the natural act of breathing, except that what is inspired is metaphorically called the "breath of life" (i.e., self-aware consciousness). As we grow in acceptance and calmness in the first stage of self-awareness, we begin to be conscious of our intuitions of being, freedom, beauty, truth, and goodness. These intuitions are beyond the awareness of the external senses but are intelligible through acceptance of the reality of the intuitions of our own internal milieu.

### Getting calm

In my clinical practice, I use brief meditation exercises to help awaken self-aware consciousness. These meditations have multiple phases, corresponding to the successive stages of self-awareness. For example, one meditation that I call "silence of the mind" begins as a simple concentrative meditation for five minutes. People are taught to relax through regular and deep abdominal breathing and closing their eyes. First, you breathe in through your nose and then out through your mouth slowly with your lips pursed like you are fogging up a mirror. Breathing should be diaphragmatic so the abdomen protrudes as you inhale. This is repeated three times slowly and quietly with the eyes open. Then you close your eyes and direct your attention to the crown of the head, which symbolizes self-awareness, and concentrate your attention on a single thought about an internal experience like love. Alternative monosyllabic words include "hope," "peace," "faith," or "joy," but "love" is particularly helpful in overcoming fears and leading to calmness. You simply let go of all criticism and struggles with your thoughts by letting any thought that emerges in consciousness flow down the stream of your consciousness. You do not try to suppress the emergence of thoughts or to escape from them because you cannot accept what you deny or renounce. You may notice what thoughts emerge but you accept their presence and simply let them go, gently bringing your attention back to the word "love" at the crown of your head. You rest calmly in that awareness and enjoy the peace and quiet. If you feel tense, you may take one or two more deep breaths while keeping your eyes closed and gently bring your attention back to love.

This meditation is continued for approximately five minutes, but no timekeeper is needed. It simply takes about five minutes for people to relax deeply and let go of the struggles with their thoughts. A longer period of relaxation is not needed and can be counterproductive because it becomes a form of escape. After extensive practice, most people can elicit an attitude of acceptance (i.e., readiness for mobile attention) and a full relaxation response by one or two deep breaths, which they can do at any time. This brief exercise can be done to help people develop calm and mobile attention before or during psychotherapy, and it can be practiced at home as much as people like without withdrawing from their responsibilities. This usually helps people become calm and experience pleasant thoughts of hope, love, and peace, which enables them to accept and adapt to problems during subsequent communication with a therapist or during meditation when alone. Only in calmness can we recognize and accept the causes and effects of our fears and other problems; otherwise our thinking is dominated by denial, blaming, and other struggles rooted in conflict. Later, a second stage of metacognition can be added to this first stage, but initially no effort is made to enter the second stage of self-awareness.

## First stage of self-aware consciousness

When people are calm and their senses are awake, they are in the first stage of self-aware consciousness, which culminates in acceptance of the partial validity of both sides of our conflicts and other problems. Self-acceptance means to let go, to stop fighting with your true self and trying to maintain a false self or ideal- ized facade. It is actually more difficult to stop fighting with our true self than to stop fighting with others. If people do not accept what they are, they fight with themselves. If they do not want to be hateful, greedy, jealous, angry, arrogant, judgmental, and so on, they fight to not be what they are. Whenever people enter the fight to be irreproachable, they are locked in self-defeating opposition with themselves. They must stop wanting to become something else and start to recog- nize and be what they are (Winnicott 1958; Thermos 2002). When people regard others with disdain, they strive to be better than other people. Consequently, it is self-centered and self-defeating to judge one's self or others and more useful to seek understanding without judging.

There is fluidity in being one's self. To be in a state of flow, you must let all the rough spots or sensitive issues appear so they can be smoothed out. Our "sensi- tivities" or "rough spots" are problems like jealousy, anger, or being judgmental. Problems mean that people are unable to face something with all of their being. Problems are things people do not understand totally. The first step to smoothing sensitivities is to see and accept that we are as we are. This is the culmination of the first stage of self-aware consciousness. Do not fight and reject or judge. Ac- cept who you are and let go of all your struggles. It is less tiring and less of a strain, but it is not at all indifference.

In the second phase of the silence of mind meditation, people are told to begin to observe the emergence of their own thoughts, rather than simply letting the thoughts go. This phase is begun after five minutes of relaxation in which at- tention has been gently and repeatedly redirected to a single word like "hope" or "love." The person is now calm. He may be ready to begin the first phase of self-awareness, which is accepting his own thoughts and feelings. I tell the per- son to observe his thoughts as they emerge. If it is too disturbing or not interest- ing, he can simply let the thoughts go down the stream of his consciousness. If a particular thought is acceptable and interesting, he is encouraged to think about the causes and effects of that thought in his life. The person should think about all the deep motivations that may contribute to the problem—sexual, material, emotional, intellectual, or spiritual. All of these motivations contribute in vary- ing degrees to problems. As long as a person is comfortable and interested in the thought, he is encouraged to try to understand it as fully as possible from all sides of the problem, rather than trying to justify any one perspective or ele- ment of the conflict. I usually say something like, "Do not try to suppress it, struggle with it, or escape from it, but recognize and understand the thought for what it actually is."

If other thoughts arise, whether different or associated with the earlier thought, the person is reminded that he is free to continue in a free flow of associations or to think about the thought that is most interesting, to grow in awareness. Usually a particular thought (or set of associated thoughts) emerges that captures the full awareness of the person. Then the mind becomes increasingly quiet, allowing growing awareness of the thought or problem of particular interest.

The acceptance of a particular thought in reflection is the end of the first stage of self-awareness, and the subsequent growth in awareness from thinking about aspects that were previously subconscious is the second stage of self-awareness. The acceptance phase of self-awareness should be short because thoughts that are one sided regarding a conflict mean that the problem is not fully understood and will be unpleasant to experience. Consequently, it is useful to combine the first and second stages of self-awareness of problems in meditation. The first phase of meditation can be focused on something calming and pleasant so that the second phase of the meditation can be a quick movement through acceptance to the more pleasant second stage of self-awareness.

How can a clinician explain acceptance to their patients? I usually say something like the following:

> What is acceptance? It is being willing to see what we are in reality without wanting to become something else. I repeat, *Acceptance is being willing to see what we are in reality without wanting to become something else.* Simply calm down so that you can accept a situation that may be painful. Do not go into an inner struggle with part of yourself. Struggle only divides you and leads to inner blockage. Instead, let go of your struggles and accept the reality of your life without tension or any effort to fight. Remember to be kind and patient with yourself, which is the natural spontaneity of all human beings. Fears and other problems are unnatural and unnecessary. The good news is that your can let go of your individual fears and other problems one by one. You do not need to try to become perfect all at once, and should not try to do so because the struggle to be irreproachable will divide, rather than integrate.

Hence, the first stage of self-aware consciousness is part of the way to seeing what is true, but it does not include full self-acceptance, direct experience of certainty about truth, or the ability to measure the interest of different experiences for our well-being. At the first stage of self-awareness, we still cannot face the full impact of problems in our life. We do not fully accept both sides of conflicts, and consequently we have difficulty cooperating with others. We do not recognize the integral nature of reality, which implies the interdependent order of all events in our life and the lives of others. In moments of tranquil union in nature, we may experience oceanic feelings of love, peace, and the inseparable unity of all things, which is a transient experience of the third stage of self-awareness. However, if something happens that is displeasing to us, we may still react as if the whole universe were disarranged, kicking us back to a lower stage of self-awareness. We seek to be rid of the problem violently or in a variety of subtle ways. We try to escape from the problem rather than to understand it.

Lacking a measure of order, our thoughts are unstable and unwise, even though we may experience transient "peak experiences" of flow and ecstasy. Then the growth of our self-awareness may stagnate if we seek to repeat such transient and private achievements (e.g., moments of happiness or creativity) instead of developing a broader awareness of the interdependent order of all things. Fortunately, repeated experience of oceanic feelings or contentment in states of psychological flow is illuminating and helps to reduce our doubts about the intelligibility of the universe.

## Second stage of self-aware consciousness

The second stage of self-awareness is the reflection on the objects of experience in the mirror of self-awareness, which is like the smooth surface of an ocean of memories. Krishnamurti described the first and second stage of self-awareness as the "foundation of meditation," which was his term for the third stage of self-aware consciousness. His description of meditation to young students at one of his schools is particularly simple and clear. He begins with calm acceptance and letting go of struggles (the first stage of self-awareness) and then moves into metacognition, that is, the mind observing itself impartially in the second stage of self-awareness.

> First of all, sit very quietly; do not force yourself to sit quietly; but sit or lie down quietly without force of any kind. . . . Then watch your thinking. Watch what you are thinking about. You find you are thinking about your shoes, . . . what you are going to say, the bird outside to which you listen; follow such thoughts and inquire why each thought arises. Do not try to change your thinking. See why certain thoughts arise in your mind so that you begin to understand the meaning of every thought and feeling without any enforcement. And when a thought arises, do not condemn it, do not say it is right, it is wrong, it is good, it is bad. Just watch it, so that you begin to have a perception, a consciousness which is active in seeing every kind of thought, every kind of feeling. You will know every hidden secret thought, every hidden motive, every feeling, without distortion, without saying it is right, wrong, good or bad. When you look, when you go into thought very very deeply, your mind becomes extraordinarily subtle, alive. No part of the mind is asleep. The mind is completely awake. That is merely the foundation. Then your mind is very quiet. Your whole being becomes very still. (Krishnamurti 1974, page 58, © KFT Ltd.)

At this second stage, people look at both sides of a conflict rather than externalizing the responsibility for the conflict to others; that is, people accept and internalize responsibility for change. The second stage of self-awareness is sometimes referred to as a "broadening of consciousness" or "growing in awareness." We are growing in awareness of information that was previously subconscious. We recognize the contributions of all the deep motivations for our feelings and thoughts, including contributions from the sexual, material, emotional, intellectual, and spiritual streams of our subconscious mind. We want to know all sides and influences on our thoughts and actions for sake of impartial understanding, rather than justification or rationalization. We want to be our true self, but conscientiousness (i.e., moral idealism) still creates tension within us as we strive to accommodate social standards.

The second stage of self-aware consciousness is the beginning of mindfulness, which is nondiscursive meditation. Attention is directed to the states of the mind as an observer with an effort to understand but not to judge or blame. Such self-witnessing is called "recollection" or "centering" because a person opens the door of perception to the subconscious in metacognition. The subconscious is a person's own inner "voice," "center," or "presence." The intention in meditation is to see the nature of thought, not to stop thinking. Such metacognition is called "bare awareness" because the primary ("bare" or "naked") intuition is observed directly without emotional conflict or intellectual judging. As direct awareness grows in meditation, a person begins to recognize that each bit of reality is part of an indivisible whole, which is truth. According to Voltaire (1980), "Better is the enemy of good," so we should "Love truth, but pardon error." When people begin to see directly that everything exists in relationship, they become more self-transcendent, letting go of the intellectual struggles of perfectionism and skepticism, and thereby growing in patience and faith. However, this insight grows by a series of steps through direct experience.

At the second stage of self-awareness, order is recognized as interdependent relationships, each of the five aspects of consciousness (sexual, material, emotional, intellectual, and spiritual) is reflected on the others, giving rise to a 5-x-5 matrix of interdependent relationships. At this stage, self-awareness can be described by a 5-x-5 matrix that is composed of 25 subplanes of thought that must be specified in an empirical psychology of self-awareness. Each subplane of thought differs in its level of self-awareness of what is spiritually interesting (i.e., contributing to our well-being by being orderly and satisfying), as described later in this chapter.

There are some truths about which we are certain at the second stage of awareness, as described by Augustine and Descartes. For example, we know we exist. We know that we know that we exist. Although we remain unsure at this stage what truly makes us happy, we also know that we wish to be happy. Even if we express doubt of any of these three statements, our doubt itself is evidence of our existence, our awareness, and our preference for happiness (Augustine 386). Hence, this second stage of self-aware consciousness is the beginning of awareness of absolute truth. At this stage, we begin to measure the spiritual interest of things, so that we can weigh the value of our thoughts and relationships in the context of what is most meaningful in our life in the sense of contributing to our true well-being (Augustine 386, pages 82–83). However, our knowledge of truth remains incomplete at the abstract idealistic stage of self-aware consciousness.

## Illuminative phase of the third stage

Like Krishnamurti, Hegel regards the abstract idealistic stage as a necessary but incomplete preliminary to the third stage of spontaneous recollection of living reality. The third stage is distinguished from the second stage by the effortless spontaneity of contemplation (Enomiya Lassalle 1974; Krishnamurti 1974; Garrigou-Lagrange 1947). In contemplation the mind is spontaneously awakened or "infused" without effort, whereas calmness is "acquired" by intentional intellectual effort in meditation. The transition to the third stage is marked by the certain recognition that the subconscious is a living reality that exists within itself, as living being or unbounded spiritual essence. In illumination, the subconscious is seen to be the presence (i.e., living being) of the individual, which exists inseparably within the universal unity of being. Therefore, only those who have experienced illumination would describe the gate to the subconscious as the Gate of God. The gate of the subconscious is recognized as the gate of the presence of living being in the third stage of self-aware consciousness, whereas it is recognized only as the gate of rational intuition in the second stage.

Hegel notes that nondualistic positive philosophers like Pascal or Spinoza may choose to set out their rational thought at this level of abstraction, but such an intellectual method is less natural, less realistic, and less satisfying than the ultimate stage of integrated rational-intuitive thinking (Godel 1961; Bjorklund 1997). In rational-intuitive thinking, logical reasoning is spontaneously integrated with recollection of personal experiences, which stimulates further intuitive leaps in logic, thereby making assumptions that go beyond the original premises (Godel 1961). For example, Bertrand Russell and Alfred North Whitehead acknowledged that their joint effort in *Principia Mathematica* (1910–1913) failed in its goal of deducing mathematics fully from a small number of self-evident logical principles. They also found the mental effort unpleasant and distressing. Russell commented (1919), "Neither of us alone could have written the book; even together, and with the alleviation brought by mutual discussion, the effort was so severe that at the end we both turned aside from mathematical logic with a kind of nausea."

Paradoxically, early in the work on *Principia Mathematica*, Russell underwent what he called a "mystic illumination," which overwhelmed him with "semimystical feelings about beauty." He and his colleague Whitehead had been "filled with anxiety" about Mrs. Whitehead's heart disease, which caused her to suffer greatly from chest pain. Russell worried that his colleague would not be able to continue productive work if Mrs. Whitehead died. One evening they went to a poetry reading without Mrs. Whitehead. In Russell's autobiography (1998, page 149, with permission of Thomson Publishing Services), he said,

> I was profoundly stirred by the beauty of the poetry. When we came home, we found Mrs. Whitehead undergoing an unusually severe bout of pain. She seemed cut off from everyone and everything by walls of agony, and the sense of the solitude of each human soul suddenly overwhelmed me. Ever since my marriage, my emotional life had been calm and superficial. I had forgotten all the deeper issues, and had been content with flippant cleverness. Suddenly the ground seemed to give way beneath me, and I found myself in quite another region. Within five minutes I went through

some such reflections as the following: the loneliness of the human soul is unendurable; nothing can penetrate it except the highest intensity of the sort of love that religious teachers have preached; whatever does not spring from this motive is harmful, or at best useless; it follows that war is wrong, that a public school education is abominable, that the use of force is to be deprecated, and that in human relations one should penetrate to the core of loneliness in each person and speak to that.

After experiencing for five minutes the oceanic feelings of the love that inseparably binds humanity, Russell was permanently transformed into a pacifist strongly opposed to British colonial imperialism. Russell's description is typical of the peak experiences or illuminations that characterize the beginning of the third stage of self-aware consciousness. In this illuminative phase, conscious thought continues in the intellectual plane but is enriched by the process of sublimation that occurs during contemplation.

However, Krishnamurti warns that even when we are aware of the conflict of opposites, we are often more concerned with escaping from the struggle rather than with understanding it. If we struggle aggressively or strive idealistically to be better, we cannot see the truth and thereby grow in goodness. The better is an obstacle to the good. Any effort to become better keeps us from entering into the full state of constant awareness. Awareness that is nonjudgmental and choiceless characterizes conscious thought in the spiritual plane, which is the unitive phase of the third stage of self-awareness. Paradoxically, we automatically grow in goodness when we recognize the truth, whereas we block growth when we try to be better. Krishnamurti (1992, Volume IV, pages 26–27, © KFT Ltd.) said,

> It is the desire to be rid of the conflict that gives strength to its continuity, and so maintains contradiction; it is this desire that must be watched and understood. Yet it is difficult to be alertly passive in the conflict of duality; we condemn or justify, compare or identify; so we are ever choosing sides and thus maintaining the cause of conflict. To be choicelessly aware of the conflict of duality is arduous but it is essential if you would transcend the problem.

## The unitive phase of the third stage

The third stage of self-awareness is the enlargement of consciousness. We begin to recognize that the coherence of the universal unity of being is the only consistent source of well-being. All particular finite goals are incomplete and imperfect means to true love. In this stage we contemplate what is good (as well as true and beautiful), so that we can grow in the depth of our love of the Truth. We see directly the difficulties of our life, our sensitivities, and our problems. We become more aware by facing reality without any judging, condemning, or struggling. We know that our individual being—body, mind, and spirit—is the recipient of the infinite love of universal unity of Being, and so we grow in our love of what is—that is, Reality, Truth, God—which is eternal, light, and good, not what is transient, heavy, and selfish. Hence, the awareness of the third stage is "choiceless" in two ways—it is nonjudging, and it is spontaneous, leading to whole-hearted growth without conflict or struggle.

In the unitive phase of the third stage of self-aware consciousness, we are conscious of thought in the plane of the spirit, which leads to understanding of the conflicts of all the lower planes. In the illuminative phase of the third stage of self-awareness, sublimation enriches our subconscious but we are not fully conscious of spiritual thoughts. In both phases of the third stage of self-awareness, the enlargement of consciousness by spiritual understanding leads to a reconciliation of the conflict of opposites so that we can "will without wanting." That is, we can act without wanting the benefits of our actions for selfish purposes. We can be ourselves without striving to become something we are not. Paradoxically, our self-awareness deepens so that we learn to orchestrate the conduct of our life in a way that is coherent and harmonious.

This third stage of self-awareness is sometimes described as the dimension of selfless love or compassion in which there is neither fear nor suffering because there is no separation into things to be feared or desired. When such compassion is conscious, we have entered the "unitive phase" of spiritual development. The unitive stage of self-awareness occurs when thought itself becomes the general object of consciousness, so that subject and object are identical. Hegel (1807) described this as the stage in which "the object is within itself, as a living being." In Krishnamurti's terms, the subject is also the object, so the observer is the observed (Bohm 1995); we realize that the whole has given everything to all, filling us with all the gifts of the spirit to the extent we are aware of our true nature. Self-aware consciousness at this third stage reaches at least partial awareness of aspects of the universal unity of being in which all being, freedom, beauty, truth, and goodness exist. Hegel refers to awareness of the universal unity of being as spirit or life itself. Thus, the third stage of self-aware consciousness is awareness of life itself. More practically, the third stage of self-awareness is what has been called "the happy life" (Augustine 386).

The coherence of relationships within the whole is the standard of truth in the unitive phase of consciousness. Correspondence between concept and reality is no longer an adequate criterion of truth because the subject and the object of study are living reality itself, which cannot be reduced fully to fixed abstract concepts. At this stage, we are aware of the three-dimensional structure of thought and its movement in time. This is what Hegel called the "triadic form" of self-awareness.

Krishnamurti described the third stage of self-aware consciousness as the transcending of time and choice. He noted that conflicts could be lastingly resolved only at this stage. In Godel's theorem, we learned that the consistency of an abstract system cannot be proved within that system. Likewise, according to Krishnamurti, we can let go of a problem only when choice in the conflict of duality has ceased:

The complete integration of the thinker with his thought cannot be experienced if there is no understanding of the process of becoming and the conflict of opposites. This conflict cannot be transcended through an act of will, it can only be transcended when choice has ceased. No problem can be solved on its own plane; it can be resolved lastingly only when the thinker has ceased to become. (Krishnamurti 1992, Volume IV, pages 26–27)

The third stage of choiceless awareness involves a person moving deeper from the foundation of calm alertness in the second stage to enlarge consciousness by sublimation in a contemplative state. Thought is shifted to the spiritual plane from the lower planes of dualistic consciousness. The only need is seen to be love of the universal unity of being. That is, sexual issues are considered from the perspective of the sexual subplane of the spiritual plane. Material needs are considered from the perspective of the material subplane of the spiritual plane. Emotional needs are considered from the vantage point of the emotional subplane of the spiritual plane. Intellectual issues are viewed from the intellectual subplane of the spiritual plane.

I use the term "sublimation" to designate the process of lifting thought up from one of the dualistic planes of consciousness to the corresponding subplane of the spiritual plane. This gives thought an elevated character or lightness while preserving the whole of our being and relationships in life. Hence, the shift of thought to the sexual aspects of the spiritual plane via sublimation leads to an understanding of hope, which reconciles the conflicts of the sexual plane. The shift of thought to the material aspects of the spiritual plane leads to an understanding of charity, which reconciles the conflicts of the material plane. The shift of thought to the emotional aspects of the spiritual plane leads to an understanding of peace, which reconciles the conflicts of the emotional plane. The shift of thought to the *intellectual* aspects of the spiritual plane leads to an understanding of faith, which reconciles the conflicts of the intellectual plane, leading to a stable and continual state of choiceless awareness or integrated intelligence. Further elevation of thought in the spiritual plane culminates in coherence of personality in which people are interested only in devotion to the unity of being.

Beginning from the foundation of the quiet of the second stage, Krishnamurti described the movement by sublimation into the living unity of the third stage as follows:

That [second stage] is merely the foundation. . . . Then go through that stillness, deeper, further. . . . To understand the whole process of your thinking and feeling is to be free from all thought, to be free from all feelings so that your mind, your whole being becomes very quiet. And that is also part of life and with that quietness, you can look at the tree, you can look at people, you can look at the sky and the stars. That is the beauty of life. (Krishnamurti 1974, page 58, © KFT Ltd.)

More specifically, living within the plane of the spirit involves freedom of the will from the attachments of the lower planes. It also involves listening to the psyche, which is essential for sublimation and the third stage of self-awareness. Choiceless self-awareness is impartial and nonjudgmental, culminating in nondual consciousness. In the serene quiet of the third stage of self-aware consciousness, Gandhi described listening to the psyche as awareness of an inner voice that enlightens the subconscious. He said, "There are moments in your life when you must act, even though you cannot carry your best friends with you. The 'still small voice' within you must always be the final arbiter when there is a conflict of duty" (Gandhi 1997, page 62). Gandhi is describing contemplation or listening to the psyche, which is not an intellectual, emotional, power-seeking, or sexual struggle to overcome conflict. Contemplation is a quiet receptivity and passive alertness in which we do not choose or seek or want anything but understanding of our whole being. Later, we may realize that we have an enlarged understanding of the solution to the conflict that was under contemplation.

In contemplation, our unconscious is lightened and our subconscious is nourished, which improves character. We increase in understanding so that we are better able to avoid self-defeating behavior and the repetition of past errors. Consequently, in the third phase of the silence of mind meditation, I encourage people to ask their psyche to inspire their subconscious in the joyful spirit of self-discovery. I say something like the following:

> When your mind becomes silent in the second phase of your meditation, you may feel you have grown in understanding of the problem. However, do not stop there. If you are calm and your mind has grown quiet, then you may ask your psyche to help you to understand yourself more deeply. You already have all the wisdom and love within you that you could ever need. Your psyche is the holder of all that love and wisdom. You can simply ask your psyche to inspire you, and your subconscious will be nourished. You may feel subtle vibrations like a gentle rain of grace at the crown of your head, or you may simply enjoy the silence while your subconscious is nourished. Simply remain calm and aware, passively receptive to an enlarging of your consciousness. Do not seek or demand any results. Simply enjoy the silence so that the light of your psyche may be added to the light of your mind and body, enriching your self-awareness of the unity of your whole being.

About thirty minutes should be reserved in a quiet place for the full sequence of the silence of mind meditation. The first phase should always be about five minutes. The second phase usually takes about ten minutes for the mind to become quiet, but this varies. At least a total of thirty minutes should be allowed for the full sequence. The meditator can be assured that there is no harm in stopping at any point. After thirty minutes, the nourishment of the subconscious may continue even while the person continues with ordinary activities or sleep. Nearly everyone has had the experience of being blocked in trying to understand a problem and then just doing something else or taking a nap, only to awaken with a deeper understanding or insight. The silence of the mind meditation is simply a systematic way to cultivate the natural processes of purifying our rational intuition.

The elevated thought of the plane of the spirit may seem unattainable, until we remember that we are all aware of the "spirit" of thoughts and relationships, although to varying degrees. If we try to be spiritual through rituals or intellectual effort, of course we will block ourselves. However, we all have a natural measure of the spirit of everything we encounter built into our central nervous system, if we will only let that operate spontaneously without tension or struggle. Whenever we experience struggle, tension, or doubt, we can be sure that we are not sufficiently self-aware. The reality of living is a highly effective biofeedback system, especially when we recognize that growth in self-awareness is the path to well-being.

## DESCRIPTION AND MEASUREMENT OF THOUGHT

### Evolutionary development

So far in this chapter, I have described self-aware consciousness qualitatively and tried to give practical descriptions about how its various phases can be experienced. However, to develop a rigorous scientific way of quantitatively measuring self-aware consciousness, it is essential to describe its developmental range. Precision in science requires quantitative measurement. To develop an appropriate scale of quantitative measurement, we must go beyond Hegel's consideration of ancient and modern history to consider the full evolution of human learning abilities throughout phylogeny. The development of individuals is known to repeat the evolutionary history of their ancestry to a substantial extent. In the famous words of Ernst Haeckel (1900), "ontogeny recapitulates phylogeny." A sound model of the development of thought must therefore take into account the evolution of learning abilities in animals. The hierarchy of the seven major steps in the evolution of human learning abilities is summarized in Table 3.1. Evidence for this evolutionary history has been documented elsewhere (Cloninger 1994). Briefly, associative conditioning of habits is well developed in bony fish and all higher vertebrates. Reptiles were the first animals able to follow their prey when out of sight and to learn an extensive repertoire of procedural skills (MacLean 1985). Mammals are the first animals who nurse their young in conjunction with maternal care, use audio-vocal communication for maintaining maternal–offspring contact, and exhibit play (MacLean 1985). Primates show reasoning ability and semantic memory (i.e., registration of personal knowledge and encoding of abstract rules) (Eccles 1989; Lewin 1998; Povinelli 2000; Wallis, Anderson et al. 2001). Great apes and early Homo developed the ability to transmit acquired knowledge within a group and between generations (Mithen 1996; DeWaal 1999; Whiten, Goodall et al. 1999). Only modern Homo sapiens have self-aware consciousness, which provides the basis for a theory of mind (i.e., metacognition or thinking about thinking)

**Table 3.1.** Hierarchy of Major Steps in the Evolution of Learning Abilities in Animals

| Evolutionary Level | Animal Group | Emergent Ability | Thought Process |
|---|---|---|---|
| 1 | Invertebrates Jawless fish | Reflex Instinct | — |
| 2 | Bony fish Amphibians | Associative habits | Habit |
| 3 | Reptiles | Procedural skills | Intention |
| 4 | Mammals | Social nurturance Play | Emotion |
| 5 | Primates | Personal knowledge | Reasoning |
| 6 | Great apes Early Homo | Cultural inheritance | — |
| 7 | Homo sapiens | Self-awareness | Intuition Creativity |

*Source*: Adapted from Cloninger, 1994.

(Povinelli 2000; Tulving 2002). Contrary to common belief, human beings do not have the largest or most convoluted brains in either absolute or relative terms (Roth 2000). Unless we accept whales and elephants as more intelligent or self-aware than human beings, the size of the human brain and the degree of its cortical convolutions cannot explain what is unique about human consciousness; therefore, either the psyche of human beings or unique brain features yet to be discovered may be necessary to account for the unique capacity of human beings for self-aware consciousness.

Each of these emergent abilities in animals is retained and modified by subsequent evolution. Five of the seven emergent abilities are particularly relevant to conscious thought processes in modern human beings. As shown in Table 3.2, these five thought processes correspond to the emergent abilities of evolutionary step 2 (habit), step 3 (intention, conation, or will), step 4 (emotion), step 5 (reasoning or intellect), and step 7 (rational intuition or self-aware consciousness). Evolutionary steps 1 and 6 do not involve a distinct process of conscious thinking. Reflexes (step 1) are modulated by conscious processes of thought but do not involve thought. Cultural transmission of personally acquired information between generations (step 6) depends on greater facility of semantic memory but not a new thought process.

The temporal sequence of processes in human thought is the reverse of the evolutionary history, as summarized in Table 3.2. The description and sequence of human thought processes have been described in detail in cognitive psychol-

**Table 3.2.** Temporal Sequence of Processes in Human Thought

| Temporal Sequence | Thought Process | (Evolved Order) |
| --- | --- | --- |
| 1. Initial perspective | Intuition | (7) |
| 2. Abstraction of ideas | Reason | (5) |
| 3. Automatic response | Emotion | (4) |
| 4. Motivated response | Intention | (3) |
| 5. Repetition of response | Habit | (2) |

ogy (Beck 1976, 1996; Bjorklund 1997). Thought depends on the initial perspective, which is the immediate apprehension of a situation or event in its spatiotemporal context. Even human infants have such intuitive recognition before they are able to reason or label their intuitions in abstract terms. However, the registration and recall of self-aware memories do not mature until about four years of age (Povinelli and Simon 1998; Povinelli, Landry et al. 1999; Tulving 2002). The immediate apprehension and recognition of a situation or event are called *intuition*, as discussed in Chapter 1. Such intuitions are also called *cognitive schemas*, which differ among individuals according to the memories and the level of development of the psyche along the path of self-aware consciousness (Augustine 388). In other words, people differ in the way they perceive events because they differ in their memories.

Second, ideas are abstracted from intuitive experience. Abstraction reduces the information to facts that may omit their spatiotemporal context. Even if spatial or temporal information is a part of the fact, it is not recollected as a living experience. The person may know that they know a fact, but a fact does not involve actual recollection of the experience of when and where the person learned it. Furthermore, the process of abstraction reduces the intuitive information to a fixed state, much like the collapse of a quantum wave function constrains many possibilities to a fixed form. The subjective judgments and choices involved in abstraction reduce the nondualistic manifold of intuitive experience to a specific dualistic object. The judgments we make and the labels we assign involve simplifying distortions of the complexity of experience, as evidenced by the inconsistencies of the accounts of witnesses. Furthermore, what we abstract from experience depends on individual differences in character, which influences the significance and meaning we assign to experience. Awareness that our character (i.e., our cognitive schemas and abstract judgments) may bias the processing of experience is an important part of cognitive and psychoanalytic therapies, even though such therapy has generally been conducted in the first or second stage of self-aware consciousness.

Third, our abstracted labels elicit automatic emotional responses, which depend on individual differences in temperament. Fourth, automatic emotional responses in turn influence our motivated behaviors, which are our intentional (willed) choices about behavior. Fifth, repetition of such procedural sequences leads to habit formation, which may reduce self-awareness. Habits are those behavioral patterns that we allow to become automated as conditioned responses to external cues, rather than flexibly directed in self-aware consciousness.

Unlike lower vertebrates, which lack self-aware consciousness, human beings can reactivate their self-awareness voluntarily at any time because their initial perspective is based on self-aware consciousness. Maintenance of the flexibility of self-aware consciousness is another way of describing the development of co-herence of personality. Recollection of the past in a state of free association with the benefit of growth in self-awareness can elevate our thoughts about problems and conflicts. However, full reconciliation can occur only through sublimation in the third stage of self-aware consciousness. To be effective in transforming per-sonality, cognitive psychology has needed a comprehensive model of the struc-ture and dynamics of human thought, as described in the next section.

## The structure of thought as a reflected object

The second stage of self-awareness involves reflection on the pattern of our thoughts. That is, thought examines a two-dimensional abstraction of itself, just like a person looking in a mirror or studying a map. In this chapter, I describe summary tables only to provide an illustrative overview of the second stage of self-awareness. The reader will soon see that the second stage of self-awareness is an abstract reduction of the third stage. All information at the second stage is only a special case of the more general model. Therefore, I will defer description of supporting empirical data until we can examine the more general structure of human thought at the third stage of self-aware consciousness.

The $5 \times 5$ matrix that I propose for describing human dualistic consciousness is shown in Table 3.3. According to this model, human thought varies widely in content, flowing across five planes that correspond to the evolutionary hierarchy of brain development. In fact, I am proposing that conscious thought is the inte-gration of five streams of subconscious thought, which correspond to the five planes of human self-aware consciousness. Each plane (i.e., each major step in evolutionary development) is concerned with the modulation of a different basic emotional conflict. Aspects of each of the five planes are also reflected in each row, giving rise to five subplanes in each plane. For example, the sexual plane of thought (plane 2) involves the modulation of the conflict between emptiness and lust, which is shown as the sexual aspects of plane 2. When unmodulated, the purely sexual aspect of sexuality leads to conflict between emptiness and lust. Likewise, the plane of material consumption (plane 3) involves modulation of the conflict between desire and aversion, which is shown as the sexual aspect of plane 3 (that is, subplane 3–2). The conflict between desire and aversion is a development of the need to eat to avoid starvation and death. When unmodulated, the sexual as-

**Table 3.3.** 5 × 5 Matrix of Elevation of Conflicts in Human Thought (Dualistic Consciousness)*

| Subplane of Thought | Plane 2 (Sexuality) | Plane 3 (Intention) | Plane 4 (Emotion) | Plane 5 (Intellect) | Plane 7 (Spirit) |
|---|---|---|---|---|---|
| Spiritual aspects (7) | {responsible} Scorn or exhibition (shy) | {purposeful} Power or sarcasm (exploratory) | {self-accepting} Contentment or relief of grief (attached) | {resourceful} [Self-actualization plus oceanic feelings] (perfectionistic) | {coherence} [Coherence seeking] |
| Intellectual aspects (5) | {sensible} Devaluation or idealization (pessimistic) | {idealistic} Pride or inferiority (impulsive) | {transpersonal} Tender-minded or tough-minded (sentimental) | {faithful} Self-transcendence and patience (eagerness of effort) | {spiritual} [Truth seeking] |
| Emotional aspects (4) | Harm avoidance— worry or denial | Novelty seeking— anger/envy or stoicism | Reward dependence— warmth or coldness | Persistence— calmness and conscience (overachieving) | [Peace seeking] |
| Material aspects (3) | {tolerant} Vulnerability or eroticism (fearful) {prejudiced} | {forgiving} Greed/competition or submission (extravagant) {revengeful} | {empathic} Sociability or aloofness (aloof) {inconsiderate} | {helpful} Cooperativeness or nonprejudice (underachieving) {unhelpful} | {charitable} [Merit seeking] |
| Sexual aspects (2) | {victimized} Emptiness or lust (fatigable) | {aimless} Desire/fight or aversion/flight (disorderly) | {approval-seeking} Succorance or rejection (dependent) | {work-hardened} Self-directedness or irresponsibility (spoiled) {inadequate} | {enlightened} [Mastery seeking] |

*Experiences that are unlikely to be fully clear in the consciousness of most people are given in parentheses. Adjectives in brackets indicate the TCI temperament subscales that provide quantitative measures of the emotional aspects of the conflict within each subplane of thought observed in dualistic consciousness. Adjectives in {} indicate the TCI character subscales that modulate that subplane, except coherence, which is the sum total of all three character scales.

pect of the material plane leads to desire or aversion when not frustrated and to fight-or-flight responses when frustrated. Plane 4 (emotion) involves modulation of the conflict between rejection and succorance (i.e., the need to love and be loved), which is the sexual aspect of emotion (subplane 4–2). Plane 5 (intellect) involves modulation of the conflict of subplane 5–2, which is the need for self-sufficiency (i.e., identity and self-directedness) versus minimizing irresponsibility and dependency. The sexual aspect of the spiritual plane is "spiritual mastery seeking," which results from the conflict between perfectionism and imperfection. Mastery seeking is an incompletely sublimated form of the wish for sexual domination. The struggle for mastery and other perfectionist needs block the elevation of thought in the plane of the spirit.

The sexual, material, emotional, and intellectual planes involve the modulation of the four temperaments, and the contents of the subplanes correspond to the subscales of the four temperaments. The Temperament and Character Inventory (TCI) subscales of temperament that provide quantitative measures of variability in the emotional conflict within each subplane of thought are indicated by the labels in parenthesis in Table 3.3. For example, the subplanes of plane 2 include the sexual subplane (measured by TCI Harm Avoidance subscale 4, fatigability), material subplane (TCI Harm Avoidance subscale 2, fear of uncertainty), intellectual subscale (TCI Harm Avoidance subscale 1, anticipatory worry and pessimism), and the spiritual subscale (TCI Harm Avoidance subscale 3, shyness). Each subscale is moderately correlated with the others in the same plane (part-whole correlations of about 0.7), and weakly or not at all with subscales related to other planes (Cloninger, Przybeck et al. 1994). Therefore, the total Harm Avoidance scale score measures the common emotional aspects, indicated as subplane 2–4. Likewise the content of the subplanes of plane 3 correspond to the subscales of Novelty Seeking: sexual (NS4, disorderliness), material (NS3, extravagance), intellectual (NS2, impulsiveness), and spiritual (NS1, exploratory excitability). The common emotional aspects of plane 3 are measured by the total score of TCI Novelty Seeking. The content of the subplanes of plane 4 correspond to the subscales of Reward Dependence: sexual (RD4, Dependence vs. independence), material (RD2, warmth vs. aloofness), emotional (total RD), intellectual (RD1, sentimentality), and spiritual (RD3, attachment). The content of the subplanes of plane 5 correspond to the subscales of Persistence: sexual (PS2, work-hardened vs. spoiled), material (PS3, ambitious vs. underachieving), emotional (total PS), intellectual (PS1, generative eagerness vs. laziness), and spiritual (PS4, perfectionistic vs. pragmatic). Table 3.3 makes explicit the matrix structure that was originally implicit in the TCI subscales for temperament.

The substructure of the character scales in relation to all five planes is also summarized in Table 3.3. A more precise description will be given in Chapter 5 after the dynamics of thought in self-aware consciousness has been described in a three-dimensional context. The elevation of thought in each of the five planes is modulated by one subscale of each of the three character dimensions. Within the two-dimensional view of Table 3.3, the overall degree of elevation of thought in each plane is defined by one of the five Self-directedness subscales. For example, Harm Avoidance in plane 2 is elevated by the Self-Directedness subscale 1 called "responsible versus victimized," so the top subplane is described as "responsible," whereas the bottom subplane is "victimized." The material aspect of Harm Avoidance in plane 2 is modulated largely by the Cooperativeness subscale 1 called "tolerance versus prejudice." The intellectual aspect of Harm Avoidance is modulated largely by the Self-Transcendence subscale 1 called "sensible versus repressive," which has also been called "self-forgetfulness." The dynamic role of the character subscales for all five planes will be examined in more detail in Chapter 5 (see Table 5.6). In brief, Self-Directedness specifies the overall degree of elevation of thought (i.e., clarity of the initial intuitive recollection and recognition of reality), Self-Transcendence specifies the degree of intellectual understanding (i.e., social radius of an individual based on his or her egocentric, allocentric, or nondual map of what is recognized intuitively), and Cooperativeness describes the degree of flexibility of movement in everyday activities within the map of reality as it is recognized and interpreted.

Initially I developed a systematic description of the content of the planes of thought by personal intuitive work that I checked empirically by having people to rank order their fears related to each of the temperaments and then to describe their thoughts when their fears were activated and when they progressed through the stages of self-aware consciousness in the meditative exercises described earlier in this chapter. This procedure provided a rank ordering of thoughts elicited transiently (i.e., over periods of seconds to hours) by a hierarchy of fears and by a hierarchy of meditative states. The TCI character scales, in contrast, were developed to quantify the degree of maturity of the usual thoughts of individuals over extended periods (i.e., months to years), rank ordering individuals from more to less severe personality disorder and increasingly mature adaptive functioning. The structure of thought is the same, nevertheless, whether the level of thought is rank ordered according to elevation of the usual level of thought over years of development or according to transient regression in thought in response to fears or transient elevation of thought in meditation. Supporting empirical data will be presented in the next two chapters after the dynamics of thought have been described. I had not expected an exact correspondence in my findings by such different approaches and was shocked to discover that the TCI scales of character provided quantitative measures of the subplanes of thought, even though the scales had been developed in 1993 before I had any idea of the matrix structure or the nonlinear dynamics of self-aware consciousness. Essentially the content of the subplanes of thought corresponded to specific TCI subscales of temperament, and the dynamics of thought in each plane corresponded to specific TCI subscales of character. The matrix structure provided a systematic dynamic order for the organization of the TCI, and the TCI provided a reliable quantification of the subplanes and the dynamics of their development. The TCI provides a reliable quantitative way to measure individual differences in the matrix substructure of human thought, which has been consistently replicated in more than a dozen cultures tested throughout the Americas, Europe, Asia, and Africa (Cloninger and Svrakic 2000).

Fortunately, the same content and structure of thought is adequate for describing the elevation and the regression of thought, suggesting that the structure of Table 3.3 may be robust regardless of the time scale for change and may describe the full range of thought that is possible among human beings regardless of their particular biopsychosocial background. However, neither the linear structure of the individual TCI dimensions nor the two-dimensional structure of Table 3.3 is completely adequate for describing or understanding the dynamics of self-aware consciousness, as we will see later in this chapter. The linear dimensions of the TCI correspond to a view of personality from the first stage of self-awareness, which is typical of ordinary adult cognition and the predominant approach to contemporary personality assessment. The reflected $5 \times 5$ matrix structure of Table 3.3 corresponds to a view of personality from the second stage of self-awareness, which allows a deeper understanding of the way character modulates the emotional conflicts of temperament. These two views, therefore, are compatible with one another and also provide a useful and essential foundation for beginning to understand the actual dynamics of human thought that is recognized in the third stage of self-awareness. Alternative five-dimensional models of personality are incompatible with the nonlinear relationships recognizable in the higher stages of awareness because they have been derived assuming linearity. For example, all the factor analytically derived models include a factor like Neuroticism which is strongly correlated with high TCI Harm Avoidance and low TCI Self-Directedness (Cloninger, Svrakic et al. 1993; Svrakic, Whitehead et al. 1993; Cloninger, Przybeck et al. 1994; Svrakic, Svrakic et al. 1996). High Harm Avoidance is closely related to low Self-Directedness in plane 2 of thought, but as Self-Directedness increases the two dimensions are dissociated. Consequently, no adequate theory of personality can be based on models that assume linearity and neglect the nonlinearity and matrix structure of personality development.

As in Freud's psychoanalytic theory, the sexual aspects of each of the planes may be regarded as "needs," "wishes," or "drives." Essentially, the perceived needs of people drive them to find a way to reconcile the conflicts between their basic wishes. However, Freud emphasized the drives for sexuality and aggression, which correspond to planes 2 and 3 here. Here other needs are also recognized: social attachment (succorance, plane 4), meaning (intellectual purpose, plane 5), and coherence (spiritual integration, plane 7). The importance of all five of these needs has been recognized by many observers of human nature. William James emphasized the "will to freedom," or the need for recognition of freedom of will, rather than determinism, as the solution to personal fears. John Bowlby and Eric Fromm emphasized the importance of social attachment. Henry Murray (1938) coined the use of the term *succorance* to refer to the need for social attachment, protection, and approval. Victor Frankl (1959, 1978) emphasized the importance of "the will to meaning," which progressively involves intellectual purpose, responsibility, compassion, patience, and self-transcendence based on his inspiring experiences in prison camps during World War II (Frankl 1959, 1978). Freud, Adler, Kant, Maslow, Erikson, Kohut, Rogers, Winnicott, and most modern cognitive psychologists have emphasized the importance of various humanistic needs in the intellectual plane of thought. Teilhard de Chardin and all of the positive philosophers emphasized the importance of the need for well-being through coherence in human life, which was for them the self-aware participation in cosmic goodness and unity.

Clearly, there are strongly felt human needs underlying each of the major steps in the evolution and development of human thought. The 5 × 5 matrix in Table 3.3 allows psychologists and psychiatrists to begin to examine the overall structure of the interactions among these needs in a systematic manner. Furthermore, I have designated each plane with a number corresponding to the step in the evolution of human learning ability. The numbering system is useful to keep the developmental perspective about the path of consciousness prominent in our thinking. The numbering system also provides a convenient way to quantify the measurement of human thought, as shown later, so that we have a metric rank of the degree of coherence of different thoughts, which indicates its value for our well-being.

There is a gap between the intellectual plane (plane 5) and the spiritual plane (plane 7). This corresponds to the large quantum jump between dualistic thought and nondualistic thought. Consequently, I have retained the phylogenetic numbering sequence; this gap appears to be meaningful psychologically.

In response to the conflict underlying each plane of thought, every human being has a need to elevate the thoughts in that plane. We all seek to reconcile our conflicts, which requires a growth in awareness about the nature of the conflict. According to psychoanalytic theory, the elevation of sexual conflicts leads to progressive increases in the creative expression of the libido. Likewise in Table 3.3, each subplane of thought increases in its lightness or coherence as there is movement from subplane 2–2 through 2–7, and then on to 3–2 through 3–7, et cetera, culminating in subplane 7–7. The elevation of thought in the sexual plane progresses from emptiness or lust (subplane 2–2) through primary narcissism and confidence expressed as scorn or exhibition (subplane 2–7), as seen in Table 3.3. The sexual drive can also be sublimated to plane 7, that is, to subplane 7–2, but first thought must be elevated to a higher level of self-awareness. It is unrealistic to try to get someone who is not highly self-aware to sublimate their sexual drives, as is shown by the frequent failure of such efforts in clergy. In the absence of sublimation, the frustration of sexuality leads to progressive degrees of anxiety, as shown by scorn (subplane 2–7), devaluation (subplane 2–5), worry (subplane 2–4), feelings of vulnerability (subplane 2–3), or emptiness (subplane 2–2).

The modulation of these emotional conflicts ("the conflict of opposites") is quantifiable in terms of the degree of the temperament dimension of Harm Avoidance, which is shown in Table 3.3 as the emotional trait associated with the sexual plane of thought. Subplane 2–4 is called Harm Avoidance because emotionality is regarded as the core of temperament traits. More precisely, we will see that Harm Avoidance is the bias in the conflict involved in responses throughout the column of thought in plane 2. In other words, high Harm Avoidance is indicated by frequency of experiencing feelings of scorn, devaluation, worry, vulnerability, and emptiness (see the high or left side of the conflicts in each subplane). In contrast, low Harm Avoidance is indicated by the frequency of experiencing exhibitionistic fantasies, idealization, denial of risk, eroticism, and lust (see the low or right side of the conflicts in each subplane). In dualistic consciousness, this conflict is partially reconciled by the process of transcendence to libido or overall vitality, which in turn may develop more fully into hopefulness when sexuality is sublimated to the sexual subplane of plane 7. The usual degree of modulation of plane 2 is measured by the Self-Directedness subscale "responsible versus victimized." If individuals are highly responsible, they are usually able to modulate Harm Avoidance, whereas they cannot if they blame others for their problems and regard themselves as controlled, abused, or victimized.

Likewise, the need for material consumption involves an emotional conflict in subplane 3–2 between what we desire (which is described as pleasant) and what we fear or dislike (which is described as unpleasant). When unopposed, our desires may lead to gluttony or addiction. When fully frustrated, desire may be replaced by shame or by sloth (aimlessness). When partially frustrated, our desires lead physiologically to the defense reflex, which is described as the "fight-or-flight" response. The defense reflex is characterized by rage, aggressive gestures, dilation of the pupils, elevation of blood pressure with cardiac deceleration, generally lower amplitude and increased rate of breathing, and changes in gastric motility and acidity (Cloninger 2002). This reflex prepares an individual for fight or flight by muscle vasodilatation, increased muscle blood flow, and decreasing sensitivity to aversive stimulation (Kelly, Richardson et al. 1973; Graham 1979; Deakin and Graeff 1991).

Plane 3 of thought involves the modulation of the defense reflex by the temperament dimension of Novelty Seeking. Plane 3 involves everyday activities and consumption of materials, such as food. The technical psychological term for such intentional activity is *conation*, which is the intentional transformation of resources in our environment for use through influential activity. When people elevate their awareness of the nature of the conflict between desire and aversion, they may feel innovative and liberal or conservative and traditional (subplane 3–5) or perhaps powerful or sarcastic (subplane 3–7). When our desire and will for power and purposeful influence is not satisfied, we become progressively proud or argumentative (subplane 3–5), angry (subplane 3–4), greedily competitive (subplane 3–3), and aggressive (subplane 3–2) if high in Novelty Seeking. Likewise, if we are low in Novelty Seeking, when our wish to be idle is frustrated, we become progressively compliant (subplane 3–5), stoical (subplane 3–4), submissive (subplane 3–3), or try to flee or escape (subplane 3–2). Alternatively, our material desires can be sublimated to the material subplane of the spiritual plane (subplane 7–3), leading to charity and work in the service of others. The degree to which Novelty Seeking is usually modulated is measured by the Self-Directedness subscale "purposeful versus aimless." If individuals are highly purposeful, they are usually able to modulate their Novelty Seeking, whereas they cannot if they feel they have little meaning or direction in their life.

It is important to recognize one of the gates of consciousness between subplane 3–3 and subplane 3–4. As thought becomes conscious of the emotional aspects of the material plane, we enter the first stage of human self-aware consciousness. Below this level, we are creatures of desire and habit, without true self-awareness of our own inner feelings and those of others. Hence, this gate may be described as the "gate of humanity." Below the gate of humanity, the behavior of people is dominated by lust, hate, gluttony, and greed. Behavioral conditioning, not self-aware consciousness, regulates thought and action below the gate of humanity.

The emotional plane of thought (plane 4) involves emotional conflicts concerning what Murray (1938) called "succorance," that is, the need to love and be loved, which leads to desire for social attachments, sympathy, and affection. When our thoughts are elevated in plane 4, we may experience empathy or detachment (subplane 4–5), or we may experience appeasement or grief (subplane 4–7). Rejection or the absence of social affiliation causes humiliation and loneliness if we are high in Reward Dependence (i.e., sociable, warm, and tender minded). In contrast, the absence of social affiliation or rejection is met by indifference if a person is low in Reward Dependence (i.e., aloof, cold, and tough minded). Alternatively, our need for immediate emotional contentment can be sublimated to the emotional subplane of plane 7, which leads to impartiality and serenity. The degree to which Reward Dependence is modulated is measured by the Self-Directedness subscale "self-accepting versus approval-seeking." If individuals are highly self-contented and self-accepting, they are usually able to modulate Reward Dependence well. If they are low in self-acceptance, they are dominated by their perceived need for approval and protection so they cannot modulate Reward Dependence.

The intellectual plane of thought involves the modulation of the need for meaning in our life. If thought remains focused on control of personal goals, our Self-Directedness can be seen to involve a conflict between self-reliance and resistance to guidance and help by others. If intellectual thoughts are further elevated to recognize the reality of the needs and freedom of others, then our thought becomes cooperative and agreeable. The recognition and acceptance of the reality of both sides of conflicts correspond to the ability to cooperate with others in "win–win" situations. Hence, subplane 5–3 (Cooperativeness) is the culmination of the first stage of self-aware consciousness. Beyond this level, we enter into the second stage of self-aware consciousness. The elevation of thought beyond subplane 5–3 (Cooperativeness) involves passage through a second gate of consciousness in which we become aware of the thought processes that were previously subconscious. This gate to metacognition or meditation can be designated as the gate of reason or, more clearly, the gate of rational intuition.

As we enter the second stage of self-aware consciousness in subplane 5–4, we become more idealistic and conscientious. That is, we grow in awareness of both sides of conflicts, so that we internalize our conflict rather than blaming problems on others. As we grow in awareness, we become more calm and impartial (emotional subplane 5–4) and then more patient and self-transcendent (intellectual subplane 5–5).

In the existential psychotherapy of Viktor Frankl (1959), the goal was to facilitate the emergence of a mature "will to meaning" as Self-Transcendence (subplane 5–5). According to Frankl, Self-Transcendence included all of the elevated features of the intellectual plane, including self-directedness, cooperativeness, persistence, patience, and faith. In Table 3.3, I limit Self-Transcendence to the intellectual and lower aspects of thought in plane 5 (i.e., subplanes 5–2 through 5–5, and not 5–7). The elevation of intellectual thought may also lead to self-actualization and oceanic feelings according to Rogers (1980) and Maslow (1962) (subplane 5–7), but the elevation of thought to subplane 5–7 involves the initial entry into the third stage of self-awareness, which involves illuminative experiences. Consequently, I have found it necessary to distinguish between all of these subplanes in a systematic empirical psychology of thought. Oceanic feelings are what Emerson (1841) described as an ecstatic participation with nature while remaining in an intellectual state. Such oceanic feelings do not necessarily involve a full awareness of cosmic unity (subplane 7–7 of thought) but allow an awareness of beauty and love that pervades nature despite a dualistic separation of subjective consciousness from objects in the external world. Alternatively, the conflicts of the intellectual plane may be sublimated to the intellectual subplane of the spiritual plane (subplane 7–5), leading to integrated intelligence or pure rational intuition.

Hence, the account of consciousness in Table 3.3 is still a description of dualistic consciousness. In Table 3.3, any thoughts in the spiritual plane (plane 7) are subconscious and still bound to the dualistic conflict involved in mastery seeking, perfectionism, or the wish for dominance. According to Spinoza (1955), perfection is synonymous with reality as a whole. If this is so, perfection cannot be achieved by anyone who thinks he or she is something separate from the rest of existence. According to Spinoza and all of the other positive philosophers, once we recognize our participation in the universal unity of being by awakening our cosmic sense, then thought begins to elevate in plane 7 and we begin to move toward coherence of personality, which leads to wisdom and well-being (subplane 7–

7). According to the paradoxical view of all positive philosophers, the beginning of wisdom and well-being is humility, not the striving for mastery or the pursuit of happiness. *When we are wise and well, we recognize that truth and love are nondual aspects of the good.*

When we do let go of all of our struggles with ourselves and with others, the content of thought about all aspects of our life is elevated. The reconciliation of the conflicts in each of the subplanes of thought is summarized in Table 3.4, which is a description of nondualistic consciousness or full coherence of thought. To be precise, these descriptors are the spiritual aspects of each of the subplanes that result from sublimation of all the conflicts to the plane of the spirit, as we examine in more detail later. Sublimated thought is always in plane 7, but what occurs effortlessly in sublimated living is shown in Table 3.4 in a way that emphasizes that sublimation does not mean the rejection of sex, food, affection, or intellectual inquiry. Rather sublimated thought involves the wise enjoyment of every aspect of life, reconciling conflicts and contradictions that occur when thought is dualistic by integrating love and truth as nondual aspects of what is recognized as good. Comparison of the content of thought in nondual consciousness (Table 3.4) with that in dualistic consciousness (Table 3.3) reveals the reconciliation of the conflict in the sexual, material, emotional, and intellectual subplanes, as well as the further elevation of thought in the spiritual subplanes. For example, in subplane 2–2, the conflict of emptiness versus lust in Table 3.3 is reconciled as "trust" in Table 3.4. Unconditional trust is actually a highly spiritual thought, which is in plane 7. In other words, the spiritual thought of trust "overcomes" or reconciles the conflict inherent in thought at subplane 2–2 while preserving the function of this aspect of life in a more elevated manner. Likewise, in subplane 3–3, "competition or submission" in Table 3.3 is reconciled as "flexibility" in Table 3.4. In subplane 4–4, "warmth or coldness" in dualistic consciousness is reconciled as "impartiality" in nondualistic consciousness. The sublimation of conflicts in the intellectual plane corresponds to what have been called the "moral virtues"— namely, moderation (temperance, subplane 5–2), justice (subplane 5–3), prudence (subplane 5–4), and perseverance (subplane 5–5). The sublimation of conflicts in the spiritual subplanes corresponds to what are called the "theological virtues", which arise from understanding of these virtues in the respective subplanes of the spiritual plane. That is, understanding of hope (subplane 7–2), understanding of charity (subplane 7–3), understanding of harmony and love (subplane 7–4), and understanding of faith (subplane 7–5) allow reconciliation of conflicts in the spiritual aspects of the corresponding lower planes. This view agrees with Christian psychology that the theological virtues (faith, hope, and love) are the result of full spiritual awareness (as in the third stage of self-awareness). Theological virtues do not arise in the second stage of self-awareness, which is like indirect awareness of objects reflected in a mirror (see 1 Corinthians 13:8–13). The subplanes of the spiritual planes correspond to what are sometimes called the gifts of the

**Table 3.4.** Matrix of Self-Awareness in Relationships (Nondual Consciousness)*

| Subplane of Thought | Plane 2 (Sexuality) | Plane 3 (Consumption) | Plane 4 (Emotion) | Plane 5 (Intellect) | Plane 7 (Spirit) | Nondual Awareness |
|---|---|---|---|---|---|---|
| Nondual awareness | [Being] | [Freedom] | [Beauty] | [Truth] | [Goodness] | [Unity] |
| Spiritual aspects (7) | Hope | Charity | Love | Faith | Coherence (goodness doing) | [Goodness] |
| Intellectual aspects (5) | Self-respect | Nonviolence | Friendship | Perseverance | Patience (truth following) | [Truth] |
| Emotional aspects (4) | Self-acceptance | Forbearance | Impartiality | Prudence | Conciliation (peace sharing) | [Beauty] |
| Material aspects (3) | Tolerance | Flexibility | Mutuality | Justice | Reverence (glory Giving) | [Freedom] |
| Sexual aspects (2) | Trust | Self-Control | Good will | Moderation | Awe of God | [Being] |

*Experiences that are unlikely to be fully clear in the consciousness of most people are given in brackets.

spirit, namely, awe of God (humility, subplane 7–2), reverence (piety or glory giving, subplane 7–3), compassion (counsel, conciliation, or peace sharing, subplane 7–4), patience (fortitude, subplane 7–5), and coherence (subplane 7–7). Coherence is the composite of all of the gifts of the spirit, including virtue, wisdom, well-being, compassion, and creativity, which all depend on the recognition of truth and love as nondual aspects of the good.

Partial awareness of the objects of the intuitive senses is indicated in Table 3.4 to be the basis for the elevation of the subplanes to the level of spirit. These objects of the intuitive senses form the basis for the emergence of nonduality, that is, for the emergence of symmetry or identity between the subject and the object of consciousness. In other words, being is the reconciliation of libido (subplane 2–7) and awe of God (subplane 7–2), freedom is the reconciliation of self-gratification (subplane 3–7) and reverence (subplane 7–3), beauty is the reconciliation of self-contentment (subplane 4–7) and love (subplane 7–4), and truth is the reconciliation of self-actualization (subplane 5–7) and pure rational intuition (subplane 7–5). Furthermore, coherence is based on the goodness of the universal unity of being. As Spinoza (1955) said in his *Ethics*, perfection is synonymous with reality. The development of nondual consciousness and coherence of personality is indicated empirically by high scores on the TCI character scales modulating thought in plane 7: hopefulness (SD5), charitable principles (CO5), and spiritual (nonlocal) awareness (ST3), which will be described in more detail in Chapter 5.

We are also now in a position to give a precise quantitative definition of the stages of self-aware consciousness, as summarized in Table 3.5. Drawing on Freud and Schiller's idea of the gates of consciousness, it is useful to distinguish three gates. The gate of humanity at thought level of 3.3 is defined as the entrance to subplane 3–4. Ordinary self-awareness is the watcher of the gate of humanity, which integrates social cues, outcomes, and behavioral contingencies of daily living. These functions are impaired if there are brain lesions in the orbital network. Lesions of the orbitofrontal cortex produce reduced empathy and social sensitivity, ethical unreliability, and poor social judgment, in which patients seem to lack principles and compassion regarding the effects of their behavior on others (Damasio 1985; Stuss and Benson 1986; Joseph 1999). This can lead to criminality, promiscuity, profane speech, and a crude, immature social manner that is inconsiderate of the feelings of others. In addition, there often is excessive eating, drinking, and hypersexuality (Joseph 1999). In other words, lesions of the orbital network result in immature thought (3.3 or lower) by disturbance of memories of the self-aware consciousness of higher cognitive needs related to emotion, intellect, and spirituality.

The gate of reason (more clearly, rational intuition) is at thought level of 5.3 at the entrance to subplane 5–4. Rational intuition is the watcher of the gate to the subconscious. Thought at 5.4 is the beginning of mindfulness, which is associated with letting go of self-centered thinking, which produces emotional conflict

**Table 3.5.** Quantitative Definition of the Stages of Self-Aware Consciousness

| Level of Thought | Description of Thought | Awareness of Conflict |
|---|---|---|
| 2.0–3.3 | Distortion of self-awareness (child like) (conscious of immediate likes and dislikes) | Repressed memory of source of conflict (strong negative emotions) (immature ego defenses dominate) (thinking is more-or-less unrealistic) |
| 3.3 | Gate of humanity | Entrance to first stage of self-aware consciousness |
| 3.4–5.3 | First stage of self-awareness (ordinary adult cognition—intention, emotion, intellect) (classic cause and effect) ("I'm right. You're wrong.") | One-sided awareness of conflicts (source of conflict externalized) (ego defense of suppression common) (thinking is more-or-less selfish) |
| 5.3 | Gate of reason (rational intuition) | Acceptance of reality of both sides of conflict |
| 5.4–5.7 | Second stage of self-awareness (metacognition, meditation, mindfulness) (conditional parental view) ("We all should be kind.") | Two-sided awareness of conflicts (calm and patient search for deeper understanding; elevation (purgation) of what was subconscious by transcendence) (thinking is judgmental and based on conditional or contingent reasoning) |
| 5.8–7.0 | Third stage of self-awareness (contemplation, self-actualization) | Impartial illumination of conflicts by sublimation (oceanic feelings of inseparable love) |
| 7.0 | Gate of the psyche | Entrance to unitive spirituality |
| 7.1–7.9 | State of constant awareness (unconditional understanding) ("Life is like that.") | No conflicts (understanding of faith) (increasing humility, serenity, wisdom, well-being, and virtue) |

and intellectual judging. Four Buddhist adepts in a meditative state of "open presence" had less activation of their orbital frontal cortex than those in ordinary states of cognition when emotionally charged sounds (e.g., laughing or crying babies) were played (Davidson 2003). The decreased activity of the orbital frontal cortex suggests a letting go of conflict and judging because the orbital frontal cortex is part of the brain circuit by which the value of stimuli is judged as pleasant or unpleasant. As thought is further elevated to self-transcendence at level 5.7, a person becomes more fully mindful, letting go of struggles and growing in compassion for others. When emotionally charged sounds were played during meditation on compassion, the same four meditators had greater activation of their left superior prefrontal cortex than others (Davidson 2003). In another study of social reasoning by nonmeditators, the left superior frontal gyrus, orbitofrontal gyrus and precuneus were activated when judgements were made about empathy and forgivability (Farrow, Zheng et al. 2001).

Rational intuition is also called speculative or theoretical reason because it is the basis of metacognition, introspection, and theory of mind, which depend on the integrity of the medial prefrontal cortex (Cloninger 2002). Patients with bilateral medial prefrontal lesions cannot anticipate future positive or negative consequences of their actions, although their behavior is influenced appropriately by immediately available contingencies (Bechara, Damasio et al. 1994, 1997, 1998). Right-sided or bilateral medial prefrontal lesions usually produce a deficit in a person's concept of temporal self-continuity in which they have difficulty thinking about themselves as having a continuity from the past to the future (Freeman and Watts 1942; Burgess, Quayle et al. 2001). Episodic memory functions, such as the ability to recollect the temporal order in which objects were initially observed, are inefficient in patients with schizophrenia, requiring selectively greater activation of the right hippocampus and medial prefrontal cortex (BA 9) in schizophrenics than in others to produce the same level of performance (Straub 2003; Heckers, Zalesak et al. 2004). When subjects engage in internal self-referential mental activity, they have greater activity of dorsal medial prefrontal cortex than they do when they direct their attention externally (Gusnard, Akbudak et al. 2001). For example, deciding whether a picture is pleasant or unpleasant activates the medial prefrontal cortex more than does deciding whether a picture is indoors or outdoors. Activity of the same region during executive functions is strongly correlated with individual differences in TCI Self-Directedness (Gusnard, Ollinger et al. 2001, 2003).

Thoughts at 5.4 are the beginning of the purification of rational intuition. The gate of the psyche at 7.0 is at the entrance to subplane 7–2. The gate of the psyche can also be called the gate of spirituality, but reference to psyche makes it clear that past this gate, individuals are in a contemplative state in which they are conscious of the functions of their psyche. In contrast, the functions of the psyche remain unconscious in the first stage of self-awareness and subconscious in the second stage of self-awareness; the psyche is the watcher of the gate to the unconscious. The efficiency of censorship of unconscious thought, the carrying out of multiple tasks simultaneously, and creativity are impaired when people are tired or stressed (Gillin, Seifritz et al. 2000). The coherence of thought, such as multitasking efficiency, depends on coherent orchestration of brain systems by the frontal polar cortex (Burgess, Veitch et al. 2000).

Sometimes people in the first stage of self-awareness strive to become someone they are not and do not understand who they are. To grow in awareness of who you are, one must enter into the second phase of self-awareness. However, individuals in Christian religious orders are encouraged to sublimate by taking vows of celibacy (i.e., sublimation of sexual plane 2), poverty (i.e., sublimation of material plane 3), divine marriage (i.e., sublimation of emotional plane 4), and obedience (i.e., sublimation of intellectual plane 5). Unfortunately, vows are ineffective as a way to sublimation without progression through the second and third phases of self-awareness. Vows in the first stage of self-awareness are forms of renunciation, not integration of sexuality and the other aspects of life into a coherent way of celebrating all the wonders of living spiritually. All aspects of life are good, if they are integrated with one another.

Likewise, individuals in Hindu and Buddhist religious orders are encouraged to transcend their conflicts by renunciation and detachment. They may follow different types of yoga as a means of transcendence, which refers to elevation of thought within a particular plane. For example, they may use tantric yoga to elevate sexual desires, karma yoga to elevate material desires to serve others, bhakti yoga to elevate their emotion to love, and jnâna yoga to elevate their intellect. However, it is psychologically impossible to elevate what we deny or renounce. Transcendence requires acceptance of our limitations, not denial or renunciation, because acceptance is the entrance into the second phase of self-awareness in which we can grow in awareness, which is the actual basis for transcendence. Traditions that encourage reliance on the individual ego, such as psychoanalysis, or that emphasize the impermanence of what is personal, such as most Zen or Buddhist sects, make radical transformation of personality difficult by blocking recognition that the personal is life that exists within itself. The failure of many psychological and religious practitioners to understand the true path of the psyche is unfortunately obvious in modern times.

The hierarchical and matrix structure of thought suggests some properties that are useful in the measurement of thought, which are summarized in Table 3.6. The matrix structure is appropriate because changes in thought are discrete events, as will be documented in Chapter 6. I suggest that a thought is a discrete packet of information and energy, much as energy is emitted in quantum-like light. We organize sets of thoughts into sentences using the theorem-like processing of language, but the components that make up language are themselves discrete. Furthermore, the hierarchical dependencies of thoughts within a plane suggest that

**Table 3.6.** Thought Moves by Quantum Steps

| |
|---|
| • Changes in thought are discrete.<br>  A thought is a packet of information and energy.<br>  Consciousness flows from one quantum of thought to another quantum.<br>• Thought can be quantified.<br>  Quantification is in terms of its hierarchy of planes and subplanes.<br>• Variability in thought can be summarized.<br>  Average and range (minimum and maximum) in each plane can be given.<br>  Global average and range (across all planes of thought) can be given. |

the subplanes can be described as varying quantitatively in their level within the hierarchy of each plane. The hierarchical nature of thought is useful in quantifying our observations (Cloninger 2002). For example, let us define thoughts of intense desire or aversion in the lowest level of plane 3 as having the coherence value of 3.0, whereas thoughts of self-gratifying power are just below 4.0. There are five subplanes dividing this interval of 1.0 unit of coherence, so on a decimal scale, each subplane encompasses an interval of 0.2. In other words, extreme desires and aversions (lower half of 3–2, from Table 3.3) can be quantified as 3.0; competition or submission is measured as 3.2 (lower half of 3–3, from Table 3.3); anger or stoicism, 3.4 (lower half of 3–4, from Table 3.3); pride or inferiority, 3.6 (lower half of 3–5); and power or sarcasm, 3.8 (lower half of 3–7). Similarly, each plane is indicated by its evolutionary rank as indicated in Table 3.3, and variation within the plane is indicated on the decimal scale from .0 to .9.

A more complete description of thoughts measured from 2.0 to 7.9 is compiled in the Appendix The Quantitative Measurement of Thought. This also indicates the sublimated thoughts that reconcile the conflict in each of the lower subplanes. These reconciling thoughts emerge from the understanding of the spiritual plane in the third stage of self-awareness, or nondual consciousness.

For example, a person who usually is thinking about the security of his warm emotional attachments would have an average thought level of about 4.5 (see Appendix and Table 3.3). Furthermore, under stress he might sometimes become worried and hypochondriacal (minimum of 2.4), and under conditions of maximum elevation of thought he might experience self-transcendent thoughts (maximum of 5.7). This person's overall distribution of thoughts could be quickly denoted as having an average of 4.5 with a range from 2.4 to 5.7. Higher levels of thought have higher spiritual interest because they are more satisfying and coherent. In other words, our level of well-being increases with the measure of our thought.

In contrast, personality is often measured in terms of scores that approximate a person's usual state, like a collapsed quantum wave function (Table 3.7). The original situational context of thought constitutes a living multiplex of limitless possibilities in space and time. However, much spatiotemporal information about

**Table 3.7.** Personality Traits Are Abstractions

---

- Personality traits are abstract factual reports that approximate an individual's "usual" state (like a collapsed quantum wave function).
- Temperament traits are averages of the bias (high or low) in responses to context-dependent conflicts in each column of the 5 × 5 matrix of dualistic consciousness.
- Character traits are averages of the level of elevation of responses to context-dependent aspects of each row of the 5 × 5 matrix of dualistic consciousness (so character is usually described at an intellectual level, as labeled in sub-plane 5–2 (Self-Directedness), sub-plane 5–3 (Cooperativeness), and subplane 5–5 (Self-Transcendence).
- Spatiotemporal information requires movement in a third dimension.

---

the situational context of thought is lost in abstract judgments that produce a fixed or static measurement about the past. The value of quantitative measures based on the quantum-like matrix structure of thought is that we are reminded that thought is not a set of fixed traits. Rather, thought is variable in level within a hierarchy. There is variation in thought within a plane, so that each plane has an average and a range (maximum and minimum value) depending on individual variation in the elevation of thought. Also, there is variation in thought between planes, in the variation of thought from one plane to another. The variation in degree of elevation of thought can be quantified in the same manner by describing the average of a person's thoughts as well as the maximum and minimum in his or her life or within a period of particular interest like an individual therapeutic session.

## MOVEMENT OF THOUGHT IN TIME

According to Hegel, the third stage of self-awareness has a three-dimensional form that is experienced when thought itself becomes the general object of consciousness. When the subject is also the object, self-aware consciousness is supposed to involve variation in three-dimensions moving freely in space and time like a living organism. The first scientist to study self-aware consciousness systematically was Wilhelm Wundt (1832–1920), who is considered the founder of experimental psychology (Boring 1957; Grastyan 1980). Wundt based his theory of emotion on a systematic analysis of introspective reports of feelings (*Gefuehlston*) elicited by sensory stimuli. Wundt (1903) concluded that all self-aware emotions could be described in terms of quantitative variation along three dimensions represented by pairs of contrasting words. The first dimension was called "*Lust* versus *Unlust*," which may be translated as "pleasantness versus unpleasantness" or as "pleasure versus displeasure." Wundt called the second dimension "*Erregung* versus *Beruhigung*," which may be translated as "arousal or excitement versus quiescence," distinguishing a state in which people feel stirred up and hypervigilant versus a state of calm attentiveness in which there is a letting go of all struggles. Wundt called the third dimension "*Spannung* versus *Loesung*," which may be translated as "tense control versus loose coping," distinguishing a state of tense struggle to dominate others and inhibit conflicts from a state of confident release from struggle ("hanging loose").

Later investigators like Pavlov (1941) retained these three dimensions in their descriptions of the physiology of "higher nervous activity." Empirical work has repeatedly confirmed Wundt's original observations about the presence of three factors of pleasure, arousal, and dominance in a person's self-aware reports of his or her internal feeling states regardless of the type of stimulus. The experimental stimuli have included ratings of words (Osgood 1952), verbal texts about common human scenarios (Mehrabian and Russell 1974; Russell 1980), a variety of nonverbal stimuli like sonar signals and aesthetic paintings (Osgood, Suci et al. 1957), and emotionally evocative pictures (Bradley and Lang 1994). The Semantic Differential Scale (Mehrabian and Russell 1974) is a widely used instrument that assesses the three-dimensional structure of self-aware emotional feelings about objects, events, and situations. It consists of a set of eighteen bipolar adjective pairs that are each rated along a 9-point scale. A 1994 study by Bradley and Lang using a standardized set of emotionally evocative pictures is summarized in Table 3.8. The three dimensions of pleasure, arousal, and dominance account for most of the variance observed in the individual eighteen ratings and are approximately independent of one another. Bradley and Lang initially called the first factor "pleasure," as had Wundt, but in more recent work they usually refer to "valence," which refers to hedonistic variation between pleasant and unpleasant feelings.

Despite the type of signal stimuli that are used, the same three-factor solution has repeatedly been obtained. This strongly suggests that the three bipolar dimensions of valence, arousal, and dominance play an important role in the modulation of self-aware consciousness. As a result, we need to recognize that the movement of self-aware consciousness in time involves a movement in three dimensions, not two as represented in Tables 3.3 and 3.4. To visualize the form of the movement of thought, it is useful to relate the three psychological dimensions to spatial relationships. Such a three-dimensional spatial representation of thought is summarized in Table 3.9.

Attention and character involve higher cognitive processes that modulate human thought. There are things that can be done without attention, and other things that cannot be done without attention. The coherence of our goals and values with what we do without effortful attention indicates our level of character development. Many routine activities in daily life are carried out in an automatized way without attention, such as riding a bicycle, typing on a keyboard, or driving our car along a familiar route. Most of these functions required attention when we first learned them, but with repetition they become habitual and automatized (Roth 2000). Such automatized or poorly attended activity is also outside of

**Table 3.8.** Contributions of Pairs of Adjectives to Three Independent Factors that Describe People's Affective Reactions to Environmental Stimuli (a Set of Emotionally Evocative Pictures)

| Adjective Pairs (Low–High) | Factor 1 "Pleasure" | Factor 2 "Arousal" | Factor 3 "Dominance" |
|---|---|---|---|
| Unhappy–happy | .91 | | |
| Annoyed–pleased | .88 | | |
| Unsatisfied–satisfied | .87 | | |
| Melancholic–contented | .73 | | |
| Despairing–hopeful | .86 | | |
| Bored–relaxed | .58 | .37 | |
| Relaxed–stimulated | | .77 | |
| Calm–excited | | .79 | |
| Sluggish–frenzied | .27 | .77 | |
| Dull–jittery | | .79 | |
| Sleepy–wide awake | | .81 | |
| Unaroused–aroused | | .83 | |
| Controlled–controlling | .26 | | −.67 |
| Influenced–influential | .29 | | −.62 |
| Cared for–in control | | | −.63 |
| Awed–important | | | −.30 |
| Submissive–dominant | | .31 | −.70 |
| Guided–autonomous | | | −.48 |
| Total of variance explained by each factor (%) | 25 | 23 | 12 |

Factor loadings below .25 were omitted (seventy-eight healthy college students rated all 18 pairs of adjectives describing their affective responses to each one of a set of twenty-one pictures that were selected from the International Affective Picture System of Peter Lang.)

*Source*: Adapted from Bradley and Lang 1994.

self-aware consciousness and poorly recollected (Moscovitch 1995). The degree to which something or an activity is recollectable (i.e., consciously recognized and recalled) indicates how self-directed the activity was when the thing or activity was experienced. The degree of self-directedness refers to the degree to which something is meaningful and purposeful, as measured by the TCI Self-Directedness scale (Table 3.9). For example, if TCI Self-Directedness is very low, individuals are unaware of their responsibility for what they do, so they blame other people and external circumstances (as in personality disorders) or deny awareness of their own agency (as in conversion disorders).

There are "shallow," "concrete," or "bottom-up" ways of processing sensory information based on selective attention to external physical features and excluding intuitively meaningful information; in contrast, there are also "top-down"

**Table 3.9.** The Movement of Thought (i.e., Recollectable Awareness and Attention) Has Three Directions in Time

1. Elevation of Awareness = Valence to Impartiality
   - Conflict between unpleasant versus pleasant (heavy, low elevation), resolved by hopeful following of the path of the psyche (light, high elevation)
   - Measured by increasingly impartial purposeful attention and recollectability (i.e., increasing TCI Self-Directedness)
   - Modulated by the brain network for Valence and Self-Directedness (especially Brodmann areas of 9 and 10 of prefrontal cortex)
2. Width of Attention = Arousal to Calm Flexible Alertness
   - Conflict between narrow egocentric attention (either overarousal if wants are frustrated or underarousal if satiated), resolved by broad allocentric (charitable) flexibility in action and calm, mobile alertness
   - Measured by the increasingly calm alertness resulting from charitable flexibility of will and voluntariness (i.e., increasing TCI Cooperativeness)
   - Modulated by the brain network for alertness and TCI Cooperativeness (especially right frontal, inferior parietal cortex, and insula)
3. Depth of Attention = Dominance to Patient Listening
   - Conflict between shallow concerns about being controlled or controlling others, resolved by faithful listening to the psyche (deep, patient listening)
   - Measured by increasingly patient, nonjudgmental, contemplative listening to the psyche and attention to meaningful information beyond shallow physical features (i.e., increasing TCI Self-Transcendence)
   - Modulated by the brain network for inhibitory control of conflict and Self-Transcendence (especially anterior cingulate, lateral prefrontal cortex, and basal ganglia)

or "deep" ways of processing information that is intuitively recognized as meaningful and purposeful (Broadbent 1958; Hirst 1995; Fell, Fernandez et al. 2003; Graboi and Lisman 2003). Shallow sensory processing based on external physical features is variously described as "objective," "externally-oriented," or "bottom-up" processing, whereas deep information processing is described as "subjective" because it involves "qualia," "internally oriented," or "top-down processing" based on intuitively recognized meaning. The deep content of consciousness is the qualitative information beyond superficial physical features to which we can attend in human self-aware consciousness, such as awareness of what it means to see the colors of a rainbow or the beauty of a painting. The depth of self-aware consciousness is measured by the TCI Self-Transcendence scale (Table 3.9). For example, individuals with Somatization disorder or alexithymia have a disturbance of affect and cognition indicated by a reduced affective and fantasy life and have difficulty in recognizing or describing their own emotions. They experience distress in terms of physical complaints and are often described as having hysterical or repressive personality traits, as measured by low Self-Transcendence, particularly low scores on the first Self-Transcendence subscale ("sensible versus repressive"). Individuals high in Self-Transcendence recognize the beauty and meaning in sensory experiences intuitively, whereas those who are low in Self-Transcendence are alexithymic, especially if they are not high in the other character dimensions. For example, scores on the Toronto Alexithymia Scale (TAS) were moderately correlated with low scores on all three TCI character scales. The strongest bivariate correlation was between the scores on the TCI Self-transcendence subscale for sensibility with the TAS subscale for externally oriented thinking ($r = -0.4$, $P < .0001$) in a sample of 644 individuals from the general population.

Attention can also be "narrow" or "narrow-minded" so that experience is egocentric and inflexible because it excludes awareness of the social context. Attention can also be "broad," "broad-minded," or "wide" when thought and behavior are flexible because they are based on an extensive allocentric context (Farrer and Frith 2002). When attention is narrow, people can be unaware of what they learned, or when and where they learned the information, or whether they are responsible for their actions. In contrast, "explicit" learning is "broad-minded" and "voluntary" in the sense that it involves flexible choices about goals and values, as measured by the TCI Cooperativeness scale (Table 3.9). Narrow learning leads to behavior that has been described as "unvoluntary" because it is inflexible and not voluntary (Jankovic 2001). For example, patients with tics have difficulty legislating their speech and behavior to be socially appropriate and cooperative. They often cannot say with certainty whether their movements are voluntary or involuntary. They are aware of their personal agency because they can suppress their movements with effortful attention or they can just let them happen; however, the distinction between voluntary and involuntary is not relevant to their natural way of attending to what happens when they utter vocal sounds or make repetitive movements (Jankovic 2001). Tics are often not preceded by a cortical readiness potential or by only a brief one, so the brain mechanisms for their production differ from ordinary voluntary movements (Karp, Porter et al. 1996). In summary, human character and attention involve the modulation of self-aware consciousness in three dissociable dimensions that can be spatially visualized as the elevation of attention ("purposeful agency" or "recollectability"), the width of attention ("flexibility" or "voluntariness"), and the depth of attention ("understanding," "selective meaning," or "subjectivity"). These dimensions are dissociable but interact in a nonlinear manner (Turner, Hudson et al. 2003); that is, the effects of the three character dimensions are partially correlated in ways that depend on the level of each of the three dimensions of character. The selective modulation of attention depends extensively on gain modulation, which is a nonlinear process by which input from one system alters the sensitivity of its target neurons to other input without modifying the selectivity or receptive field properties of the target neurons (Salinas and Sejnowski 2001). In this way, we can focus attention selectively to increase our self-awareness without altering the perceptual representation of the reality given in experience.

## BRAIN REGULATION OF ATTENTION AND AFFECT

The fundamental nature of the three dimensions of valence, arousal, and inhibitory control is supported by their apparent identity with three well-known brain networks involved in the modulation of attention, affect, and cognition. Michael Posner and his colleagues have identified three specific brain networks that regulate different aspects of human attention. Each network regulates different processes of attention, and each has its own functional anatomy, cellular structure, and neurotransmitter circuitry (Posner and Fan 2003). The system for orienting to sensory events is the most basic of these developmentally beause it is mature at birth. The modulation of the orienting response appears to be more closely related to individual differences in temperament than to self-aware consciousness (Cloninger 2002). However, the other two systems that Posner has characterized are the alertness brain network and the inhibitory control brain network, which appear to correspond directly to individual differences in arousal and dominance, respectively. In addition, other investigators have studied the neuroanatomy of valence and cognitive processes that are measurable as character traits, such as awareness of intention and control of actions (Frith, Blakemore et al. 2000). Hence the three factors of valence, arousal, and dominance appear to correspond directly to three well-known brain networks, as noted in Table 3.9.

Substantial evidence suggests that valence and arousal are regulated by different neural networks (Lane, Reiman et al. 1997; Lang, Bradley et al. 1998; Bradley and Lang 2000). Pleasant and unpleasant emotions are each distinguished from neutral emotion conditions by increased blood flow in the medial prefrontal cortex, thalamus, hypothalamus, and midbrain in studies of healthy volunteers using positron emission tomography (PET) (Lane, Reiman et al. 1997). Other work using functional magnetic resonance imaging showed that the evaluation of internal emotions (pleasant or unpleasant pictures) was associated with increased activity of the medial prefrontal cortex (Gusnard, Akbudak et al. 2001). Individual differences in activation of the medial prefrontal cortex are also strongly correlated with TCI self-directedness (Gusnard, Ollinger et al. 2001). Therefore, the brain areas that are activated with both pleasant and unpleasant emotions are characteristic of the level of self-aware consciousness, not the differentiation of pleasant stimuli from unpleasant stimuli. The medial prefrontal cortex allows mental state representations to be distinguished from physical state representations, thereby allowing a theory of mind or "mentalizing" (Frith and Frith 2003). This mentalizing ability is shown by mirror recognition of oneself at about 18 months of age in humans, as well as implicit attribution of intentions and other mental states. Between the ages of 4 and 6 years explicit mentalizing becomes possible, and from this age children are able to explain the misleading reasons that have given rise to a false belief, thereby facilitating reality testing and self-directedness (Frith and Frith 2003).

The valence network is expected to distinguish pleasant stimuli from neutral stimuli. In PET studies of healthy volunteers, responses to pleasant pictures were distinguished from the response from neutral but not unpleasant pictures by activation of the head of the left caudate nucleus (Lane, Reiman et al. 1997). There is additional evidence to suggest that the valence factor may be related to another well-known system involved in regulating the expectation of pleasant experiences in human beings (Cloninger 2002; Gusnard, Ollinger et al. 2003) and the prediction of rewards in other primates (Schultz, Tremblay et al. 1998). The reward prediction network is a distributed circuit in the brain involving the ventral striatum, the anterior cingulate (Brodmann area 24), and the orbitofrontal cortex (Brodmann area 47), all bilaterally (Gusnard, Ollinger et al. 2003). Differences between human individuals in the activity of this circuit have been correlated with their tendency to rate pictures as pleasant instead of rating them as neutral. This suggests that the greater the activity in this circuit, the greater is bias toward pleasantness in self-aware consciousness. Furthermore, the personality trait of Persistence was highly correlated ($r = 0.8$) with these differences in circuit activity and the bias toward pleasant ratings of pictures from the International Affective Picture System (Gusnard, Ollinger et al. 2003). The conflict between biases for unpleasant and pleasant stimuli is resolved by the elevation of thought to allow impartial purposeful actions, which requires reality-testing and a sense of following a meaningful direction in one's life regardless of the hedonic valence of one's context, as measured by increasing TCI Self-Directedness (see Table 3.9) (Guillem, Bicu et al. 2002). The coherence of such self-directed behavior requires prospective autobiographical memories that depend on the medial and rostral prefrontal cortex (Brodmann areas 9 and 10)(Burgess, Quayle et al. 2001; Maguire, Henson et al. 2001; Burgess, Scott et al. 2003), which are highly correlated with TCI Self-Directedness (Gusnard, Akbudak et al. 2001; Gusnard, Ollinger et al. 2001; Gusnard, Ollinger et al. 2003).

Likewise, the alertness (arousal) brain network is another well-known distributed brain network that involves primarily the right frontal and right parietal cortex, as well as noradrenergic projections from the locus coeruleus in the brainstem (Marrocco and Davidson 1998; Davidson and Marrocco 2000; Posner and Fan 2003). Drugs like clonidine, which block the activity of norepinephrine, reduce or eliminate the normal effect of warning signals on reaction time, but have no effect on orienting to the target location. The alertness brain network seems to continue to mature well into adulthood according to Posner's developmental studies (Posner and Fan 2003). The development of the ability to modulate arousal is impaired in individuals with neuropsychiatric disorders involving the right inferior parietal cortex and anterior insula (Bottini, Karnath et al. 2001; Farrer and Frith 2002). The posterior superior temporal sulcus region nearby the insula is also consistenly activated during both implicit and explicit mentalizing tasks, and it has been proposed as the site for the detection of agency (i.e., the qualia of voluntariness or free will) (Frith and Frith 2003). Being aware of wanting or voluntarily intending to cause an action is associated with activation of the anterior insula, whereas being aware of external control of an action is associated with activation of the inferior parietal cortex (Bottini, Karnath et al. 2001; Farrer and Frith 2002). These two regions are thought to be involved in the perception of complex representations of an individual and interactions with the external world. The anterior insula integrates all the concordant multimodal sensory signals associated with voluntary movements, thereby representing an egocentric representation of space. The inferior parietal, in contrast, represents voluntary actions in an allocentric coding system that can be applied to the actions of others as well as the self. Such an allocentric representation is necessary for cooperative behavior, which requires flexibility of choice in representations of self–other relationships. The three brain networks modulating character development are partially overlapping, so they are dissociable but may also function coherently. For example, the inferior parietal cortex is a prominent part of the networks proposed here to be associated with cooperativeness and self-transcendence. The inferior parietal cortex is hyperactive in individuals who feel they are being externally controlled, such as schizophrenics with delusions of passivity or alien control or normal individuals under constrained experimental conditions (Spence, Brooks et al. 1997; Frith, Blakemore et al. 2000; Frith, Blakemore et al. 2000; Nathaniel-James and Frith 2002; Blakemore, Oakley et al. 2003). The representations of the current and predicted state of the motor system are encoded in the parietal cortex, whereas the representations of intended actions are found in the prefrontal and premotor cortex (Frith, Blakemore et al. 2000). The awareness of internal control of when an action is initiated is associated with the activation of the anterior cingulate and dorsolateral prefrontal cortex, whereas actions that are externally triggered do not activate these brain regions (Jahanshahi, Jenkins et al. 1995; Paus 2001; Stephan and Schall 2002).

The control aspect of agency (i.e., awareness of the control of motor responses) is associated with the activation of the anterior cingulate and dorsolateral prefrontal cortex, and it is involved in the selective sculpting of motor responses (Farrer and Frith 2002; Nathaniel-James and Frith 2002). Likewise, the inhibitory control network of attention described by Posner depends on the same brain regions and is involved in the suppression or inhibition of conflicts, such as the inhibition of conditioned responses that are no longer adaptive. For example, a typical conflict test is measured by the Stroop task. The Stroop task requires the subject to learn to respond to the color of ink (e.g., red) when the target is a competing color word (e.g., blue). Conflict is present when the cues are incongruent rather than when they are congruent. Such conflict tasks activate a distributed brain network, including the basal ganglia, the lateral prefrontal cortex, and the anterior cingulate gyrus (Spence, Brooks et al. 1997; Nathaniel-James and Frith 2002; Fan, Fossella et al. 2003; Posner and Fan 2003), just as does awareness of the control of internally initiated movements. The lateral prefrontal cortex is particularly involved in holding in mind information that is relevant to the task, which is called *working memory*. The anterior cingulate is a place of convergence for motor control, homeostatic drive, emotion, and cognition (Spence, Brooks et al. 1997; Paus 2001). The anterior cingulate is part of the limbic system, which regulates emotional responses, such as separation and play, in reptiles and all higher vertebrates (MacLean 1985). In humans and great apes, however, there is a unique cell type that is not present in other primates (Nimchinsky, Gilissen et al. 1999; Allman 2001). The inhibitory control system matures in late childhood along with self-aware consciousness, increasing substantially from ages four to seven years and then stabilizing (Posner and Fan 2003). Other work shows that flexibility and efficiency in carrying out multiple tasks develop around four years of age along with the emergence of self-aware consciousness (Povinelli and Simon 1998; Povinelli and Giambrone 2001).

Hence, the information available about the brain networks regulating valence, arousal, and conflict control correspond well with psychological findings that have been repeatedly observed for more than a century. These three brain networks can also be experimentally activated, demonstrating predictably their role in the modulation of sensory, motor, emotional, cognitive, and integrative functions, which can be reliably measured by the three character dimensions of the TCI and their subscales. The convergence of the psychological results and the brain imaging results suggests that self-aware consciousness is not two-dimensional as represented in Tables 3.4 and 3.5 but is truly three-dimensional and modulated by the character traits of TCI Self-Directedness, Cooperativeness, and Self-Transcendence.

## THE SPIRAL PATH OF CONSCIOUSNESS

With this descriptive information about self-aware consciousness, we are now in a position to specify its form. The available facts about the path of self-aware consciousness are that the form varies in three dimensions, corresponding to Self-Directedness increasing with height, Cooperativeness increasing with width, and Self-Transcendence increasing with depth, as described in Table 3.10. In addition, this hierarchical progression in the level of self-awareness should also specify a succession of five planes of thought, as in a spiral. Furthermore, the spiral should be narrow at its base (plane 2) where the three regulatory brain systems are independent, and then the spiral should expand progressively in diameter with increasing coherence. In other words, the correlation among self-directedness, cooperativeness, and Self-Transcendence necessarily increases with increasing coherence and diameter of consciousness.

Thoughts may spiral up or down, as described in Table 3.10. Essentially, a downward spiral is evoked by any incoherent attitude, such as lust, gluttony, or

**Table 3.10.** Thoughts May Spiral Up or Down

A. Downward Spiral of Distress and Addiction (initiated by any incoherent attitude—lust, gluttony, envy, apathy, greed, hate, pride)
  • Increasingly hedonistic and narcissistic
    —Heavy = seeking pleasure and avoiding displeasure
    —Wishful thinking or see only problems, lacking satisfying purposefulness
    —Conflict = unpleasant versus pleasant events
    —Lowering of Self-Directedness
  • Increasingly aroused and fearful
    —Aroused = narrow egocentric focus
    —Inflexible because overaroused if wants frustrated or underaroused if wants satiated
    —Conflict = frustrated wants versus restful satiation
    —Lowering of Cooperativeness
  • Increasingly controlled and impatient
    —Shallow = superficial, externally oriented understanding
    —Struggling to control conflicts by force due to lack of immersion in contemplative listening to the psyche
    —Conflict = controlled versus controlling relations
    —Lowering of Self-Transcendence
B. Upward Spiral of Well-Being and Awareness (initiated by any coherent attitude—hope, charity, love, responsibility, generosity, kindness, humility)
  • Increasingly impartial, purposeful, and hopeful
    —Enlightened = impartial, purposeful, hopeful
    —Effortless awareness and inner-directed order, which is mental expression of following the path of the psyche
    —Understanding of hope and Self-Directedness
    —Conflict between unpleasant versus pleasant events resolved by hopeful and realistic purposefulness
  • Increasingly calm, flexible, and charitable
    —Broad = calm allocentric awareness
    —Spontaneous kindness, the mental expression of free will
    —Understanding of charity and Cooperativeness
    —Conflict between frustrated wants versus restful satiation resolved by charitable principles
  • Increasingly patient, nonjudgmental, and faithful
    —Deep = patient, nonjudging understanding
    —Patiently letting go of all struggles, which is mental expression of contemplative listening to the psyche
    —Understanding of faith and Self-Transcendence
    —Conflict between controlled versus controlling relations resolved by faithful listening to psyche

other attitudes that are sometimes called "vices." This simply means that these attitudes elicit increasing dissatisfaction, arousal, and struggle to restrain conflicts. For example, downward spirals occur with incoherent attitudes in any plane of thought, such as fears of annihilation or sexual abuse (plane 2), eating disorders and substance dependence (plane 3), social rejection (plane 4), intolerant judgments (plane 5), and mastery seeking or perfectionism (plane 7).

In clinical practice, there are three distinguishable pathways that lead to a downward spiral. The first is the loss of flexibility (i.e., freedom of will and lowering of TCI Cooperativeness) from conditioning of maladaptive habits, as in various forms of gluttony, such as substance dependence. To be cooperative, a person must adopt an allocentric perspective rather than an egocentric perspective. From the allocentric perspective, a person may choose freely whether to act selfishly or charitably, whereas truly cooperative choices are inconceivable from an egocentric perspective. The second pathway is catastrophic and impatient thinking, which involves a loss of faith in struggles between being controlled and seeking to control others). When we catastrophize or become impatient and judgmental, there is a decrease in Self-Transcendence and we become preoccupied with struggles against problems and obstacles over which we have no control, as in posttraumatic stress disorders. The third pathway is ignoring reality by illusory or distorted thinking, as in borderline, narcissistic, or psychotic disorders in which there is a decrease in, or underdevelopment of, TCI Self-Directedness.

The downward spiral of thought from reduction in freedom of will by conditioning of maladaptive habits is illustrated for substance dependence in Figure 3.1. This figure (Koob and LeMoal 2001) was prepared to describe the developmental process of addictive behaviors generally based on the *DSM-IV* diagnostic criteria for substance dependence (American Psychiatric Association 1994). Preoccupation with getting drugs for oneself involves low freedom of will and low Cooperativeness in the material plane (i.e., hostility and revengefulness, as measured by low scores on CO subscale 4). The desire for drugs leads to preoccupation with the problem of the need for an ever-increasing supply due to increasing tolerance, increasing negative affects (anxiety, irritability, loneliness, and so on), and an ambivalent struggle to stop self-defeating behaviors. For example, a drug-dependent patient of mine said, "I cannot stop . . . I need it." When asked if she wanted to stop, she explained, "I wish I could stop, but I just can't. I've tried to stop hundreds of times, but I just feel miserable whenever I do and restart within a few hours. I need to continue despite all the problems with doing so." Notice that the self-justification is self-centered, self-defeating, and backward—that is, it begins with what cannot be done (lack of freedom) because of misunderstood problems, rather than defining hopeful goals and going on to identify both internal and external resources to help accomplish them. Instead of developing greater awareness, increasing resourcefulness, and getting help, real work on personal change is delayed by

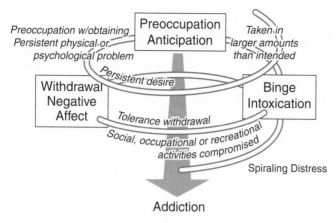

Figure 3.1. The criteria for substance dependence as a downward spiral of thought. (Reprinted with permission from Koob and LeMoal 2001.)

denial, rationalization, and blaming other people and external circumstances (e.g., "I'm addicted," "I cannot stop," "Everything I do is a failure," "There is no way out of this mess"). Once this backward processing of information begins, progressive decreases in flexibility and awareness lead to a vicious downward spiral of recurrently narrowing interests and of increasingly dissatisfying and stereotypic (ritualistic) behaviors. Struggle with desires leads to more arousal, more problems, and less hope, which in turn lead to further increases in cravings. Arousal is greatest when selfish desires are frustrated, but may remain high even when a person feels empowered by having their desires temporarily satisfied. Consequently, the cycle of increasing inflexibility, struggle, and hopelessness repeats itself with increasing intensity. Eventually, the preoccupation with drugs pervades every aspect of a person's life. The conflict between frustrated wants and restful satiation (i.e., jittery versus dull, frenzied versus sluggish) is only really resolved by elevation of thought to be calmly and flexibly alert in charitable and compassionate activity.

Similarly, a downward spiral of thought can occur without any initial loss of free will. When a person becomes preoccupied with an unpleasant situation, problem, or obstacle, then they numb their general awareness of opportunities by reducing their listening to their psyche. For example, consider a situation in which you are bicycling down a mountain road and notice a rock on the path ahead. If you continue to focus on the rock, you are likely to hit it. On the other hand, if you simply focus on where you now want to go, then you will automatically avoid the obstacle. Likewise, reduced listening to the psyche leads to reduced awareness of what is opportune and pleasant, which leads to a downward spiral of thought as in the anxiety states that occur after severe stress or disasters like terrorist attacks.

For example, a patient with posttraumatic stress disorder (PTSD) is like a bicyclist thinking about obstacles on his or her path rather than where he or she really wants to go. The diagnosis of PTSD requires the occurrence of trauma that results in the downward spiral of thought, as indicated by feelings of fear, helplessness, or horror. The development of PTSD has been carefully studied in large-scale population-based studies (North, Nixon et al. 1999). Some people attempt to control the emergence of their feelings of distress and conflict by avoidance behavior and a numbing of general responsiveness, which I propose involves an effort to reduce listening to their psyche because of the unpleasantness of their recollections. Low listening to the psyche in the sexual plane is indicated by low Self-Transcendence in plane 2 (i.e., repression or low sensory responsivity as measured by ST subscale 1). Intense arousal and unpleasant recollections occur in most people after a severe disaster, but the presence of avoidance and numbing symptoms occurs in only a minority of people in a general population. Therefore the diagnosis of PTSD, which requires symptoms in all three groups, depends on the presence of symptoms of intense inhibitory control leading to avoidance behavior and a numbing of general responsiveness. For example, nearly all people (94%) with avoidance and numbing symptoms met the full criteria for PTSD after the Oklahoma City bombing (North, Nixon et al. 1999). Overall 34% of exposed individuals developed PTSD after the Oklahoma City bombing. The best predictor of PTSD was the diagnosis of a personality disorder, which indicates low overall self-awareness. Numbing and avoidance symptoms were moderately correlated with low scores on TCI Self-Directedness ($r = -.33$, $p < .01$) and higher scores on TCI Harm Avoidance ($r = .42$, $p < .01$) and TCI Self-Transcendence ($r = .22$, $p < .05$) in 107 people exposed to the Oklahoma City disaster (North, Nixon et al. 1999). These TCI scores show that worrying about obstacles (high Harm Avoidance) and failure to look where you want to go (low Self-Directedness) are moderately associated with a downward spiral of thought.

Likewise, individuals who frequently ignore reality inevitably confront problems and obstacles for which they are not prepared, which leads to a downward spiral. On the other hand, individuals who are mature in all three aspects of their character are unlikely to develop psychiatric disturbance, even after a severe disaster. Coherent attitudes, like hope and kindness, are uplifting, as described in Table 3.10, so individuals who maintain such coherent attitudes are resilient despite challenges that even threaten their life. A coherent attitude (i.e., a "virtue") is an attitude that elicits increasing personal satisfaction, sublimation, and flexibility regardless of external circumstances. A simplified form of the spiral path of consciousness is illustrated in Figure 3.2. My formerly dependent patient changed in her perspective and began to mature in her personal and social life while maintaining abstinence. She declared, "I realized I was killing myself and knew I had to change my life. I felt a surge of hope and knew things would get better. I just decided what I wanted to do and did it. I didn't feel hopeless or helpless anymore." With such a positive perspective,

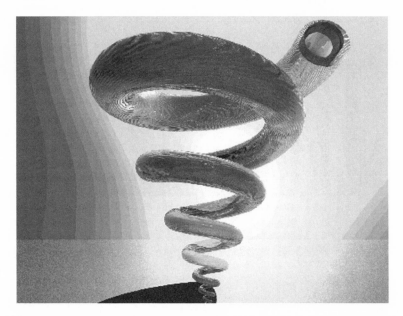

Figure 3.2. The spiral path of consciousness. The successive levels of the spiral represent successive planes of increasingly elevated thought. (Reprinted with permission of C. R. Cloninger, Center for Psychobiology of Personality, Washington University.)

challenges are not insurmountable problems; rather they are opportunities for growth and adaptation that initiate an upward spiral toward coherence of personality.

These observations about the movement of thought in the development of well-being are strongly supported by observations in a sample of 804 individuals representative of the general population of the St. Louis area (Cloninger, Bayon et al. 1998). We related quantitative measures of positive emotionality and negative emotionality to individual differences in personality. Well-being, as measured by the presence of positive emotions (e.g., cheerful, happy, contented) *and* the absence of negative emotions (sad, distressed, dissatisfied), occurred only if people had coherence of character. Coherence of character was measured by the presence of high scores on all three of the TCI character traits of Self-Directedness, Cooperativeness, and Self-Transcendence. Our findings are illustrated in Figure 3.3. One of six people were classified as "sad" based on high scores on the depression scale of the Center for Epidemiological Studies (Radloff 1977). One of six people were classified as "happy" based on high scores on positive emotionality scale of the Inventory of Personal Characteristics (Tellegen, Grove et al. 1990). Character was rated using the TCI, distinguishing those who were in the top third of Self-Directedness (S), Cooperativeness (C), and self-Transcendence (T), from those in the lowest third of Self-Directedness (s), Cooperativeness (c), and Self-Transcendence (t), or in the middle third on each test (–). As can be seen

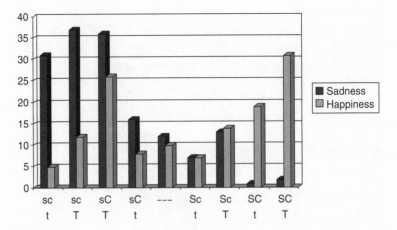

Figure 3.3. The percentages of individuals who are happy or sad according to their TCI character configuration.

in Figure 3.3, 12% of people who are near average on all three traits of character report being depressed and 10% report being happy. In contrast, about a third (31–37%) of people who are low in Self-Directedness are depressed (see first three sets of bars on the left in Figure 3.3). The percentage of those low in Self-Directedness who are happy is 5% if people are also neither cooperative nor transcendent and increases to 26% if they are both cooperative and transcendent. Furthermore, if Self-Directedness or Cooperativeness is high, but not both, then people do not differ much in mood from those with average character profiles (see middle three bars in Figure 3.3). If both Self-Directedness and Cooperativeness are elevated, then happiness is much more frequent than sadness (19% versus 1%). Finally, people who are elevated on all three aspects of character have the highest percentage of happiness (26%). In other words, the development of well-being (i.e., presence of positive emotions and absence of negative emotions) depends on the combination of all three aspects of self-aware consciousness. Lack of development of any one of the three factors leaves a person vulnerable to the emergence of conflicts that can lead to a downward spiral of thought into a state of depression.

The relationship of well-being to character types was further examined using Reed's self-transcendence scale, which is a well-validated measure of well-being, self-awareness, and coherence of personality in both healthy and terminally ill people (Coward and Reed 1996; Ellerman and Reed 2001). We studied this measure of well-being together with the TCI in a community sample of 915 people representative of the general population of St. Louis. As predicted, well-being is lowest in individuals who are low in all three TCI character dimensions and highest in those who are high in all three TCI character dimensions. In addition, we found that variability in well-being was inversely related to the mean value of the different character types in Figure 3.3. That is, the standard deviation in Reed's Self-transcendence score was low in character types who had high mean scores in coherence, whereas the standard deviation was high in character types who had low mean scores in coherence (Table 3.11). This supports the relationship of well-being to coherence, which implies that stability increases along with positive emotions.

My recent clinical work has confirmed my research observations that the state of readiness for character development can be understood as a succession of stages in self-aware consciousness. These three stages of the development of self-aware consciousness, summarized in Table 3.5, have been described in detail in studies of spiritual development by many positive philosophers, such as Plato, Clement of Alexandria, Augustine, al-Ghazali, and Hegel, as reviewed elsewhere (Garrigou-Lagrange 1947; Cloninger and Svrakic 1997). The paleoanthropologist Teilhard de Chardin also describes the development of consciousness in three corresponding stages, which he calls the neocosmic, ultrahuman, and panChristic stages (Teilhard de Chardin 1959, 1978). The stages of cognitive development have also been described as the ego-states typical of the "child" (stage 0), "adult" (stage 1), and "parent" (stage 2) in Eric Berne's transactional analysis of dysfunctional social relationships, neglecting the stage of coherent well-being (stage 3) important in healthy therapeutic relationships (Berne 1977). Of course, such simplified stepwise descriptions are abstractions of the fluid interaction of multiple interdependent processes, including obstacles and experiences that are unique to each individual. Each step in the path reflects all three stages in microcosm, as in the three-fold path of Buddhism in which change always involves cultivation of (*1*) elevation of moral values, (*2*) broadening of awareness in mindful meditation,

**Table 3.11.** Mean values (in Standard Form as Z Score) and Standard Deviations of Reed's Self-Transcendence Scale, a Measure of Well-Being and Coherence of Personality, in Different Character Types Measured with the TCI in 915 People from the General Population

| TCI Character | Type | n | Reed's Self-Transcendence Score | | | |
| --- | --- | --- | --- | --- | --- | --- |
| | | | *Mean* | *SD* | *Minimum* | *Maximum* |
| Melancholic | (sct) | 171 | −0.84 | 1.04 | −4.36 | 1.57 |
| Disorganized | (scT) | 116 | −0.34 | 0.97 | −2.88 | 1.88 |
| Dependent | (sCt) | 48 | −0.36 | 0.85 | −2.33 | 0.87 |
| Cyclothymic | (sCT) | 50 | 0.02 | 0.87 | −2.18 | 1.80 |
| Average | (—) | 13 | 0.10 | 0.79 | −1.79 | 1.18 |
| Autocratic | (Sct) | 99 | 0.07 | 0.80 | −3.50 | 1.80 |
| Fanatic | (ScT) | 32 | 0.25 | 0.73 | −1.63 | 1.41 |
| Organized | (SCt) | 164 | 0.33 | 0.75 | −2.49 | 1.88 |
| Creative | (SCT) | 163 | 0.74 | 0.76 | −3.89 | 1.88 |

and (*3*) wisdom born from deeper understanding. These three processes lead to stepwise increases in a hierarchy of five levels of mental powers and coherence: (*1*) confidence/trust, (*2*) energy/power, (*3*) concentration/contentment, (*4*) mindfulness/clarity, and (*5*) insight/joy (Levey and Levey 2003). Stepwise descriptions are misleading unless it is recognized that they are only averages of abstractions that crystallize what is actually a nonlinear complex of adaptive life processes. Therefore we must test the clinical use of the concepts and methods described in this chapter through examination of well-documented examples of the development of self-aware consciousness.

## REFERENCES

Allman, J. M. (2001). "The anterior cingulate cortex: The evolution of an interface between emotion and cognition." *Annals of the New York Academy of Sciences* 935: 107–117.

American Psychiatric Association (1994). *Diagnostic and Statistical Manual of Mental Disorders*. Washington, DC, APA.

Augustine (386). *The happy life; Answer to skeptics; Divine providence & the problem of evil, soliloques*. New York, Cima Publishing Co., 1948.

Augustine (388). The magnitude of the soul. *Writings of Saint Augustine*. New York, Cima Publishing Co.: 51–59, 1947.

Bechara, A., A. R. Damasio, et al. (1994). "Insensitivity to future consequences following damage to human prefrontal cortex." *Cognition* 50: 7–15.

Bechara, A., A. R. Damasio, et al. (1998). "Dissociation of working memory from decision making within the human prefrontal cortex." *Journal of Neuroscience* 18: 428–437.

Bechara, A., H. Damasio, et al. (1997). "Deciding advantageously before knowing the advantageous strategy." *Science* 275: 1293–1295.

Beck, A. T. (1976). *Cognitive therapy and the emotional disorders*. New York, International Universities Press.

Beck, A. T. (1996). Beyond belief: A theory of modes, personality, and psychopathology. *Frontiers of cognitive therapy*. P. M. Salkovskis. New York, Guilford Press: 1–25.

Berne, E. (1977). *Intuition and ego states: The origins of transactional analysis*. San Francisco, California, TA Press.

Blakemore, S. J., D. A. Oakley, et al. (2003). "Delusions of alien control in the normal brain." *Neuropsychologia* 41(8): 1058–1067.

Bjorklund, D. F. (1997). "In search of a metatheory for cognitive development (or, Piaget is dead and I don't feel so good myself)." *Child Development* 68: 144–148.

Bohm, D. (1995). Interview about Krishnammurti. *Krishnammurti: 100 years*. E. Blau. New York, Stewart, Tabori & Chang.

Boring, E. G. (1957). *A history of experimental psychology*. New York, Appleton-Century-Crofts.

Bottini, G., H. O. Karnath, et al. (2001). "Cerebral representations of egocentric space: Functional-anatomical evidence from caloric vestibular stimulation and neck vibration." *Brain* 124(Pt 6): 1182–1196.

Bradley, M. M. and P. J. Lang (1994). "Measuring emotion: The self-assessment manikin and the semantic differential." *Journal of Behavioral Therapeutics and Experimental Psychiatry* 25: 49–59.

Bradley, M. M. and P. J. Lang (2000). "Affective reactions to acoustic stimuli." *Psychophysiology* 37: 204–215.

Broadbent, D. E. (1958). *Perception and Communication*. London, Pergamon.

Burgess, P. W., E. Veitch, et al. (2000). "The cognitive and neuroanatomical correlates of multitasking." *Neuropsychologia* 38: 848–863.

Burgess, P. W., A. Quayle, et al. (2001). "Brain regions involved in prospective memory as determined by positron emission tomography." *Neuropsychologia* 39: 545–555.

Burgess, P. W., S. K. Scott, et al. (2003). "The role of the rostral frontal cortex (area 10) in prospective memory: a lateral versus medial dissociation." *Neuropsychologia* 41(8): 906–918.

Cloninger, C. R. (1994). "The genetic structure of personality and learning: A phylogenetic perspective." *Clinical Genetics* 46: 124–137.

Cloninger, C. R. (2002). Functional neuroanatomy and brain imaging of personality and its disorders. *Biological psychiatry*. H. D'haenen, J. A. den Boer and P. Willner, eds. Chichester, England, John Wiley & Sons, Ltd.: 1377–1385.

Cloninger, C. R. (2002). Implications of comorbidity for the classification of mental disorders: The need for a psychobiology of coherence. *Psychiatric Diagnosis and Classification*. M. Maj, W. Gaebel, J. J. Lopez-Ibor, and N. Sartorius, eds. Chichester, England, John Wiley & Sons, Ltd.: 79–106.

Cloninger, C. R., C. Bayon, et al. (1998). "Measurement of temperament and character in mood disorders: A model of fundamental states as personality types." *Journal of Affective Disorders* 51: 21–32.

Cloninger, C. R., T. R. Przybeck, et al. (1994). *The Temperament and Character Inventory: A guide to its development and use*. St. Louis, MO, Washington University Center for Psychobiology of Personality.

Cloninger, C. R. and D. M. Svrakic (1997). "Integrative psychobiological approach to psychiatric assessment and treatment." *Psychiatry* 60: 120–141.

Cloninger, C. R. and D. M. Svrakic (2000). Personality Disorders. *Comprehensive Textbook of Psychiatry*. B. J. Sadock and V. A. Sadock. New York, Lippincott Williams & Wilkins: 1723–1764.

Cloninger, C. R., D. M. Svrakic, et al. (1993). "A psychobiological model of temperament and character." *Archives of General Psychiatry* 50: 975–990.

Coward, D. D. and P. G. Reed (1996). "Self-transcendence: A resource for healing at the end of life." *Issues Mental Health Nursing* 17: 279–288.

Csikszentmihalyi, M. (1991). *Flow: The psychology of optimal experience*. New York, HarperCollins.

Csikszentmihalyi, M. (1993). *The evolving self*. New York, HarperCollins.

Damasio, A. R. (1985). The frontal lobes. *Clinical Neuropsychology*. K. M. Heilman and E. Valenstein, eds. New York, Oxford University Press: 339–375.

Davidson, R. J. (2003). *Investigating the Mind: Studies of emotion*. Mind & Life Conference, Massachusetts Institute of Technology, Cambridge MA.

Davidson, R. J. and R. T. Marrocco (2000). "Local infusion of scopolamine into intraparietal cortex slows covert orienting in rhesus monkeys." *Journal of Neurophysiology* 83: 1536–1549.

Deakin, J. F. W. and F. G. Graeff (1991). "5-HT and mechanisms of defense." *Journal of Psychopharmacology* 5: 305–315.

DeWaal, F. B. M. (1999). "Cultural primatology comes of age." *Nature* 399: 635–636.

Eccles, J. (1989). *Evolution and the brain: Creation of the self.* London, Routledge.

Ellerman, C. R. and P. G. Reed (2001). "Self-transcendence and depression in middle-age adults." *Western Journal of Nursing Research* 23: 698–713.

Emerson, R. W. (1841). The Method of Nature. *The American Transcendentalists: Their prose and poetry.* P. Miller. Garden City, NY, Doubleday & Company: 49–68.

Enomiya Lassalle, H. M. (1974). *Zen meditation for Christians.* La Salle, Illinois, Open Court.

Fan, J., J. Fossella, et al. (2003). "Mapping the genetic variation of executive attention onto brain activity." *Proceedings of the National Academy of Sciences USA* 100: 4706–7411.

Farrer, C. and C. D. Frith (2002). "Experiencing oneself vs another person as being the cause of an action: the neural correlates of the experience of agency." *Neuroimage* 15(3): 596–603.

Farrow, T. F., Y. Zheng, et al. (2001). "Investigating the functional anatomy of empathy and forgiveness." *NeuroReport* 12(11): 2433–2438.

Fell, J., G. Fernandez, et al. (2003). "Is synchronized gamma activity relevant for selective attention." *Brain Research—Brain Research Reviews* 42(3): 265–272.

Frankl, V. E. (1959). *Man's search for meaning: An introduction to logotherapy.* New York, Simon & Schuster.

Frankl, V. E. (1978). *The unheard cry for meaning: Psychotherapy and humanism.* New York, Pocket Books.

Freeman, W. and J. W. Watts (1942). *Psychosurgery: Intelligence, emotion, and social behavior following prefrontal lobotomy for mental disorders.* Springfield, Illinois, C. C. Thomas.

Freud, S. (1900). *The interpretation of dreams.* New York, MacMillan Company.

Frith, C. D., S. Blakemore, et al. (2000). "Explaining the symptoms of schizophrenia: abnormalities in the awareness of action." *Brain Research—Brain Research Reviews* 31(2–3): 357–363.

Frith, C. D., S. J. Blakemore, et al. (2000). "Abnormalities in the awareness and control of action." *Philosophical Transactions of the Royal Society of London-Series B: Biological Sciences* 355(1404): 1771–1788.

Frith, U. and C. D. Frith (2003). "Development and neurophysiology of mentalizing." *Philosophical Transactions of the Royal Society of London-Series B: Biological Sciences* 358(1431): 459–473.

Gandhi, M. (1997). *All men are brothers: Autobiographical reflections.* New York, Continuum.

Garrigou-Lagrange, R. (1947). *The three ages of the interior life.* London, B. Herder Book Co.

Gillin, C., E. Seifritz, et al. (2000). Basic science of sleep. *Comprehensive Textbook of Psychiatry.* B. J. Sadock and V. A. Sadock, eds. Philadelphia, PA, Lippincott Williams & Wilkins: 199–209.

Godel, K. (1961). The modern development of the foundations of mathematics in the light of philosophy. *Collected works.* New York, Oxford University Press.

Graboi, D. and J. Lisman (2003). "Recognition by top-down and bottom-up processes: the control of selective attention." *Journal of Neurophysiology* 90(2): 798–810.

Graham, F. K. (1979). Distinguishing among orienting, defense, and startle reflexes. *The orienting reflex in humans.* H. D. Kimmel, E. H. Van Olst, and J. F. Orlebeke, eds. Hillsdale, New Jersey, Lawrence Erlbaum Associates: 137–167.

Grastyan, E. (1980). "Emotion." *Encyclopedia Brittanica* 6: 757–566.

Guillem, F., M. Bicu, et al. (2002). "The dimensional structure of schizophrenia and its association with temperament and character." *Schizophrenia Research* 56: 137–147.

Gusnard, D. A., E. Akbudak, et al. (2001). "Medial prefrontal cortex and self-referential mental activity: Relation to a default mode of brain function." *Proceedings of the National Academy of Sciences USA* 98: 4259–4265.

Gusnard, D. A., J. M. Ollinger, et al. (2003). "Persistence and brain circuitry." *Proceedings of the National Academy of Sciences USA* 100: 3479–3484.

Gusnard, D. A., J. M. Ollinger, et al. (2001). "Personality differences in functional brain imaging." *Society of Neuroscience Abstracts* 27: 11.

Haeckel, E. (1900). *The riddle of the universe at the close of the nineteenth century.* New York, Harper & Brothers.

Heckers, S., M. Zalesak, et al. (2004). "Hippocampal activation during transitive inference in humans." *Hippocampus.*

Hegel, G. F. W. (1807). *Phenomenology of spirit.* Oxford, England, Oxford University Press.

Hegel, G. F. W. (1981). *The Berlin phenomenology.* London, Reidel Publishing Company.

Hirst, W. (1995). Cognitive aspects of consciousness. *The Cognitive Neurosciences.* M. S. Gazzaniga. Cambridge, Massachusetts, MIT Press: 1307–1321.

Jahanshahi, M., I. H. Jenkins, et al. (1995). "Self-initiated versus externally triggered movements. I. An investigation using measurement of regional cderebral blod flow with PET and movement-related potentials in normal and Parkinson's disease subjects." *Brain* 118: 913–933.

Jankovic, J. (2001). "Tourette's syndrome." *New England Journal of Medicine* 345: 1184–1192.

Joseph, R. (1999). "Frontal lobe psychopathology: Mania, depression, confabulation, perseveration, obsessive compulsions, and schizophrenia." *Psychiatry* 62: 138–172.

Karp, B. I., S. Porter, et al. (1996). "Simple motor tics may be preceded by a premotor potential." *Journal of Neurology, Neurosurgery and Psychiatry* 61: 103–106.

Kelly, D., A. Richardson, et al. (1973). "Stereotactic limbic leucotomy: Neurophysiological aspects and operative techniques." *British Journal of Psychiatry* 123: 133–140.

Kohut, H. (1984). *How does analysis cure?* Chicago, Illinois, University of Chicago Press.

Koob, G. F. and M. LeMoal (2001). "Drug addiction, dysregulation of reward, and allostasis." *Neuropsychopharmacology* 24: 97–129.

Krishnamurti, J. (1974). *On education.* London, Krishnamurti Foundation Trust Ltd.

Krishnamurti, J. (1992). *Complete collected works of J. Krishnamurti.* Ojai, California, Krishnamurti Foundation of America.

Lane, R. D., E. M. Reiman, et al. (1997). "Neuroanatomical correlates of pleasant and unpleasant emotion." *Neuropsychologia* 35: 1437–1444.

Lang, P. J., M. M. Bradley, et al. (1998). "Emotion, motivation, and anxiety: Brain mechanisms and psychophysiology." *Biological Psychiatry* 44: 1248–1263.

Levey, J. and M. Levey (2003). The fine arts of relaxation, concentration, and meditation. Boston, Wisdom Publications.

Lewin, R. (1998). *Principles of human evolution: A core textbook.* London, Blackwell Science.

MacLean, P. D. (1985). "Brain evolution relating to family, play, and the separation call." *Archives of General Psychiatry* 42: 405–417.

Maguire, E. A., R. N. Henson, et al. (2001). "Activity in prefrontal cortex, not hippocampus, varies parametrically with the increasing remoteness of memories." *Neuroreport* 12(3): 441–444.

Marrocco, R. T. and R. J. Davidson (1998). Neurochemistry of attention. *The attention brain*. R. Parasuraman, ed. Cambridge, Massachusetts, MIT Press: 35–50.

Maslow, A. (1962). *Toward a psychology of being*. Princeton, D. Van Nostrand.

Mehrabian, A. and J. A. Russell (1974). *An approach to environmental psychology*. Cambridge, Massachusetts, MIT Press.

Mithen, S. (1996). *The prehistory of the mind: The cognitive origins of art, religion, and science*. London, Thames and Hudson, Ltd.

Moscovitch, M. (1995). Models of consciousness and memory. *The Cognitive Neurosciences*. M. S. Gazzaniga. Cambridge, Massachusetts, MIT Press: 1341–1356.

Murray, H. A. (1938). *Explorations in personaolity*. New York, Oxford University Press.

Nathaniel-James, D. A. and C. D. Frith (2002). "The role of the dorsolateral prefrontal cortex: evidence from the effects of contextual constraint in a sentence completion task." *Neuroimage* 16(4): 1094–1102.

Nauta, W. J. H. and M. Feirtag (1986). *Fundamental neuroanatomy*. New York, W. H. Freeman.

Nimchinsky, E. A., E. Gilissen, et al. (1999). "A neuronal morphologic type unique to humans and great apes." *Proceedings of the National Academy of Sciences USA* 96: 5268–5273.

North, C. S., S. J. Nixon, et al. (1999). "Psychiatric disorders among survivors of the Oklahoma City bombing." *Journal of the American Medical Association* 282: 755–762.

Osgood, C. (1952). "The nature and measurement of meaning." *Psychological Bulletin* 49: 172–237.

Osgood, C., G. Suci, et al. (1957). *The measurement of meaning*. Urbana, Illinois, University of Illinois.

Pavlov, I. P. (1941). *Conditioned reflexes and psychiatry*. New York, International Publishers.

Paus, T. (2001). "Primate anterior cingulate cortex: where motor control, drive and cognition interface." *Nature Reviews Neuroscience* 2: 417–424.

Posner, M. I. and J. Fan (2003). Attention as an organ system. *Neurobiology of perception and communication: From synapse to society*. J. Pomerantz, ed. Cambridge, England, Cambridge University Press.

Povinelli, D. J. (2000). *Folk physics for apes: The chimpanzee's theory of how the world works*. New York, Oxford University Press.

Povinelli, D. J. and S. Giambrone (2001). "Reasoning about beliefs: A human specialization?" *Child Development* 72: 691–695.

Povinelli, D. J., A. M. Landry, et al. (1999). "Development of young children's understanding that the recent past is causally bound to the present." *Developmental Psychology* 35: 1426–1439.

Povinelli, D. J. and B. B. Simon (1998). "Young children's understanding of briefly versus extremely delayed images of the self: Emergence of the autobiographical stance." *Developmental Psychology* 34.

Radloff, L. S. (1977). "The CES-D scale: A self-report depression scale for research in the general population." *Applied Psychological Measurement* 36: 749–760.

Rogers, C. R. (1980). *A Way of being*. Boston, Houghton Mifflin.

Roth, G. (2000). The evolution of consciousness. *Brain evolution and cognition*. G. Roth and M. F. Wullimann. New York, John Wiley & Sons: 555–582.

Russell, B. (1919). *Introduction to mathematical philosophy*. New York, MacMillan.

Russell, B. (1998). *Autobiography*. London, Routledge.

Russell, J. (1980). "A circumplex model of affect." *Journal of Personal and Social Psychology* 39: 1161–1178.

Salinas, E. and T. J. Sejnowski (2001). "Gain modulation in the central nervous system: where behavior, neurophysiology, and computation meet." *Neuroscientist* 7(5): 430–440.

Schultz, W., L. Tremblay, et al. (1998). "Reward prediction in primate basal ganglia and frontal cortex." *Neuropharmacology* 37: 421–429.

Spence, S. A., D. J. Brooks, et al. (1997). "A PET study of voluntary movement in schizophrenic patients experiencing passivity phenomena (delusions of alien control)." *Brain* 120(Pt 11): 1997–2011.

Spinoza, B. (1955). *Works of Spinoza*. New York, Dover Publications.

Stephan, V. and J. D. Schall (2002). "Neuronal control and monitoring of initiation of movements." *Muscle Nerve* 26: 326–339.

Straub, R. E. (2003). *Dysbindin, cognitive and fMRI phenotypes in schizophrenia*. Integrating progress in the genetics and neuropharmacology of schizophrenia, Banbury Center, Cold Spring Harbor Lab, New York.

Stuss, D. T. and D. F. Benson (1986). *The frontal lobes*. New York, Raven Press.

Svrakic, D. M., C. Whitehead, et al. (1993). "Differential diagnosis of personality disorders by the seven factor model of temperament and character." *Archives of General Psychiatry* 50: 991–999.

Svrakic, N. M., D. M. Svrakic, et al. (1996). "A general quantitative theory of personality development: Fundamentals of a self-organizing psychobiological complex." *Development and Psychopathology* 8: 247–272.

Teilhard de Chardin, P. (1959). *The phenomenon of man*. New York, Harper & Row.

Teilhard de Chardin, P. (1978). *The heart of matter*. New York, Harcourt Brace Jovanovich.

Tellegen, A., W. Grove, et al. (1990). *Inventory of personal characteristics No. 7*. Minneapolis, Minnesota, Department of Psychology, University of Minnesota.

Thermos, V. (2002). *In search of the person: "True" and "false" self according to Donald Winnicott and St. Gregory Palamas*. Montreal, Canada, Alexander Press.

Tulving, E. (2002). "Episodic memory: From mind to brain." *Annual Review of Psychology* 53: 1–25.

Turner, R. M., I. L. Hudson, et al. (2003). "Brain function and personality in normal males: a SPECT study using statistical parametric mapping." *NeuroImage* 19:1145–1162.

Voltaire (1980). Familiar quotations. *Bartlett's familiar quotations*. J. Bartlett. Boston, Little, Brown and Company: 343.

Wallis, J. D., K. C. Anderson, et al. (2001). "Single neurons in prefrontal cortex encode abstract rules." *Nature* 411: 953–956.

Whitehead, A. N. and B. Russell (1910–1913). *Principia Mathematica*. Cambridge, UK, Cambridge University Press.

Whiten, A., J. Goodall, et al. (1999). "Culture in chimpanzees." *Nature* 399: 682–685.

Winnicott, D. (1958). *Collected papers: Through pediatrics to psychoanalysis*. New York, Basic Books.

Wundt, W. (1903). *Characteristics of physiological psychology*. Leipzig, Austria, W. Engelmann.

# 4

# THE SOCIAL PSYCHOLOGY
# OF TRANSCENDENTALISM

## THE CULTURAL ATMOSPHERE OF EARLY AMERICA

American transcendentalism emerged as a liberal flowering of intuitive spirituality in New England in reaction against Unitarianism, which at that time had grown to be conservative and uninspiring. Earlier Unitarianism had been a response to an even more oppressive form of Calvinism. Emerson (1880, page 5) began his classic autobiographical description of the transcendentalist movement with the simple but profound statement, "There are always two parties, the party of the Past and the party of the Future, the Establishment and the Movement." Emerson is referring to the recurrent conflict between conservative and liberal factions in church and state. To understand the cultural atmosphere of the American transcendentalists and the significance of what they said and did, we need to understand the psychological issues underlying the developmental history of Calvinism and Unitarianism.

The history of these religious developments closely parallels the development of conservatism and liberalism in politics and economics. In fact, conservation of religious practices has always been a major force in maintaining stability and continuity of established social traditions. According to historians, the attitudes of conservatives in politics and economics are based on the assumption that men are not born naturally free or good but are naturally predisposed to anarchy, aggression, and evil (Viereck 1965). As the conservative George Washington said, "Few men have virtue to withstand the highest bidder." The conservative belief in an innate human tendency to depravity corresponds to the religious belief in "original sin." The conservative belief in the human tendency to sin is strongly rooted in the assumptions of the early American colonists, who were called either Puritans or Calvinists. The Puritans wished to practice a "pure" Protestant religion characterized by hard work, social conformity, and strict discipline enforced by elders. The Puritans wanted to be free of any Catholic influence and free of persecution by the Church of England, which they thought retained too much of Catholic practices.

In view of the conservative orientation of later Calvinist practice, it is ironic that John Calvin converted to Protestantism as a result of his study of the Stoic philosopher Seneca's essay *Concerning Clemency*. In classical Greek and Roman times, Stoicism was created by the Syrian philosopher Zeno of Citium during the third century BC as a liberal democratic philosophy opposed to control by a conservative aristocracy. According to the Stoics, the basis of human happiness is to live a life of self-control (i.e., self-aware virtue) because wealth and possessions do not ensure happiness. In 1536, after reading the work of Seneca, John Calvin (1509–1564) wrote *Institutes of the Christian Religion*. This was a systematic manual of Protestant dogma, but it left open many questions of interpretation. His follower Theodore Beza made Calvinism much more legalistic than it had been originally. In particular, Beza reverted to an emphasis on the predestination of human beings, rather than acknowledging any awareness of the importance of gifts of grace and freedom of will along the path of the psyche. Beza also emphasized the literal interpretation of the Bible by presbyters (i.e., local church elders) rather than by episcopals (i.e., bishops). Both Beza and John Knox (1514–1572) were extremely conservative and insisted on the strict maintenance of traditions by church elders. Deviations from strict obedience were taken as evidence that a person was not one of the chosen elect. This was tantamount to condemnation to Hell because the Calvinists believed that Christ died only for a few elect, not for the salvation of all human beings. The chosen were responsible to respond in dutiful obedience to divine commandments as interpreted by local church elders. Furthermore, there was a pietistic and pragmatic concern for one's personal salvation among English Puritans, rather than interest in charitable service to others.

Besides Calvinism, another line of thought that led to the American Protestant Ethic (Weber 1958) was the philosophy and example of Benjamin Franklin. According to private correspondence with the president of Yale College, Ezra Stiles, Franklin said that he believed in Deism but doubted the divinity of Jesus Christ and regarded the reports of his miracles as absurd. Like Franklin, the first three U.S. presidents (Washington, Adams, and Jefferson) were all Deists, despite their differing in conservative and liberal ideas. *Deism* refers to what Hume and others sometimes called "natural religion," that is, the acceptance of a small number of religious beliefs that are inborn in every person or can be acquired through reason alone (Cassirer 1955). According to the British deist Lord Herbert, five religious ideas were recognized as innate in the mind of all human beings as a result of divine illumination: the belief (1) in a supreme being, (2) in the need for worship of the divine, (3) in the pursuit of a pious and virtuous life as the most desirable form of worship, (4) in the need of repentance for sins, and (5) in rewards and punishments in the next world. According to Herbert, these ideas were innate in the first human being and underlie all positive religion since that time. However, Deism is specifically opposed to acceptance of other religious knowledge that is supposed to be acquired either through divine revelation or through the teachings of any organized church supported by evidence of miracles rather than reason. Franklin's personal creed, as described to Ezra Stiles, was the same as Herbert's five fundamental beliefs of Deism (Brands 2000, pages 706–707).

Franklin created a self-image of success through intelligent hard work and moral development, based on the principles of rationalism and Deism that were popular among free thinkers at the time. As a result, he defined the concept of the "American dream" of going from "rags to riches" by means of personal merit and reason, which has inspired many people in the United States. Likewise, Illuminism was a Deistic movement associated with the Freemasons in Europe and the United States to replace Christianity with a religion of reason, acknowledging divine providence but not Christ. Its roots were in British Deism of the seventeenth century, described by Lord Herbert. When Deism spread to Germany, France, Italy, and other parts of Europe during the eighteenth century, it was called Illuminism. Its symbol is the "all-seeing eye" of Providence, which is associated with some nonChristian religions, such as Unitarianism. Franklin, who was the Grand Master of the Pennsylvania Freemasons, recommended that the "all-seeing eye" be added to the Seal of the United States (Brands 2000). As a result, this deistic symbol still appears at the top of the pyramid on the United States one-dollar bill.

Doubt about the divinity of Jesus and his miracles was based on the Deistic belief that God created the world but then left it alone without any personal intervention through divine revelation, miracles, or incarnation. The transcendent God of Deism is much more remote than the personal incarnation of God in Christian religions. As a result of the remoteness of God in Deism, it is often impossible to distinguish the Providence of Deism from fatalistic predestination and rational materialism. Essentially, Deists deny the effective role of human free will and charismatic gifts, such as prophecy, in the ongoing evolution of human understanding and social relationships along the path of the psyche. Self-reliance on the illuminated reason of the individual requires salvation through intelligent hard work and obedience of traditional authorities, rather than the theological virtues of faith, hope, and love.

These unorthodox interpretations of Christian doctrine have occurred intermittently since the second century. The Calvinist and Deist doctrines are efforts to deal with recurrent human dilemmas based on fears that a particular person may have no hope of salvation (because of predestination) or that the responsibility for personal salvation rests largely on his hard work and obedience to commands. Are we one of the chosen few? Are we strictly obedient to what is demanded of us by authority? According to positive philosophers, such as Augustine and Albert the Great, strict determinism by predestination involves the error of denial of hope for many, as well as lack of awareness of freedom of will as a gift of grace. Likewise, emphasis on personal hard work to merit salvation is a denial of divine love, as well as a lack of awareness of the grace involved in charitable service to others. Submission of the individual's will to external authorities is a denial of faith that each human being has a divine soul with freedom of will that needs to be trusted and exercised to develop along the path of the psyche. According to the positive philosophy, service to others, not preoccupation with self-salvation, is the only way a human being can show gratitude as a free expression of his or her love of God. That is, service of the universal unity of being necessarily involves respect for the personal freedom of all people combined with loving service to others, not preoccupation with personal salvation to the neglect of the needs of others.

From the time of Franklin to the present time, many people have become wealthy and influential through intelligent, hard work in America. However, the Protestant Ethic of Calvinism and Deism placed a great burden on the individual Calvinist or Deist and posed difficult and serious theological questions for Christianity as a whole. This oppressive burden is still prominent today in the contrasting stereotypes of the Victorian Englishman and the romantic Frenchman. The caricature of the Anglo-Saxon is a cold, conservative, almost lifeless robot who works endlessly to accumulate more material and social security with little or no real joy in life. In contrast, there is the "French Paradox," in which the jovial French people enjoy wine, food, and sex liberally but nevertheless have health and longevity.

Freedom from the oppressive and unpromising Calvinist traditions was sought in the emergence of rationalism during the Enlightenment. Unitarianism emerged in England and the United States during the eighteenth and nineteenth centuries as a Deistic commitment to the rational advancement of scientific truth. Unitarianism emphasizes that God is One and denies the doctrine of the Trinity. More specifically, Unitarians deny that Jesus Christ was the incarnation of God.

Unitarianism is the same doctrine that was taught by Arius of Alexandria in the fourth century. Early Christian theologians like Clement of Alexandria and Augustine understood the teachings of Jesus in terms of the universal unity of being of positive philosophy. However, many logical problems arise about the relations of "the one and the many" when Christian teachings are viewed from a dualistic perspective. For example, if God created man, how could any man, such as Jesus, be co-equal with God? The resolution of these problems by Augustine based on the universal unity of being was adopted as Catholic orthodoxy by the Council of Nicaea in 325. According to Augustine, God is the eternal "One who is" and Christ as the divine Logos ("Word"), who is the image of God and the co-equal bridge that enables man to become one with God.

Arius, a fourth-century priest in Alexandria at the time of Augustine, taught that Christ was Son of God only as a created being and was not co-equal or co-eternal with God. Athananius, the orthodox opponent of Arius, said that a subordinate Christ could not save man. Augustine provided a deeper synthesis, emphasizing the universal unity of being, whose essential nature was the good, which has the nondual aspects of truth and love. When the Catholic Church officially adopted Augustine's synthesis, the teachings of Arius were referred to as the "Arian heresy." Augustine's synthesis took the perspective that the Arian heresy (and later Unitarianism) involved lack of awareness and denial of the universal presence of love and of the grace to recognize truth. From the perspective of the positive philosophy, Arius failed to recognize that he had reduced his view of the world to rational materialism, which does not recognize the mind's ability to know itself and thereby to become one with the universal unity of being, which is God or the good.

Reformers of Christianity, such as Luther, Calvin, and Zwingli, were devout men who tried consistently to reaffirm orthodoxy. However, when they set out to describe orthodoxy as dogma written in terms of rational materialism, their systems were not completely logical. Reformers like Calvin refused to draw logical conclusions from their materialistic assumptions because of their devotion to orthodoxy, which was given priority over logical consistency. Less devout followers often extended the logical implications of rational materialism, which inevitably leads to deviations from the positive philosophy.

For example, Unitarian theology was historically based on the philosophy of John Locke, who was a rational materialist, as we discussed in Chapter 1. The implication of a rational materialistic philosophy is that human personality is reduced to temperament, as we discussed in Chapter 2. In fact, the English and American Unitarians were greatly influenced by two scientists, Joseph Priestley and David Hartley, who laid the foundation for rational materialism in modern behavioral psychology. Hartley and Priestley provided Unitarianism with the philosophical basis for divorcing religious practice from metaphysics. Both were close friends of Franklin.

David Hartley was trained to be an Anglican minister but refused to take holy orders because of his belief in the strictly materialistic basis of psychology. From *Essay Concerning Human Understanding* (Locke 1690), Hartley developed the first formulation of behaviorism, which he called associationism. According to Hartley, even complex psychological processes (e.g., reasoning and recollection) might be reduced to sequences of elementary sense impressions.

Priestley was a Unitarian minister who came to the United States from England at the encouragement of his friend Benjamin Franklin. Priestley was well respected as a medical scientist and is still well known as the discoverer of oxygen. He settled in the United States and was a friend of both John Adams and Thomas Jefferson. He was heavily influenced by John Locke and incorporated the principles of the rational materialism in all aspects of his life; this included work as a clergyman, political theorist, educator, and scientist. He carried out rigorous empirical research on human respiration, which led to his discovery of oxygen, and he investigated electricity with Franklin.

The Unitarianism of Hartley and Priestley was intended to free people from the oppressive traditions of Calvinist Puritanism through commitment to scientific advance based on rational materialism. The three main assumptions of Unitarianism were Calvin's doctrine of the absolute providential rule of God, Newton's mechanical universe, and Locke's plea for rational common sense. These three assumptions influenced many Presbytyerian or moderate dissenters in the English church. These "dissenting" preachers taught that God was the sole creator of the universe and ruler of the world. God was best worshipped by a moral life as described by his messenger Jesus Christ. Although Jesus was not co-equal with God, his authority was authenticated by his miracles and his resurrection. These beliefs correspond exactly to the teaching of Arius of Alexandria.

When these dissenters were challenged to define their faith in orthodox terms, they used only the words of scripture in their preaching. This gave them substantial freedom. Nevertheless, an evangelical revival, led by the Methodist John Wesley, caused a renewal of orthodoxy, so that the dissenters split again into orthodox and unorthodox factions. When old congregations began to shrink, many became Unitarians. This unorthodox faction included Joseph Priestley, who began to preach the Arian scheme with open enthusiasm. Priestley was strongly committed to the primacy of what he saw as reason over orthodoxy.

Likewise in the United States, William Ellery Channing of Boston challenged the orthodox doctrine of the atonement of sin by the death of Jesus. He taught the loving fatherhood and unity of God. The American Unitarian Association was founded in Boston in 1825. The Unitarians quickly grew conservative in their adherence to literal rationalistic interpretations of the Bible. As the Unitarians spread to the U.S. West, the doctrine changed from an emphasis on Christ and the Bible to emphasize human self-determination and the empiricism of natural and applied science. In 1838, Emerson delivered a lecture at the Harvard Divinity School, in which he proclaimed the radical belief that innate ideas "transcend" all sense experience. This shocked the Unitarians into evaluating the assumptions underlying their rational materialism. The Unitarian church was irreconcilably split, and the Transcendentalist Movement spread beyond it (Miller 1957).

## EMERSON AND THE AMERICAN
## TRANSCENDENTALIST MOVEMENT

### Overview

When the American Transcendentalist Movement is studied in depth psychologically, it provides a rich illustration of the clinical methods described in Chapter 3 and illustrates the conditions needed for transformation of personality and some aspects of the course of change. In addition, the movement produced classical literary works that continue to inspire a deeper understanding of the way to freedom, well-being, and wisdom.

The founder of the movement, Ralph Waldo Emerson, was a liberal Unitarian minister who published his first book, *Nature*, in 1836. Emerson's three main points in *Nature* were that (*1*) all necessary truth is its own evidence, (*2*) no doctrine about God needed to appeal to a book, and (*3*) Christianity is a rule of life, not a system of intellectual doctrines; each religious sect is an imperfect crystallized form of the one perennial philosophy that all the great souls of every widespread religion have spoken. From this perspective, Emerson concluded that God is immanent in every person and that the purpose of life is the cultivation of self-awareness and freedom from past conditioning. Later, such self-cultivation was called "self-actualization" in humanistic psychology (Rogers 1980) or the development of integrity and authenticity (Winnicott 1958; Erikson 1964; Kohut 1984). Emerson's suggested method of self-actualization was the intuitive study of nature in which every human being participates as an interdependent element of the whole. According to Emerson, the observation of nature with the physical senses was inadequate for the perception of living truth. Nature must be studied in relation to oneself with the intuitive senses to appreciate beauty, truth, and goodness.

Initially, the leader of the Unitarians, William Ellery Channing, was supportive of Emerson and facilitated his interactions with others in their intellectual community, which was centered at Harvard College in Boston. Then in 1838, Emerson made clear in his address to the Harvard Divinity School that he believed that human beings have knowledge through their intuitive senses that transcends the experience of their physical senses. This was an aspect of the rational idealism of Kant and the English romanticist Coleridge that challenged the assumptions of Unitarian belief. Moreover, Emerson spoke with personal conviction from his own experience, so he was not engaging in an intellectual discussion without personal certainty. Emerson had experienced an illumination in 1833. He transiently experienced oceanic feelings of participation in the universal unity of being by means of communion with nature. The authenticity of his faith in recollection and communion with what was beautiful, true, and good in nature inspired and awakened elevated recollections in others. Some of these awakened admirers were chosen by Emerson as disciples to learn his "method of nature" as a way to union with the universal unity of being (Emerson 1841). His disciples were also intended to help Emerson transform American culture, as he described in his address *The American Scholar* in 1837, which began what is now known as the American Renaissance.

Emerson's transcendentalism split the liberals in the community from the conservatives, such as Emerson's most outspoken opponents, Nathaniel Frothingham and Andrews Norton (Miller 1957). These opponents doubted Emerson's notion of innate ideas and the self-evident nature of truth to each individual, preferring to rely on the Bible and church traditions. Nevertheless, many people were drawn to Emerson by virtue of his outstanding intellect and charismatic authenticity as a lecturer. By 1867 he was internationally acclaimed as "the sage of Concord" and "the wisest man in America." Emerson was widely honored, including receiving an honorary doctorate and election as overseer of Harvard University.

Movements in psychosocial development always have at least four phases. The first phase is the *debut*, which is the starting point by the founder. The second phase is the initial *diffusion* to others, who are close and faithful disciples of the founder. The third phase is a broader *popular spread* to a larger number of participants in which the movement is most well known to the general public although usually with less commitment than the original disciples. The fourth and final phase is the *stagnation* or *end* of the movement. In each of these phases are different influences that may facilitate or block the further growth of self-aware consciousness. We will see that the development of self-aware consciousness involves a variety of relationships, including the founder, other people, and the world as a whole, just as there are three dimensions of the movement of self-aware consciousness and three dimensions of mental self-government. Accordingly, we will begin by studying the life experiences of the founder and then his relationships with his disciples.

The historical record that made the following study possible is enormous. For example, Emerson kept a personal journal with regular entries from the time he was seventeen years old until he was more than seventy-two years old. Following Emerson's example and encouragement, many of his disciples also kept journals, in addition to extensive records of letters, lectures, and published works of literature. This made it possible to evaluate the same events and relationships through the eyes of multiple observers over many years. Here I will only summarize the essential observations that describe the psychological development of Emerson and his disciples, to illustrate a systematic method of describing thought and human relations, which I began describing in Chapter 3. The materials used in creating the ratings of thought and relationships are well-documented records, so interested readers may deepen their understanding of the method through direct comparison of my ratings with the quotations, published works, and cited historical records. I believe that the analyses described here add psychological depth to the already extensive biographical studies of the American transcendentalists. However, some readers may only want to see an illustration of the clinical approach or to better understand the variables that facilitate or obstruct the development of self-awareness in its social context or to see what is a typical course of personality change after an illuminating experience. The same analysis serves all of these purposes.

## The early life of Ralph Waldo Emerson

Major public events in the life of Ralph Waldo Emerson are summarized in Table 4.1. Waldo, the second of five sons of a Unitarian Minister, was born in Boston. Tuberculosis was pandemic at the time and claimed the lives of Emerson's father, two brothers, first wife, and later his most outstanding disciple, Henry Thoreau. Emerson himself had tuberculosis, which required him to travel to warmer areas for rest before his first marriage, when he was twenty-six years old. After his father's early death, his mother took in boarders to support the family and continued to emphasize the importance of education. She managed for all of her sons to graduate from Harvard College except for one who was mentally retarded.

Waldo was encouraged to become a Unitarian minister by his father's sister Mary, who wanted the Emerson line of ministers to continue. Mary Moody Emerson was nicknamed the "angel of death" because she was a highly religious eccentric who always dressed in black, symbolizing her readiness for death. She had been a Calvinist but described herself as an "Arian" in her beliefs, providing an example of free-thinking Unitarianism. Aunt Mary served as a muse to Waldo until he married. She encouraged his love of everything intellectual and religious but related to him in an autocratic manner. The autocratic relationship with his "angel of death" became Emerson's model of friendship. He thought that a friend should serve an adversarial role "forever a sort of beautiful enemy, untamable, devoutly revered, and not a trivial conveniency to be soon outgrown and cast aside" (Baker 1996, page xiv). Hence, Emerson saw friends as engaged in a noble dialectic of thesis, antithesis, and synthesis, pushing them ever onward toward truth and happiness. Emerson had a need for social warmth and approval; that is, he was moderately high in Reward Dependence. However, he often restrained this because of his shyness and his autocratic style of relating to many, but not all, people.

All of his life, Emerson would struggle with the conflicts between his need for social recognition and approval on the one hand and his need for solitude and privacy on the other hand. Emerson's emphasis on self-reliance was a way of asserting that he could not be rejected "because he held the universe within himself" in the words of Virginia Woolf (Richardson 1995, page 95). In Emerson's case, however, the recognition of the "infinitude of the private man" was not just a way of overcoming neurotic conflicts. His recognition of the infinitude of the psyche arose from awareness in contemplation of oceanic feelings, as we shall see later.

**Table 4.1.** Chronology of Major Public Events in the Life of Ralph Waldo Emerson

| Year | Event |
|---|---|
| 1803 | Born in Boston, May 25, second of five sons |
| 1813 | Father, William, a Unitarian minister, dies; mother, Ruth takes in boarders for income |
| 1813–1817 | At Boston Latin School |
| 1817–1821 | At Harvard College, graduates thirtieth of fifty-nine |
| 1821–1828 | Teaching and studying at Harvard Divinity |
| 1829 | Pastor at 2nd Church of Boston; married to Ellen Tucker |
| 1831 | Death of his wife from tuberculosis in February |
| 1832 | Resigned pastorate in September; sails for Europe in December |
| 1833 | Returned from Europe in October |
| 1834 | Death of younger brother Edward from tuberculosis |
| 1835 | Married to second wife, Lidian, in September; resided in Concord and resumed preaching and lecturing to support wife, mother, and family in November |
| 1836 | Brother Charles died in May. *Nature* published in September. Son Waldo born in October. |
| 1837 | Gave Phi Beta Kappa address at Harvard University (*The American Scholar*) |
| 1838 | Gave *Harvard Divinity School Address* (July 15) |
| 1839 | Called "infidel" by conservative Harvard theologians; daughter Ellen born |
| 1841 | Published *Essays. First Series* (*Self-Reliance, Over-Soul*); daughter Edith born |
| 1842 | Son Waldo died. Edits *Dial* (1842–1844) |
| 1844 | Published *Essays. Second Series* (*The Poet*); son Edward born |
| 1847 | Published *Poems*. Made second visit to Europe. |
| 1850 | Published *Representative Men* |
| 1853 | Mother, who still lived with him, died |
| 1856 | Published *English Traits* |
| 1859 | Retarded brother Bulkeley died |
| 1860 | Published *Conduct of Life* |
| 1863 | Aunt Mary died |
| 1867 | Published *May Day* (poems). Received honorary doctorate at Harvard University and elected overseer of University |
| 1868 | Older brother William died |
| 1870 | Published *Society and Solitude* |
| 1871 | House burned; made third visit to Europe |
| 1872 | Published *Letters and Social Aims* |
| 1882 | Died at Concord on April 27 |
| 1892 | Wife Lidian died |

The role of minister in the Emerson line fell to Waldo when his older brother William decided to become a lawyer and his younger brother Edward gave up the ministry after studying the newly emerging biblical criticism in Germany. Edward also had many features of bipolar mood disorder. His mood varied from "preternatural energy" to sad withdrawal, and he was hospitalized at McLean Asylum in Charleston for a "nervous breakdown" in which he was first unable to work because of fainting and anxiety. After a month Edward became "violently deranged," requiring physical restraint. The mentally retarded brother, Bulkeley, was also irritable, loud, and episodically overtalkative, requiring recurrent hospitalization at McLean Asylum.

As a young man, Waldo Emerson was vulnerable to feelings of inadequcy and discouragement. He was usually shy, reserved, and cautious—moderately harm avoidant. For example, when he proposed to his second wife, Lidian, he wrote a letter rather than speaking to her directly. He explained that in the "gravest acts" of his life he always trusted more to his pen than his tongue (Baker 1996, page 37). He frequently ruminated about decisions. With his twenty-first birthday approaching while teaching and studying at Harvard Divinity School, he continued to ruminate in his journal about whether to pursue theology or literature as a profession. At this time, he felt sad and self-deprecating, weak, worthless, and sometimes inferior. In an overly critical mood, he regarded himself as weak in reasoning, indolent, self-indulgent, and lacking in social warmth. He was also keenly aware of his strong need for recognition: "Shall I embroil my short life with a vain desire of perpetuating its memory when I am dead and gone in this dirty planet?" (Emerson 1960–82, Volume 2, page 231, March 1824). Emerson's conflict between pride versus feelings of inferiority would plague him throughout his life. As a step toward resolution of this conflict, he decided to become a minister based on a commitment to growth in self-awareness. On making this decision, his mood immediately improved along with his sense of self-direction.

While studying the Bible in divinity school, he continued to read widely and passionately in philosophy and literature (Richardson 1995). At this time, the Harvard Divinity School was dominated by Unitarian ideas, but Emerson was even more liberal than the Unitarian faculty. Emerson was intensely curious and exploratory of all that was new, but this was primarily expressed in his intellectual pursuits, presumably because of his high intelligence and his high harm avoidance. One of his earliest friends, Dr. William H. Furness, wrote about Emerson that "I don't think he ever engaged in boys' plays; not because of any physical inability, but simply because, from his earliest years, he dwelt in a higher sphere. My one deep impression is, that, from his earliest childhood, our friend lived and moved and had his being in an atmosphere of letters, quite apart by himself" (Emerson and Forbes 1914, Volume 1, page 2).

Emerson's intellectual interests were broad. Although Unitarianism was founded on Locke's ideas and a philosophy of rational materialism, Emerson was actively examining the ideas of many positive philosophers (e.g., Plato, Montaigne, and

Augustine), rational idealists (e.g., Kant, Coleridge), and mystics like Swedenborg. He was particularly impressed by Coleridge's *Aids to Reflection* and integrated the ideas of Plato and Montaigne into those of Coleridge, who emphasized the distinction between understanding (i.e., intellect) and reason (i.e., rational intuition). From Coleridge, he recognized that reason is intuitive (Richardson 1995, page 104). Even in divinity school, Emerson was interested in the Bible only as an example for emulation in writing his own ideas, rather than as a sacred object of study. He was highly rationalistic and skeptical of the "frivolous mythology" and "gross superstition" in the Bible. Nevertheless, after he was 21 years old he closed the school where he had been teaching and took up residence at the divinity school to complete his studies.

Early in his time at divinity school, Emerson's reliance on rationality was threatened by the radical skepticism of the negative philosopher David Hume. Emerson found the answer to his doubts about how to reconcile materialism and idealism in reading the works of the hopeful skeptic and positive philosopher Montaigne. Montaigne's *Apology for Raimonde de Sebonde* was a defense of both natural theology and Christianity. According to Montaigne, human beings are an integral part of the universal natural order and awareness of this unity and reality inspires awe and reverence, and leads to wisdom and well-being. After reading *The Essays of Montaigne*, Emerson said, "No book before or since was ever so much to me as that" (Richardson 1995, page 69). Montaigne's message expressed Emerson's thought so well that he wrote, "It seemed to me as if I had written the book myself in some former life" (Emerson 1889, page 29).

Emerson was consciously eager to accept and assimilate Montaigne's positive philosophy as his own, thereby elevating his own thoughts and eliminating the problems caused by Hume's negative philosophy. After assimilating Montaigne's uplifting message, Emerson confided to his Aunt Mary on June 15, 1826, that "I know that I exist, and that a part of me, as essential as Memory or Reason, is a desire that another being exist" (Emerson and Forbes 1914, Volume 2, page 105). A growing awareness of the positive philosophy provided Emerson with a foundation of certainty on which his self-awareness and faith would develop rationally and authentically.

## Emerson as lecturer and pastor

Emerson was initially self-conscious about lecturing. He carefully studied style and decided that he would always speak with certainty based on his personal experience, rather than relying on external authority. In this way, he cultivated an outstanding oratorical manner, becoming an eloquent and charismatic speaker. According to a typical description,

> The originality of his thoughts, the consummate beauty of the language in which
> they were clothed, the calm dignity of his bearing, the absence of all oratorical ef-

fect, and the singular directness and simplicity of his manner, free from the least shadow of dogmatic assumption, made a deep impression on me. . . . His voice was the sweetest, the most winning and penetrating of any I ever heard. (Baker 1996)

Many people who heard Emerson speak were "lifted to higher thoughts" by listening to his philosophical idealism (Baker 1996).

His reputation as a lecturer and preacher resulted in his being offered the pastorate at the Second (Unitarian) Church of Boston when he was twenty-six years old. His father had been the pastor at the First Church of Boston, but Reverend Nathaniel Frothingham already held that position. The pastorate would provide the steady financial support much needed by Emerson's family. Waldo had become the principal supporter of his extended family, caring for his mother and mentally retarded brother and assuming the role of patriarch vacant since the death of his father "in whose stead Waldo has risen up." The role of pastor represented professional success and financial security, but it also represented restraint on his intellectual curiosity and freedom. Waldo described his ordination to his brother William as the approach of his "execution day."

Although Emerson was an eloquent speaker, he was not good at pastoral work. He was charismatic when speaking from the pulpit or lectern, and he could be charming and courteous in social settings. He was considerate of others, but he was never effective at pastoral work because he had difficulty communicating social warmth in most intimate situations (Richardson 1995, page 90). Consequently, he preferred the solitude of his private study to pastoral work and social interaction despite his need for social approval and recognition.

While preaching in 1827, he impressed the sixteen-year-old Ellen Tucker with his eloquence and charm. Ellen was pretty, open, lively, and warm; she loved nature and people; and she thought that she had a gift for poetry. They met, were engaged within a year, and married in 1829. The relationship with the vivacious Ellen brought out the warmth in Waldo's personality, similar to the effect that some other women (e.g., Margaret Fuller and Caroline Sturgis) would have on him after Ellen's death of tuberculosis in 1831. For example, Ellen Sturgis dedicated a poem to Waldo describing him as a cool intellectual, lacking the heat of social warmth—a "dry lighted soul" whose "blood doth miss the heat which ofttimes breeds excess" (Sturgis 1957). Emerson would struggle with his needs to restrain excess and his needs for warmth and approval throughout his entire life.

Ellen died in February of 1831 from chronic tuberculosis. Waldo had felt a strong love and fidelity for Ellen. The relationship with Ellen brought out Emerson's capacity for sympathy with others (Baker 1996, page 98). When she died, he wrote, "The aroma of my life is gone like the flower with which it came" (Emerson and Forbes 1914, Volume 2, page 388, June 20, 1831). On her deathbed, Ellen lovingly told Waldo that she could do him "more good by going than by staying" (Baker 1996, page 11). In fact, her estate provided Emerson with independent income throughout the rest of his life, which gave him the freedom to pursue his work as a lecturer and writer with a secure financial foundation.

Within two years of Ellen's death, Emerson resigned his pastorate because he could not accept the ritual practice of communion. This disagreement was not merely a casual intellectual disagreement. Ever since reading Montaigne, Emerson had felt that every moment should be a prayer in celebration of life and that "all that can be done for you is nothing to what you can do for yourself" (Richardson 1995, page 69). He felt that people should commune with life at all times, not in an artificial ritual that depended on a minister as intermediary. After careful reflection, Emerson resigned his pastorate over this issue in September 1832.

After resigning his pastorate, he made responsible provisions for his family and set sail for Europe on Christmas Day, 1832. Because Emerson was now financially independent (Myerson 1995, page 31), he literally left the weights of his emotional and spiritual past behind him on his voyage. The visit to Europe would open a new door in his consciousness, bringing about the debut of the American Transcendentalist Movement.

In terms of average or usual personality traits, Waldo Emerson can be described as having a sensitive temperament with many conflicts throughout his life. Emerson was "conscientious to a fault, ever vigilant, always considerate" (Baker 1996, page 13). In other words, he was high in all four temperaments (Harm Avoidance, Novelty Seeking, Reward Dependence, and Persistence), which gave him a complex set of emotional conflicts. Specifically, Emerson had a persistent conflict between pride and inferiority, which was related to his being high in both Novelty Seeking and Harm Avoidance. In addition, he had a prominent and persistent conflict between his needs for recognition and solitude, which was related to his being high in both Harm Avoidance and Reward Dependence. Emerson also had a conflict between liberal innovation and conservative tradition, which was related to his being high in both Novelty Seeking and Reward Dependence. Nevertheless, Emerson regulated his emotional conflicts fairly well most of the time throughout his life, and the coherence of his character increased in a stepwise manner as he matured. He was average in character development during college except that he was more introspective than most people. He had grown in self-directedness by age twenty-two in 1825, when he felt a clearer calling to the ministry. After his experiences in Europe at age thirty in 1833, he had become a creative character who was more fully developed in all three dimensions of character than most people. Nevertheless, Emerson suffered from his conflict between feelings of superiority and inferiority throughout his life. In coping with this major conflict, Emerson emphasized particular aspects of his character to varying degrees. Specifically, Emerson took particular pride in his self-directedness, which he described as self-reliance. He regarded "the infinitude of the private man" as his gospel. He preferred to look inwardly rather than outwardly for inspiration. In other words, he was less cooperative than he was self-directed and self-transcendent in most situations as a mature adult.

Such a sketch of Emerson or any person does not fully describe the unique variability in personality and thought at different times and situations or in different interpersonal relationships. The same person may have qualitatively different patterns of thought, feeling, and action with different people at the same time. Furthermore, the thoughts and relationships of a person may vary over time; the description of someone's usual personality traits is merely an average that provides an approximate beginning to a full description of people and the path of their self-aware consciousness.

Sometimes we supplement these averages traits by adding descriptions of episodes of depression or other problems when they become prominent, such as changes in interpersonal relationships or major events like the death of a wife or conflicts with friends and associates. However, the actual structure of thought is much more dynamic and multidimensional than can be explained by average traits supplemented by episodes of disorder. When a thorough description of Emerson's thought and relationships is made, we will see that his range of thoughts and relationships was stable throughout his life except for one permanent change after his "illumination" when he was thirty years old.

## MEASURING EMERSON'S THOUGHTS

Fortunately, the limitations of traditional personality assessment can be overcome in our assessment of Emerson and the transcendentalist movement. The development of Emerson's thoughts across most of his lifespan can be examined in a wealth of detail in the personal journals he kept from 1820 through 1875. The basis for assessment can also be expanded to include his extensive correspondence, lectures and sermons, and publications. Collateral accounts by others can also be compared with what Emerson himself recorded.

The chronology of Emerson's thoughts is summarized in Table 4.2 for the even years from 1820 (age seventeen) through 1874 (age seventy-one) using the measuring system for rating thought described in Chapter 3. The qualitative descriptions of thought are presented in Tables 3.3 and 3.4 and related text. The quantitative descriptions of thought are shown in the Appendix on measurement of thought. At Harvard College, his average thoughts reflected his identification of himself as a purposeful and industrious person. At age sixteen as a junior at Harvard College, he already foresaw his future as an eloquent pulpit orator.

> Let us suppose a pulpit Orator to whom the path of his profession is yet untried, but whose talents are good and feelings strong, and his independence, as a man, in opinion and action is established. . . . Let him come to them in solemnity and strength, and when he speaks he will claim attention with an interesting figure and an interested face. (Emerson and Forbes 1914, Volume 1, page 14, February 1820)

**Table 4.2.** Chronology of Mean and Range of Ralph Waldo Emerson's Thoughts as Recorded in His Journals for the Even Years from 1820 (Age Seventeen) through 1874 (Age Seventy-One)

| Journal Year | Mean | Minimum | Maximum |
|---|---|---|---|
| COLLEGE | | | |
| 1820 | 3.9 [Powerful] | 2.9 [Confident] | 5.0 [Self-reliant] |
| DIVINITY SCHOOL | | | |
| 1822 | 3.9 | 3.1 [Obsessive] | 5.0 |
| 1824 | 3.9 | 3.1 | 5.1 [Purposeful] |
| 1826–28 | 3.9 | 3.1 | 5.2 [Helpful] |
| BOSTON PASTOR, DEATH OF WIFE | | | |
| 1830 | 3.9 | 3.0 [Shameful] | 5.4 [Conscientious] |
| 1832 | 3.8 [Power seeking] | 3.0 | 5.4 |
| CONCORD WRITER, LECTURER, SAGE | | | |
| 1834 | 4.0 [Sympathy seeking] | 3.5 [Curious] | 5.8 [Oceanic feelings] |
| 1836 | 4.1 [Approval seeking] | 3.6 [Inferior] | 5.8 |
| 1838–74 | 4.2 [Recognition seeking] | 3.6 | 5.8 |

Emerson's average thoughts from the beginning of his journal until 1932 are rated as 3.9, indicating his personal sense of power and purpose. In Table 3.3, this rating corresponds to the descriptor of subplane 3–7, "power versus sarcasm," as well as the descriptions for 3.9 in the Appendix. The applicable descriptor of purposefulness for Emerson is "power," because he is high in Novelty Seeking, whereas "sarcasm" is characteristic of purposeful thought at the same level in individuals who are low in Novelty Seeking.

In addition to measuring average thoughts, we need to know the range of a person's thoughts during a particular period. The range of thought is defined by the maximum and minimum thoughts. In college, Emerson's most elevated thoughts involved his rationalistic thinking and ambition to establish his identity and self-sufficiency through the use of his rationality rather than dependence on emotionality or mysticism. Therefore, his maximum thoughts are rated as 5.0, which is summarized as "self-reliant" in Table 4.2. In Table 3.3, 5.0 corresponds to "self-directedness" in subplane 5–2, and in the Appendix this level of thought is usually described as "need for self-sufficiency and sense of identity." For example, in college Emerson's view of the bounds of the intellect was that of a rational materialist, not a transcendentalist:

> It is a singular fact that we cannot present to the imagination a longer space than just so much of the world as is bounded by the visible horizon; so that, even in this stretching of thought to comprehend the broad path lengthening itself and widening to receive the rolling Universe, stern necessity bounds us to a little extent of a few miles only. (Emerson and Forbes 1914, February 1820, Volume 1, page 13)

In contrast, his minimum thoughts recorded in his journal in college involve his romantic fantasies of honor and chaste virtue as a scholar. On March 11, 1820, he described his elevated sexual fantasy of his literary investigations, which is rated as 2.9:

> Could I seat myself in the alcove of one of those public libraries which human pride and literary rivalship have made costly, splendid and magnificent, it would indeed be an enviable situation. I would plunge into the classic lore of chivalrous story and of fairy-land bards, and unclosing the ponderous volumes of the firmest believers in magic and in the potency of consecrated crosier or elfin ring, I would let my soul sail away delighted into their wildest phantasies. . . . I stand in the fair assembly of the chosen, the brave and the beautiful; honour and virtue, courage and delicacy are mingling in magnificent joy. Unstained knighthood is sheathing the successful blade in the presence of unstained chastity. (Emerson and Forbes 1914, Volume 1, pages 18–19)

Such grandiose and romantic fantasy is elevated to the spiritual subplane of sexuality (i.e., subplane 2–7), but the sexual nature of the imagery is clear. In Table 4.2, the term "confident" (thought level 2.9) is used to refer to such exhibitionistic fantasy, but individual words are merely incomplete labels for the distinctions being made about intuitions that cannot be fully reduced to words.

From a methodological perspective, ratings of thoughts are guided by comparing the content of personal statements, such as journal entries, with the content of the qualitative descriptors in Table 3.4 and more detailed quantitative descriptors in the appendix on measurement of thought. However, the rater cannot simply depend on intellectual interpretation of the words alone. The ratings require an intuitive awareness of thoughts, not just an intellectual judgment. In making such ratings, we allow ourselves to enter into a transcendental (i.e., sympathetic and transpersonal) relationship using our rational intuition so that we can directly experience or recollect the thought of the communicator in our own being. Using the distinction of Kant and later Coleridge, such measurement is based on reason (i.e., rational intuition) rather than merely understanding (i.e., intellect). When making ratings, we need to be beyond the first stage of self-awareness; we need to be calm, impartial, and patient to recollect the thoughts and feelings of those with whom we really communicate (see Table 3.10). Possible examples of rational intuitive communication include compassionate listening to our patients, sympathetic listening to music, vicarious enjoyment of reading books, or, in this case, intuitively reading journals and other historical records.

To evaluate the reliability and validity of measurement of thoughts as recorded by Emerson and his associates, I carried out a systematic study to determine whether my ratings were reproducible by others.

## RELIABILITY AND VALIDITY OF MEASURING THOUGHT

The method for the diagnosis of the frequency of thought (DFT) was taught to a group of thirty native English speakers. They were healthy college graduates who were interested in the development of increased self-awareness through a deeper understanding of the measurement of human thought. They learned about the DFT in a seminar over two days, much as described in chapter 3.

After training, the thirty measurers were given a set of twenty quotations drawn primarily from the writings of the American transcendentalists but also including individuals quoted by them, such as Montaigne. They were told only that the possible range of the quotations was from 2.0 to 7.9, omitting 6.0 to 6.9 as described in Chapter 3. The twenty quotations were each rated independently by the thirty raters. There was no set time limitation because they were encouraged to be calm, impartial, and patient, as is expected in the second or third stage of self-aware consciousness. Nevertheless, the ratings were completed in less than one hour by each measurer. Most contemporary psychologists would describe the process as "coding," but I will use the term "measuring" to emphasize that the precise assessments require a person to use their rational intuition as an internal standard of measurement.

The measurers were independently rated by me on their level of serenity, which was quantified by mental status examination of the degree of calmness and appropriateness of affect of each person at the beginning of the measurement period. Serenity was rated independent of any information about their DFT measurements, which were collected independently by my associate.

This design allowed me to compute the correlation between my ratings of the quotations, which I will designate as the standard, and those of the thirty other measurers. This procedure provided a test of bias in the standard in comparison to the mean ratings of the other measurers, as well as a test of the individual measurers in relation to the standard. It was possible to take into account the serenity of the measurer and the putative level of the thought of the quotation according to the standard.

The distribution of the correlation between the thirty measurers with the standard is shown in Figure 4.1. The range of correlation with the standard was 0.32 to 0.95. All except four of the thirty measurers correlated with the standard 0.7 or better, which is considered "strong" agreement in clinical reliability studies. The most frequent level of agreement was .85 to .89 (sixteen of thirty individuals).

The relationship between the serenity of the measurers and their correlation with the standard is shown in Table 4.3. More serene measurers had closer agreement with the standard.

The possibility of a consistent pattern of bias (high or low values) across the twenty quotations was evaluated in relation to the serenity of the measurers. The overall bias, which was computed as the difference between the measure and the standard, was negligible (−0.1) overall. The percentage of those who were biased increased as serenity decreased, as shown in Table 4.4. One of the ten most serene was biased, compared with half of the least serene.

The possibility of a consistent pattern of bias depending on the level of the standard was also examined. There was a slight tendency to overrate quotations in planes 2 or 3 and to underrate quotations in higher planes, as shown in Table 4.5. However, overall there was a negligible bias between the standard and other measurements across all thirty measurers and all twenty quotations.

These results indicate that thought can be reliably measured as described here. The agreement of the standard with mean measurements of thirty independent measurements also supports the ordinal ranking of thought across the five planes described in Chapter 3.

Learning to measure is similar to learning to play a musical instrument. Substantial progress can be made by nearly everyone in a short time, and further

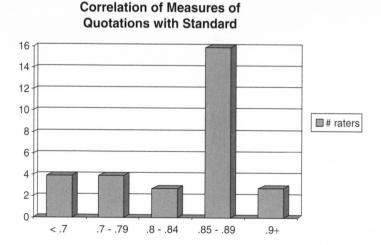

Figure 4.1. Distribution of correlation of individual measurers with the standard for all quotations.

**Table 4.3.** Correlation of DFT Measures of Twenty Quotations by Thirty Independent Raters with the Standard According to an Independent Rating of the Serenity of the Measurer

| Serenity of Measurer | No. of Measurers | Correlation with Standard | | | |
|---|---|---|---|---|---|
| | | Mean | SD | Minimum | Maximum |
| High | 10 | .88 | .03 | .86 | .95 |
| Intermediate | 10 | .84 | .06 | .74 | .91 |
| Low | 10 | .72 | .19 | .32 | .90 |
| Total | 30 | .81 | .13 | .32 | .95 |

progress depends on various differences between individuals and on practice. In the case of measurement, the development of coherence of personality and serenity of the psyche is an important variable, which depends on personal work to grow in depth of self-aware consciousness. Fortunately, work on understanding the measurement and movement of thought is helpful in developing self-awareness.

Emerson and the other transcendentalists were skilled communicators in their prose and poetry, so much of the "life" or "spirit" of their thought is conveyed in their poetic choice of descriptors. Hence, it is both feasible and fitting to apply a system for transcendental measurement (i.e., measurement based on rational intuition) to the study of the American transcendentalists. In fact, the goal of Emerson and the other transcendentalists was to draw on nature as the source of effective imagery and appropriate language for communicating through rational intuition in writing and speech. Likewise, the method of rating thought that I am describing here is based on a natural lexicon of rational intuition. The best way to learn to use such a lexicon is to immerse oneself in it, as when learning a language or a musical instrument.

Remember that the maximum level of thoughts that Emerson recorded in his journal during college involved rationalistic self-reliance, which is rated as 5.0, involving thoughts in subplane 5–2. Remember also from Chapter 3 that there are five planes and five subplanes within each of these; therefore, on a decimal

**Table 4.4.** Mean Bias of Raters on Twenty Quotes (i.e., Estimate – standard) by Serenity of Rater

| Serenity of Measurer | No. of Measurers | Raw Deviation from Standard | | | | |
|---|---|---|---|---|---|---|
| | | Mean | Minimum | Maximum | SD | Biased (%) |
| High | 10 | 0.1 | −0.2 | +0.6 | 0.8 | 10 |
| Intermediate | 10 | 0.0 | −0.6 | +0.5 | 0.9 | 30 |
| Low | 10 | −0.3 | −1.1 | +1.2 | 1.0 | 50 |
| Total | 30 | −0.1 | −1.1 | +1.2 | 1.0 | 30 |

Biased = significantly different from zero.

**Table 4.5.** Deviation of Measures for Each Quotation from Standard for All Respondents (i.e., Estimate − Standard) According to the Level of Standard, Showing Negligible Bias from Standard Overall

| Level of Standard | No. of Quotes | Mean Bias for Quotes Across All Raters | |
|---|---|---|---|
| | | Mean of Means | Mean of SDs |
| 2.0–2.9 | 3 | 0.6 | 0.6 |
| 3.0–3.9 | 4 | 0.4 | 0.8 |
| 4.0–4.9 | 5 | −0.4 | 0.8 |
| 5.0–5.9 | 4 | −0.4 | 1.0 |
| 7.0–7.9 | 4 | −0.4 | 0.9 |
| 2.0–7.9 | 20 | −0.1 | 0.8 |

system from .0 to .9, the integer refers to the plane and the decimal point refers to degree of elevation in the subplanes. The lowest level of plane 5 is designated as 5.0, where 5 refers to plane 5 (intellect) and .0 refers to the lower half of the lowest subplane (i.e., rational materialism).

## MEASURING EMERSON'S SOCIAL RELATIONS

### Emerson's illumination

As shown in the ratings of his journal entries in Table 4.2, Emerson's average thoughts increased from 3.9 in college to 4.2 by 1838 (age thirty-five years) and stabilized at that level. In other words, Emerson's average thoughts throughout his adult life after the success of his first book in 1836 involved his conflict between the needs for recognition and privacy. His book *Society and Solitude* refers precisely to this conflict. In fact, Emerson was internationally acclaimed, which served to satisfy his continuing need for recognition. During 1832, there was a transient drop in average thoughts to 3.8 ("power seeking") during the period of conflict with his church about communion, but this improved after his resignation and visit to Europe during 1833 (see in Table 4.1).

Emerson's maximum thoughts rose slightly in steps from 5.0 to 5.2 during his divinity training, as he became more idealistic and less materialistic in his assumptions about rationality. This rise began in 1824 when his faith increased and he decided to enter divinity school full time, as discussed earlier in sketching his early life. Then, as a regular preacher and pastor, his maximum thoughts entered the second stage of self-awareness, as he began more consistently to observe his own thoughts in a calm and impartial manner. His maximum thoughts are rated as 5.4 during the period from 1830 to 1832 before his trip to Europe. He was conscientious and growing in self-awareness, as he meditated on the meaning of communion. This eventually led him to resign his pastorate out of conscience. He then conscientiously arranged provisions for his family and made arrangements for himself to continue his growth in awareness by a visit to Europe.

While Emerson was visiting the Garden of Plants (Jardin des Plantes) in Paris on July 13, 1833, he had an illuminating realization that had a profound impact on his thought immediately and ever afterwards. The effect of the visit was a transformation or awakening of contemplative thought. The Jardin des Plantes was a botanical garden that had been managed by three successive generations of one family, the Jussieus, from the middle of the eighteenth century to the middle of the nineteenth century. The exhibits in the botanical garden were organized according to the natural system of classification of plants of Antoine Laurent de Jussieu (1748–1836). There was an excellent Cabinet (i.e., museum) of Natural History within the Garden. In Emerson's words,

> How much finer things are in composition than alone. It is wise for man to make cabinets. . . . The Garden itself is admirably arranged. They have attempted to classify all the plants *in the ground*, to put together, that is, as nearly as may be, the conspicuous plants on each class on Jussieu's system. (Emerson and Forbes 1914)

The proximity of arrangement implied evolutionary connections, which elevated Emerson's thoughts and stimulated the wish that he change from a minister to a naturalist. Emerson reported, "I say continually, 'I will be a naturalist.'"

Emerson's thoughts were uplifted as he experienced oceanic feelings. Entering the third stage of self-aware consciousness, he had transient awareness of plenitude, providence, and unity, as described in the upward spiral of thoughts in Chapter 3. He recorded the experience of his thoughts being elevated by the pleasant awareness of the abundance of life. This pleasant growth in awareness is what Teilhard de Chardin later called the "sense of plenitude" (1978), which elevates thought like a light in darkness. For example, regarding his visit contemplating the displays in the museum of natural history in the Garden, he recorded

> Here we are impressed with the inexhaustible riches of nature. The Universe is a more amazing puzzle than ever as you glance along this bewildering series of animated forms, the hazy butterflies, the carved shells, the birds, beasts, fishes, insects, snakes, and the upheaving principle of life everywhere incipient in the very rock aping organized forms. (Emerson and Forbes 1914)

Emerson also experienced the broadening of the width of his consciousness as a calmness and trust in the benevolence and order of Providence, which Teilhard de Chardin later called the "sense of convergence" (1978), which creates strong social bonds like strong nuclear forces bind material particles. He said, "It is very pleasant to walk in this garden" (Emerson and Forbes 1914). Furthermore, in describing the lightness of his mood in the exhibit of birds in the garden, Emerson recorded

> When I was come into the Ornithological Chambers I wished I had come only there. The fancy-coloured vests of these elegant beings made me as pensive as the hues and forms of a cabinet of shells, formerly. It is a beautiful collection and makes the visitor as calm and genial as a bridegroom. The limits of the possible are enlarged, and the real is stranger than the imaginary.

The analogy to "a bridegroom" is frequent in contemplative literature (e.g., St. John of the Cross, St. Teresa of Avila). At such times, consciousness is filled with the hope, kindness, and faith of a person newly entering—and growing in awareness of—an ocean of love. Hence, Emerson also experienced an increased depth of consciousness as a loving bond or sympathy that connects all things as free but integral parts of the universal unity of being. This increased depth of consciousness is what Teilhard de Chardin later called the "unitive sense" (1978), which attracts the psyche like gravity attracts matter. Emerson recorded

> Not a form so grotesque, so savage, nor so beautiful but is an expression of some property inherent in man the observer,—an occult relation between the very scorpions and man. I feel the centipede in me,—cayman, carp, eagle, and fox. I am moved by strange sympathies. . . .

Before coming to Paris, he had written in complaint to his Aunt Mary, "The wise man—the true friend—the finished character—we seek everywhere and only find in fragments. . . . I want instructors. God's greatest gift is a Teacher and when will he send me one, full of truth and of boundless benevolence and heroic sentiments" (Baker 1996, page 26). In Jussieu's Cabinet of Natural History in the Jardin des Plantes, Emerson met his teacher with the three qualities of fullness with truth, boundless benevolence, and heroic sentiments: "Ah! said I, this is philanthropy, wisdom, taste,—to form a cabinet of natural history" (Emerson and Forbes 1914).

In view of Emerson's family history suggestive of bipolar mood disorder and his own recurrent periods of low mood, it is important to point out that there is no indication that Emerson was manic or hypomanic at the time of his change in self-aware consciousness. There was no grandiosity, impulsiveness, or other signs of mania and excessive inflation of ego functions. Furthermore, the change in Emerson's self-aware consciousness was a permanent change, rather than an episodic event.

From his awakening in the Jardin des Plantes, Emerson took nature as his teacher. He began lecturing on natural science, recruiting disciples with similar interests, and in 1836 published his first book *Nature*, which announced to the world the vision of his newly transformed consciousness. After he returned from Europe, Emerson was aware that his conduct could best be guided by listening to his psyche, which he sometimes called his "inner light," as described by Quakers and most contemplative groups. More frequently, Emerson and the transcendentalists referred to awakening and listening to their "genius." Emerson had written before his visit to Europe, "No man can write well who thinks there is any choice of words for him. In writing there is always a right word, and every other word than that is wrong" (Emerson and Forbes 1914, July 8, 1831, Volume 3, page 401). After his illumination, Emerson recognized that listening to the psyche provided a means to live in intuitive awareness so that intellectual choice was unnecessary. He now saw that the way to truth was best recognized by each person listening to their psyche (i.e., spirit, inner light, inner voice), not the Bible or authorities of any church. "Can you believe, Waldo Emerson," he wrote, "that you may relieve yourself of this perpetual perplexity of choosing, and by putting your ear close to the soul, learn always the true way?" (Emerson and Forbes 1914, February 12, 1834, Volume 3, page 260)

By August 1835, Emerson had concluded in his journal that the study of nature alone was not adequate to satisfy the desire for beauty. "Natural history by itself has no value. It is like a single sex. But marry it to human history, and it is poetry . . . is truth at once." The same year Emerson explained his idea of a poet as living in choiceless awareness and harmony with the world. Writing to his future wife Lidian, he said: "Still am I a poet in the sense of a perceiver and a dear lover of the harmonies that are in the soul and in matter, and specially of the correspondences between these and those" (Emerson 1939, February 1, 1835, Volume 1, page 435). In 1836, in his first book *Nature*, he explained that nature both educates human beings and satisfies their need for beauty. As he expressed this concept in his first book, *Nature*, "The world thus exists to the soul to satisfy the desire for beauty. This element I call an ultimate end. No reason can be asked or given why the soul seeks beauty. Beauty, in its largest and profoundest sense, is our expression for the universe." The essential act of Emerson's ethical poet was the harmonious resonance between the psyche and nature, which resulted in the loving recognition of beauty by the intuitive senses.

In 1838 in his Harvard *Divinity School Address*, Emerson had concluded that human beings are born with memories that are recollected in later experience. The idea of recollection of innate ideas was not new. Originally Plato described recollection in *Phaedo* to explain the differences between people in their intuitive responses to experience (Plato 1986). According to Plato's view, what Emerson had experienced in the Jardin des Plantes was the awakening of dormant elevated memories. Other recollections of Emerson were clearly based on specific life events. For example, Emerson's poem *Earth and Sea* is based on an actual experience recorded in his May 16, 1834, journal entry about his visit to a beach as a boy. Emerson's notion of recollection in self-aware consciousness had to cover experiences such as he had in the Jardin des Plantes in which there was no known earlier life event and others in which there was an earlier life experience. The transcendentalist view of Emerson was based on the distinction of Kant between the ordinary consciousness of the intellect (the "mind") and the rational intuition of the psyche (the "heart" or "pure reason"). On May 16, 1834, recalling a childhood visit to the seashore, Emerson wrote in his journal (Emerson and Forbes

1914), "The sun illumines the eye of mind, but the eye and heart of the child. His heart is in the right place. Many eyes go through the meadow, but few see the flowers in it." In the words of transcendentalism, the self-aware consciousness of human beings "transcends" the finitude of the individual self when the poet's heart is pure in its love for the universal unity of being (i.e., when the "heart is in the right place"). Our rational intuition can be purified by the mind growing in awareness of itself. Such thinking about thought is the second stage of self-aware consciousness, which involves calm and patient listening to the psyche. Listening to the psyche opens the door to the superconsciousness of each person's psyche, which Emerson called the "infinitude of the private man."

It is noteworthy that Emerson chose the term "private" man because privacy has a dual meaning. Privacy or being alone can refer to a feeling of isolation and separate alienation. It can also refer to the seeking of awareness of universal unity of being by quieting the mind's distractions by external attachments so that we become aware of our infinitude. Emerson was hopeful that his method would improve his life. On May 5, 1838, he commented,

> I complain in my own experience of the feeble influence of thought on life, a ray as pale and ineffectual as that of the sun in our cold and bleak spring. . . . It takes a great deal of elevation of thought to produce a very little elevation of life. How slowly the highest raptures of the intellect break through the trivial forms of habit. Yet imperceptibly they do. Gradually, in long years, we bend our living toward our idea. . . . (Emerson and Forbes 1914)

Emerson's recognition of the genius and light of intuition made it possible for him to emphasize self-reliance while maintaining a reverence for the divine in all things. In the Jardin des Plantes in 1833, Emerson saw that the divinity and unity of the "upheaving principle of life" was abundantly expressed in the "inexhaustible riches of nature." By 1839, when transcendentalism was at its "full dawn," Emerson was asked to describe his religion by a relative, David Haskins. He replied that he was "more of a Quaker than anything else. I believe in the 'still small voice' and that voice is Christ within us" (Haskins 1887, page 118). Emerson's new acceptance of the divinity of Christ was a radical departure from his earlier Unitarianism, which had denied the infinitude of Christ and need for Christ as the link between mankind and God. Jesus and other human beings could be fully one with the infinity of all things under only one condition—if and only if all things were integral aspects of the universal unity of being. Hence, when Emerson was also asked to describe the core idea of Transcendentalism around the same time, he wrote,

> In all my lectures, I have taught one doctrine, namely, the infinitude of the private man. This the people accept readily enough, and even with loud commendation, as long as I call the lecture Art; or Politics; or Literature; or The Household; but the

moment I call it Religion,—they are shocked, though it be only the application of the same truth. (Baker 1996, pages 136–137)

A more detailed analysis of Emerson's thoughts before, during, and after his visit to the Jardin des Plantes is presented in Table 4.6. For this analysis, Emerson's journals were supplemented with records of his letters, sermons, lectures, and publications. In this more detailed DFT, the average and range of thoughts are examined within each of the five planes of thought. In other words, variability is described among those thoughts that involved each particular plane. For example, consider plane 5 (intellectual thoughts) before the illumination. Emerson's thoughts before the visit to Europe in plane 5 usually involved his being helpful, which is rated as 5.2. His minimum thoughts in this plane involved his need for rationalistic control or the struggle to be intellectually self-sufficient, which is rated as 5.0. His maximum thoughts in plane 5 involved being meditative, which is rated as 5.6. In plane 7 (coherence or spirituality), all his thoughts are at 7.0, which means that he is a perfectionist who is seeking spiritual mastery when he has spiritual thoughts at all. Essentially, Emerson's goal in life at this point was to write his own bible or to found his own religion.

The global maximum of 5.4 is the overall average of the maximum thoughts in the five planes. For example, in 1830 Emerson's most elevated thoughts are about being conscientious, which is level 5.4. On June 2, 1830, he wrote,

**Table 4.6.** Ralph Waldo Emerson's Thoughts Before, During, and After His Illumination during His Visit to the Botanical Garden in Paris on July 13, 1833, Based on His Journals and Other Available Sources: DFT

|  | *Plane of Thought Frequency* | | | | | | |
|  | *2* | *3* | *4* | *5* | *7* | *Global* | *Descriptor* |
|---|---|---|---|---|---|---|---|
| A. DFT IN EARLY 1833 BEFORE ILLUMINATION | | | | | | | |
| Average | .4 | .4 | .5 | .2 | .0 | 3.8 | "Power seeking" |
| Maximum | .7 | .6 | .6 | .6 | .1 | 5.4 | "Conscientious" |
| Minimum | .2 | .1 | .0 | .0 | .0 | 3.2 | "Competitive" |
| B. DFT ON JULY 13, 1833, DURING ILLUMINATION | | | | | | | |
| Maximum | .7 | .7 | .7 | .8 | .2 | 5.8 | "Oceanic feelings" |
| C. DFT AFTER ILLUMINATION (TYPICAL 1834–1874) | | | | | | | |
| Average | .6 | .6 | .5 | .3 | .0 | 4.2 | "Recognition seeking" |
| Maximum | .7 | .7 | .7 | .8 | .2 | 5.8 | "Oceanic feelings" |
| Minimum | .3 | .3 | .1 | .1 | .0 | 3.6 | "Inferiority" |

Intelligence . . . knows when men speak in simplicity, and when they speak conventionally. . . . It needs also a tender conscience, which shall lead men to improve themselves, to keep the ear and soul open to receive truth, and then this straightforwardness
shall make them act and utter the truth. (Emerson and Forbes 1914)

Similar thoughts are typical of Emerson's elevated thinking at this time, so his
global maximum is measured as 5.4. However, in meditating on this theme, there
are infrequent thoughts at 5.6, which are noticeable when only intellectual thoughts
are examined. Consequently in the detailed DFT, Emerson's maximum in plane
5 is 5.6 in 1830. For example, on February 28, 1830, while meditating on "What
is prayer?" Emerson recorded in his journal a thought at 5.6 that God is "the most
elevated conception of character that can be formed in the mind. It is the
individual's own soul carried out to perfection." However, his conclusion integrating his meditations defined *prayer* as a conscientious effort. He concluded
that "prayer is the effort of the soul to apply itself in all its length and breath to
this sovereign idea, is the attempt to bring home to the thoughts so grand a mind
and converse with it, as we converse with men." Similarly, on December 10, 1830,
he clearly described his maximum thoughts in a way characteristic of the second
stage of self-aware consciousness, with a global maximum at 5.4 in the emotional
aspect of the intellectual plane:

God is the substratum of all souls. Is not that the solution of the riddle of sympathy? . . . It has often occurred to me that a man was a reflection of my own self. I
understand his smile and his scowl. So far we go along together and have one nature. The moment I do not understand him, the moment he departs from me, I am
pained, for I feel that either he is wrong or I am. As long as that difference subsists,
so long will our uneasiness on that point. It is an unshaken conviction of both, that
both cannot be right.

Emerson's average thoughts were in the emotional aspects of planes 2–4, as
shown in Table 4.6. That is, his average thoughts in the sexual plane involve
"worry" (2.4), those in the material plane involve anger or aggravation (3.4), and
those in the emotional plane involve his being considerate or supportive (4.5).
However, he has a wide range of thoughts in each plane, indicating many interests and conflicts.

His thought pattern changed substantially in Paris on July 13, 1833. During his
illumination he experienced oceanic feelings, which is rated as 5.8, referring to
the spiritual aspects of intellectual thinking. As quoted earlier from his journal,
Emerson's thoughts in the Jardin des Plantes involve romantic idealization (2.7),
thrilled exhilaration (3.7), empathy (4.7), oceanic feelings or ecstasy (5.8), and
philanthropic kindness (7.2). Throughout the rest of his life, there was a substantial elevation in most aspects of his thought, as indicated in Table 4.6 C. The main
change was the sense of resourcefulness in his maximum thoughts, but there also

was some increase in his average thoughts. His minimum thoughts increased to 3.6, indicating that he continued to feel inadequate and inferior at times, as previously described.

## The initial diffusion to Emerson's disciples

When Emerson returned to the United States, he gave lectures and sermons as a guest preacher in New England. His presentations were often inspiring. In 1834, Lydia Jackson found herself "so lifted to higher thoughts" that she "regarded him with reverence as an angelic being" (Baker 1996). All of his disciples were stimulated to recollect "higher thoughts" by Emerson, whereas others had no such recollections and remained neutral or hostile toward him. Within a year, Lydia Jackson had become both Emerson's disciple and his wife. Emerson renamed her "Lidian," and they settled in Concord together in 1835.

Initially, Emerson and his followers met for discussions in what came to be called the "Transcendentalist Club" or the "Hedge Club"—the meetings were often called when Hedge visited from Maine. Emerson hoped to attract young people to his views who would transform American culture. In 1837, Emerson gave the Phi Beta Kappa lecture to Henry Thoreau's graduating class at Harvard College. In this lecture, called *The American Scholar*, Emerson called on the Harvard graduates to free themselves from European models and to devote themselves to a life of the mind through nature, books, and action. A visit from Alcott and Hedge two weeks before the lecture stimulated Emerson to set out his theory of the scholar's function in his journal on August 18, 1837.

> The hope to arouse young men at Cambridge to a worthier view of their literary duties prompts me to offer the theory of the Scholar's function. He has an office to perform in Society. What is it? To arouse the intellect; to keep it erect and sound; to keep admiration in the hearts of the people; to keep the eye open upon its spiritual aims. How shall he render this service? By being a soul among those things with which he deals. Let us look at the world as it aids his function.
>
> One thing is plain, he must have a training by himself. The training of another age will not fit him. He himself, and not others, must judge what is good for him. Now the young are oppressed by their instructors. . . . Meek young men grow up in colleges and believe it is their duty to accept the views which books have given and grow up slaves.

Emerson felt strongly that a scholar's power came from the freedom of his own experience and understanding. On August 13, 1837, he wrote, "God never meant that we should learn Language by Colleges or Books. That only can we say which we have lived. Life lies behind us, as the quarry from whence we get tiles and cope-stones for the masonry of to-day" (Emerson and Forbes 1914).

By the summer of 1839, Emerson had more than a dozen followers who were faithful to him and his vision of transcendental scholarship. As a result, the summer of 1839 was called the "full dawn of the transcendental movement" by one of the disciples, William H. Channing (Miller 1957, page 36). One of the original fifteen disciples, Orestes Brownson, became a dissenter in 1844, but Ellery Channing had become a disciple in the meantime, keeping the number of close disciples around 15.

The disciples are listed and briefly described in Table 4.7. The disciples were idealistic intellectuals from New England. Many were friends and classmates at Harvard College in Boston. Henry James described them as a "young band of the ardent and uplifted" (Miller 1957, page 275). Emerson's disciples included six Unitarian preachers and scholars: Orestes Brownson, Frederick Hedge, William Channing, Theodore Parker, and Christopher Cranch. Orestes Brownson became a Catholic convert in 1844, preferring the structure of an organized church (Brownson 1957). Father Edward Taylor was a Methodist preacher in the Boston seaport. Bronson Alcott was an educational reformer. Sam Ward was a painter. Nearly all were poets or prose writers. Only Emerson received inter-

**Table 4.7.** Close Disciples of Ralph Waldo Emerson in the Initial Diffusion of American Transcendentalism (1834–1846)

| Name | Lifespan | Distinctions |
|---|---|---|
| Father E. T. Taylor | 1793–? | Inspiring preacher, pastor in Boston seaport |
| Bronson Alcott | 1799–1888 | Educational reformer, Platonic scholar |
| Lidian Emerson | 1802–1892 | Occasional poet, Emerson's second wife |
| Orestes Brownson | 1803–1876 | Preacher, writer, and early disciple but dissented from Emerson and in 1844 became a Catholic priest |
| Frederick Hedge | 1805–1890 | Preacher in Maine, German literary scholar |
| Margaret Fuller | 1810–1850 | Feminist, book writer, literary critic, died in shipwreck fleeing revolution in Italy |
| William H. Channing | 1810–1884 | Preacher, co-edited Fuller's memoirs, later socialist reformer |
| Theodore Parker | 1810–1860 | Scholar, preacher, social reformer |
| Ellen Sturgis | 1812–1848 | Transcendental poet, elder sister of Caroline |
| Jones Very | 1813–1880 | Mystical poet, essayist |
| Christopher Cranch | 1813–1892 | Preacher, poet, humorist, musician |
| Elizabeth Hoar | 1814–1878 | Close family friend, Emerson called her "sister" because she was engaged to his brother Edward, who died before the wedding |
| Henry Thoreau | 1817–1862 | Naturalist and author of classic books and poetry about nature and freedom |
| Ellery Channing II | 1817–1901 | Frequent companion and friend of Emerson and Thoreau in Concord |
| Caroline Sturgis | 1818–1888 | Free-spirited poet, friend of M. Fuller |
| Samuel Gray Ward | 1818–? | Painter and art historian, friend of Fuller |

national acclaim during their lifetime. Thoreau's later works, particularly *Walden* and *Civil Disobedience*, now have the status of classics that have had enduring significance for the appreciation of nature, freedom, and civil rights. Margaret Fuller has been lionized as an early feminist of notable intellect and journalistic accomplishment.

The individuals in Table 4.7 are described as disciples because their relationship with Emerson was most frequently on an intellectual level. As we will see later, the "modal" or "most frequent" relationship does not convey the full range of interactions that occur in a relationship that has aspects in each of the five planes. Sometimes people falsely conclude that a relationship has deteriorated, when in actual fact conflicts that were always present are simply activated under relevant conditions. For example, later we will examine some detailed descriptions involving all five planes for Emerson and Thoreau, who had a complex relationship. However, it is better to begin by considering the dominant influence of the modal level of relationship.

My diagnoses of the human relationships (DHR) of the disciples and Emerson around August 1839 are summarized in Table 4.8. The relationships were rated on the same quantitative scale as used previously to describe thoughts because the relationship can be characterized in terms of the thoughts and feelings produced by

**Table 4.8.** Diagnosis of Human Relationships (DHR) of Disciples to Ralph Waldo Emerson and of Emerson to His Fifteen Disciples at End of Summer of 1839, which Was Described by William Channing as the "Full Dawn of Transcendentalist Movement"

| Name | Modal DHR in August 1839 | | | |
|------|------|------|------|------|
| | *Disciples to Emerson* | | *Emerson to Disciples* | |
| Taylor | 5.0 | "Reliable" | 5.0 | "Reliable" |
| Alcott | 5.2 | "Helpful" | 5.2 | "Helpful" |
| Lidian | 4.9 | "Comfort" | 5.1 | "Executive" |
| Brownson | 5.0 | "Reliable" | 5.0 | "Reliable" |
| Hedge | 4.9 | "Comfort" | 5.1 | "Executive" |
| Fuller | 4.9 | "Comfort" | 5.2 | "Helpful" |
| Channing | 5.0 | "Reliable" | 5.1 | "Executive" |
| Parker | 5.0 | "Reliable" | 5.1 | "Executive" |
| E. Sturgis | 5.1 | "Ambitious" | 5.0 | "Reliable" |
| Very | 5.1 | "Ambitious" | 5.0 | "Reliable" |
| Cranch | 5.1 | "Ambitious" | 5.2 | "Helpful" |
| Hoar | 5.0 | "Reliable" | 5.2 | "Helpful" |
| Thoreau | 5.0 | "Reliable" | 5.0 | "Reliable" |
| C. Sturgis | 5.1 | "Ambitious" | 5.2 | "Helpful" |
| Ward | 5.1 | "Ambitious" | 5.0 | "Reliable" |

the relationship. The level of the modal DHR of the disciples to Emerson was 4.9–5.1. Similarly, Emerson's modal DHR to his disciples ranged from 5.0 to 5.2, as shown in Table 4.8. Emerson himself did not use the term *disciple*. He referred to them as "my platoon" (Emerson 1939, August 18, 1848, Volume 4, page 107; Baker 1996, page 325), which is consistent with the executive role he assumed in relation to most of them to cultivate them as scholars and artists. Emerson described Margaret Fuller as "one of my luminaries" in introducing her to Thomas Carlyle, which is consistent with his helpful relationship (i.e., 5.2) with her (Baker 1996).

Table 4.8 also shows that the relationships between Emerson and his disciples were closely concordant. Such symmetry in the modal relationships means that they were mutually satisfying most of the time (but not always, as we shall see). Emerson was the charismatic founder and most accomplished writer of the group. He had an uplifting effect on their thoughts. Some felt highly elevated emotional contentment, which is rated as 4.9. This group includes Emerson's wife Lidian, Margaret Fuller, and Frederick Hedge, Emerson's long-term associate who traveled regularly from Maine to see Emerson. Most disciples looked to Emerson for a sense of intellectual identity, as indicated by ratings of 5.0–5.1. In return, Emerson's relationships to his disciples were that of the executive director (5.0–5.1) or one who helps himself by helping others (5.2). Some people, including Caroline Sturgis and Margaret Fuller, were able to bring out Emerson's social warmth, as we will discuss later. However, Emerson deliberately tried to maintain some emotional distance from his disciples. Consequently, he was frequently perceived as a cold and detached intellectual. As Ellen (Sturgis 1957) said in the poem she dedicated to Emerson as a "dry lighted soul":

> Thou art the mountain where we climb to see
> The land our feet have trod this many a year.
> Thou art the deep and crystal winter sky,
> Where noiseless, one by one, bright stars appear.

It is interesting to compare Emerson's relationships with his disciples to those with his friends and opponents, as summarized in Table 4.9. Here I am describing "friends" as those whose modal relationship is essentially based on emotional attachment, that is, 4.0–4.7. William Channing I was Emerson's warm and supportive mentor in divinity school. In his relationships with peers who were friends, Emerson was most frequently considerate and support-giving (modal DHR of 4.5). For example, Emerson's gave recognition and advice to Walt Whitman, which solidified a supportive emotional attachment between them. Emerson had an empathic relationship with his Concord neighbor Nathaniel Hawthorne (4.7) that was somewhat asymmetric. Hawthorne was a slightly taciturn but friendly neighbor. Emerson was affirming and comforting in his modal DHR with James Freeman Clarke, whom he asked to help him edit Margaret Fuller's memoirs. However, Clarke was more a friend of Fuller than a disciple of Emerson.

**Table 4.9.** Diagnosis of Human Relationship (DHR) of Friends and
Opponents to Ralph Waldo Emerson and of Emerson to His Friends and
Opponents at the Full Dawn of the Transcendentalist Movement

| | *Modal DHR in August 1839* | |
| *Name* | *Associate to Emerson* | *Emerson to associate* |
|---|---|---|
| FRIENDS | | |
| William E Channing I | 4.6 | 4.4 |
| | "Warm" | "Support seeking" |
| Nathaniel Hawthorne | 4.2 | 4.7 |
| | "Recognition seeking" | "Empathic" |
| Oliver Wendell Holmes | 4.4 | 4.5 |
| | "Support seeking" | "Support giving" |
| Thomas Carlyle | 4.3 | 4.5 |
| | "Pleasing" | "Support giving" |
| Charles Newcomb | 4.3 | 4.5 |
| | "Pleasing" | "Support giving" |
| Walt Whitman | 4.2 | 4.5 |
| | "Recognition seeking" | "Support giving" |
| James F. Clarke | 3.9 | 4.8 |
| | "Influential" | "Giving comfort" |
| | | |
| OPPONENTS | | |
| Andrews Norton | 3.1 | 3.3 |
| | "Opposing" | "Reserved" |
| N. L. Frothingham | 2.9 | 3.1 |
| | "Scornful" | "Offended" |

Another person who might superficially appear to be a disciple was Charles Newcomb. The relationship of Emerson to Newcomb, however, was a conditional emotional attachment. Charles Newcomb had shown early promise to Emerson "with his fine perceptions, his excellent instincts, his beautiful learning, his catholic mind." However, in 1848 Emerson met Charles and learned he had not written any literary work in the prior three years for fear of disturbing his feelings of contentment from reading other great writers. Emerson's friendship with Charles ended when Emerson recorded in his journal a final psychological farewell, at a DHR of 3.6:

> He has become the spoiled child of culture, the *roué* of Art and Letters, *blasé* with too much Plato, Dante, Calderon, and Goethe. . . . Farewell, my once beautiful genius. . . . I have learned a sordid respect for uses and values. . . . Are we to say a man shall not go out to the shed to bring an armful of wood, lest this violence of action hurt the balance of his mind? (Richardson 1995, page 461)

Emerson also had opponents who were highly critical of him. The relations with opponents are rated with modal DHRs below the Gate of Humanity, that is, they range from 3.3 to 2.9. Reverend Nathaniel Frothingham was the pastor of the First Church in Boston, having succeeded Emerson's father in that position. Emerson had initially regarded him positively as a scholar, as shown in Emerson's journal entry on August 9, 1837. Nevertheless, after Emerson gave his Divinity school address, Frothingham became a scornful critic of Waldo (modal DHR of 2.9). Likewise, Andrews Norton, the Dexter Professor of Sacred Literature in the Harvard Divinity School, stigmatized Emerson's as an "infidel" (Miller 1957). Emerson was restrained but deeply offended by such condemnation.

## The stable pattern of Emerson's social relations

Emerson's thoughts ranged from 5.2 to 3.1 before 1833, and from 5.8 to 3.6 after 1833. Likewise, there was always variability in the state of his relationships with his disciples. The modal relationships among Emerson and his disciples were from 4.9 to 5.2, which are all below 5.4, which is below the Gate of Rational Intuition. None of the relationships developed past 5.3 at any time. In other words, although these interpersonal relationships were fairly elevated, they were all conditional and based on one-sided (selfish) judgments. Consequently, there were frequent conflicts, strains, and disappointments in these relationships, which were manifest by the variation in the thoughts of Emerson and his disciples. What I described in Table 4.7 were the "modal" or most frequent relationships. These modal relations were what sustained the relationships, but there were many problems and sensitivities that became manifest on occasion. In the case of Emerson's disciples, the emergence of such problems did not mean that the modal relationship had changed. Nevertheless, the conflicts in the relationships became prominent at times.

Nearly all the disciples became frustrated and disappointed with Emerson at times, much as he expected they would. For example, Fuller's attitude toward Emerson is encapsulated in a letter to William Story, which she wrote shortly before her death in 1850. She arrogantly refers to some poems of friends of Emerson as follows: "They are of the Emersonian kind, entirely out of all rule, not of high power, but genuine though imperfect reflexes of the higher life of their writers" (Baker 1996, page 317).

Likewise, Thoreau wrote in 1851 about Emerson that "I enjoy thee more than other men, yet I am more disappointed with thee than with others." Thoreau wrote in his journal (Broderick 1981) that Emerson "offered me friendship on such terms that I could not accept it, without a sense of degradation. He would not meet me on equal terms, but only be to some extent my patron. He would not come to see me, but was hurt if I did not visit him. He would not readily accept a favor, but would gladly confer one."

Ellery Channing, who was a frequent walking partner of Emerson and Thoreau, and remained loyal to Emerson, nevertheless had moments in which he felt highly defensive and uncomfortable with his mentor. On one occasion in 1849 (Baker

1996, page 329), Ellery called Emerson "a terrible man to deal with—one has to be armed at all points. He threshes you out very soon; is admirably skillful, able to go anywhere and do anything. Those nearest to him feel him hard and cold; no one knows even what he is doing or studying. . . . Nobody knows what his real philosophy is; his books do not tell it. I have known him for years intimately and I have not found it out. Women do not like him; he cannot establish a personal relation with anyone, yet he can get on agreeably with everyone."

Alcott also had a wide range of feelings about Emerson. At times, he felt that Emerson "always kindles a sublime sentiment. . . . A solemn and supernatural awe creeps over one as the serene pathos of his manner and the unaffected earnestness of his bearing come upon the senses" (Baker 1996, page 90). At other times, he regarded Emerson as a "high and commanding" genius, but felt that he was not always "fully in earnest" and often wrote and spoke "for effect" (Baker 1996, page 90). Hence, Alcott's relationship to Emerson was based more on Alcott's admiration of Emerson's intellect than on Emerson's spirituality. Alcott wrote about Emerson: "Fame stands before him as a dazzling award, and he holds himself somewhat too proudly. . . . His life has been one of opportunity, and he has sought to realize in it more of the accomplished scholar than the perfect man.—A great intellect, refined by elegant study, rather than a divine life radiant with the beauty of truth and holiness. He is an eye more than a heart, an intellect more than a soul."

The criticism by Emerson's disciples was only a belated recognition of limitations that Emerson had long acknowledged. In April 1834, he had already recognized that "the whole secret of the teacher's force" might be "in the conviction that men are convertible. And they are. They want awakening." In other words, a teacher must approach others with hope, kindness, and patience founded on the awareness that each person has a freedom of will that can be awakened, even if it is currently dormant. However, "The wise man must be wary of attaching followers. He must feel and teach that the best of wisdom cannot be communicated; must be acquired by every soul for itself" (Baker 1996, page 31). Later, on April 14, 1842 (Emerson and Forbes 1914), "If I should write an honest diary, what should I say?" Emerson wrote, "Alas, that life is halfness, shallowness. I have almost completed thirty-nine years; and I have not yet adjusted my relations to my fellows on the planet, or to my own work. Always too young or too old, I do not justify myself; how can I satisfy others?" Once again Emerson's needs for recognition and solitude were a persistent source of conflict and doubt for him.

Likewise, his disciples were gradually realizing what Emerson had long known—social interaction and the example of someone who had already "seen the light" may help to prepare a person for the awakening of their own self-aware consciousness, but *no one can transform the consciousness of another person*. Thoreau and the other disciples were often mocked for their effort to emulate Emerson, which provoked ambivalent feelings in them about their leader. Whatever he did for his disciples, and he did much, Emerson could never satisfy all their wishes. Even if he had wanted to try to satisfy their wishes, and he needed his own solitude too much to do that, he could not allow them to be dependent on him. Each disciple needed guidance and encouragement, but Emerson also had to maintain the detachment necessary for their self-actualization. No one can give another person self-awareness. Emerson could only point the way to his disciples and encourage each to trust himself or herself so that they could listen to their own psyche impartially, calmly, and patiently.

These strains in the relationships of Emerson and his disciples show the complexity of human social relationships. A thorough description of human relationships requires measurement of the relationship in each of the five planes. I will describe such an analysis later for Emerson and Thoreau. However, first it is useful to describe a detailed analysis of Emerson's thoughts, which reflect the complexity of his relationships.

## The stable pattern of variability in Emerson's thoughts

When Emerson was forty-three to forty-four years old (in 1847–1848), he was coping with a variety of conflicts. His son Waldo (1836–1842) had died at age five. He and Lidian had three other children: Ellen (1839–1909), Edith (1841–1929), and Edward (1844–1930). However, Lidian, Waldo, and their eldest daughter never fully recovered from their grief at little Waldo's death. At the same time, Emerson became impatient with what he perceived as the failure of his spiritual children (i.e., his disciples) to distinguish themselves by their creative works. In his essay *Experience*, he says "We see young men who owe us a new world, so readily and lavishly they promise, but they never acquit the debt; they die young and dodge the account: or if they live, they lose themselves in the crowd."

Emerson's thoughts spiraled up to oceanic feelings (i.e., thoughts at 5.8) in contemplation and spiraled down to feelings of pride versus inferiority (i.e., self-aware or secondary narcissism, thoughts at 3.6) in times of conflict throughout all the years after 1834. For example, in 1847 Emerson felt dissatisfied with his disciples and himself. He arranged a visit to England to try to get away from these problems and give lectures, which was a frequent mode of relief for him. While in England he was treated royally and was gratified by admirers and their worldly success. Emerson wrote to Carlyle, "England is the country of success, and success has a great charm for me, more than for those I talk with at home" (Emerson 1964, October 2, 1848, page 442).

Coincidentally, the year of 1848 was a time of political revolution in Europe. In February 1848, the weak French king Louis Philippe was overthrown, and a provisional government composed of the middle class and socialists established a republic. Metternich's Viennese government fell apart in March. Italian partisans led by Mazzini opposed the rule of the Austrians. Venice declared itself independent. Monarchs throughout Europe suddenly agreed to constitutional changes. In the midst of all these upheavals, in May 1848, Emerson visited France from England. He visited the Jardin des Plantes again but was more impressed on this visit by the shops and abundance of books in Paris. "Everything odd and rare and rich can be bought in Paris" (Emerson and Forbes 1914, May 1848, Volume 7, page 472).

Emerson heard a lecture by the great transcendental poet Alphonse Lamartine, who was playing a prominent role in the provisional French government. Emerson was sympathetic to the French revolutionaries. Emerson was impressed by Lamartine's wisdom but was not inspired by Lamartine's application of the positive philosophy to social and political reform.

Lamartine was the living synthesis of the positive philosophy during Emerson's time, as we saw in the quotations from Lamartine's work in Chapter 2. Lamartine enacted the abolition of slavery in France. He established a democratic government by refusing to accept appointment as president. As a transcendental poet and a philosopher of great depth, Emerson's communication with Lamartine could have led to a great climax in Emerson's spiritual development. However, the light of Lamartine's spirit was overshadowed in Emerson's clouded mind by the emerging violence and confusion of the Revolution of 1848. The provisional government established in February 1848 in which Lamartine held a major position had been comprised of both the middle (or bourgeois) class and the socialists. However, by May elections had been held in which the bourgeois had won heavy majorities and the socialists had suffered large defeats. Emerson visited a club run by the leader of the socialists on May 14 and saw the fanatical fervor of the socialists. The next day, May 15, the socialists overran the National Assembly in Paris, in a prelude to a more serious revolt later that summer. Emerson saw first hand much violence and confusion in the streets of Paris (Richardson 1995, pages 454–456). In Emerson's current discouraged mood, this confusion only confirmed his personal lack of hope and confidence in applying transcendental philosophy to social reform in the way that Lamartine was doing. On June 8, 1848, Emerson remarked in his journal, "The world is always childish, and with each gewgaw of a revolution or a new constitution it finds, thinks it shall never cry any more. . . . It is always becoming evident that the permanent good is for the soul only and cannot be retained in any society or system."

For Emerson, this meant that he would not enjoy the personal guidance of the greatest positive philosopher of his time, Lamartine. Shortly afterwards, Lamartine would decline appointment as head of the French government and insist on a popular vote to maintain the principle of democratic equality. He was not elected and happily withdrew from political activity to write without distraction. Unfortunately, Lamartine and Emerson never spoke personally and did not correspond with one another.

Emerson had benefited spiritually from his first visit to Paris in 1833, but he sensed he had lost something important during his visit to England and France in

1848. Emerson had a conflict between liberal innovation and conservative traditions. Although he was himself revolutionary in his thinking at times, he also wished for order and control of his life. The confusion of the French Revolution of 1848 led him to conclude that the way of transcendentalism had no place in challenging established laws and government. He did not recognize that the perennial philosophy that he loved—the philosophy of Plato and Montaigne that had always inspired him—was a perpetually revolutionary philosophy, as exemplified by the activities of Lamartine and Emerson's own disciples Fuller and Thoreau. Emerson failed to see the application of his own principles to political life and social reform through nonviolent nonconformity in the way that his disciples Fuller and Thoreau had already seen. Thus the tensions Emerson had had for many years with Thoreau and Fuller would remain unreconciled on Emerson's return from Europe.

A vivid example of Emerson's narcissism (Svrakic 1990) and occasional unhappiness is revealed by the list he made during his return voyage in July 1848 of his "intellectual poverties." As recorded in his journal, these inadequacies included "weak eyes . . . no animal spirits, an immense and fatal negative with our Anglican race. No Greek, no mathematics, no politics," which I rate as indicating a sense of inferiority and inadequacy, or lack of power" (i.e., thought level 3.6).

Emerson's sense of inadequacy in 1848 was typical of his minimum thoughts after the success of his publication of *Nature* in 1836. Such thoughts of inadequacy had been recurrent throughout Emerson's life. Such low thoughts are similar to the feelings of inadequacy that Emerson had experienced just before his twenty-first birthday, as previously described in describing him during divinity school. Emerson always felt he was "a bore" who by skill made others believe that he was witty and agreeable. He had dreams mixed with anger and sadness in which he was an unhappy, toothless old man, or a show horse that could not really run forward. However, even at such times, he usually was able to elevate his thoughts to an intellectual level by meditation, or even higher in contemplation.

When Emerson's thoughts did fall, he was often impatient with himself and others. For example, upon his return from Europe he was impatient with Henry Thoreau and Charles Newcomb. The young English intellectuals also had looked to him for leadership, but Emerson did not feel up to the role of spiritual visionary (Richardson 1995, page 444).

Emerson was usually self-assured but had a strong need for recognition (average thoughts of 4.2 after 1833). With his sensitive temperament, he always needed much evidence of appreciation by others. However, by 1848, the fervor and frequency of admiration by his original disciples had diminished. Hedge and Parker were influential in their writing about German philosophy during the 1830s but remained at a distance and less active after 1840. In 1840, Jones Very went into seclusion for the remainder of his life (Miller 1957, page 278). After 1841, Lidian was often sick and Emerson felt shackled by the permanence of their marriage

(Richardson 1995, pages 330–331). In 1942, Margaret resigned as editor of the *Dial*, moved away, and became increasingly independent. In 1847, Caroline Sturgis married and moved to Europe for many years, corresponding only intermittently. Thoreau became increasingly independent after 1844, when Emerson criticized the poetry he had written prior to that time. Thoreau threw much of it away and later regretted it (Miller 1957, page 229), but Emerson's criticism appears to have been justified from what survived, as we will see later. Alcott, "Sister" Elizabeth, Ellery, and Sam were the only disciples Emerson was seeing frequently on his return from Europe. However, Emerson was quite busy giving public lectures, which were well received. Emerson's lectures and publications led to broad popularity but no deepening of his thought.

The days of ecstasy in contemplation following Emerson's illumination in 1833 were largely recollections of his past before 1842. The reduced activity of Emerson's contemplative life after 1842 had fateful consequences for everyone involved in the transcendentalist movement. Pessimism and increasing frustration formed a vicious cycle in Emerson's relationships with his disciples. The formerly liberal Emerson was becoming a part of the conservative establishment, which further strained his relationships to his disciples, particularly Margaret Fuller and Henry Thoreau. Emerson later opposed slavery with fervor, which was certainly an affirmation of the importance of freedom of will and action in opposition to determinism. However, the opposition to slavery had long been an established intellectual tradition in New England. Emerson nevertheless was comfortable with abolitionists who continued to support the federal government. Emerson was critical of Thoreau for his refusal to pay taxes because of the government's support of slavery, and he was critical of Margaret Fuller for her involvement with Italian partisans revolting against Austrian rule.

Emerson's own spiritual stagnation and his difficulties with his disciples were rooted in his limited vision of personality development. Emerson remained an elite intellectual who wanted only to be "the head of his order." In his journal entry for April 30, 1838, he saw only an "inextinguishable dualism" that despite "the broadest assertions of the One nature, we must yet admit always the co-presence of a superior influx; must pray, must hope, (and what is hope but affirmation of two)." Emerson supported meritocracy as an intermediate position between extreme individualism and extreme socialism. He saw his relationship to others as "armed neutrality." According to Emerson, some people are naturally born leaders, geniuses, heroes, and men of honor as gifts of Nature. Such heroes and geniuses were a self-reliant elite "raised above themselves" by awareness of beauty in nature, which gives them "a sense of delicious liberty and power" (Miller 1957, pages 299–300). Furthermore, Emerson did not expect such geniuses to be saints or virtuous or coherent. He saw the true aristocrat as someone "who is at the head of his own order" (Miller 1957, page 302). Consequently, Emerson criticized the humble positive philosopher Ali for not acting to attain success and power. As

Alcott said, Emerson was excessively driven by his own pride and desire for mastery, rather than awakening to full coherence in which there is understanding and respect for the freedom of all.

Emerson discussed coherence at an intellectual level, but he never sought to live it spiritually, contenting himself with his perception of fame reinforced by steadfast effort to deny the preeminence of any other figure in literature during his time. Consequently, he remained divided by his desire for the "divine life" on the one hand and his desire for status and social recognition on the other hand. The search for unity in oneself, in society, and in God is not easy, and many lose their way in egoism or elitism.

Emerson and his disciples helped one another to keep from entirely losing sight of the true way. Emerson was aware of his own conflicts, which divided his heart between love of society and of God in solitude, and tried to stay on the transcendentalist's path of the psyche toward divine unity. In June 1852, he wrote in his journal, "Thoreau gives me in flesh and blood and pertinacious Saxon belief, my own ethics. He is far more real, and daily practically obeying them, than I; and fortifies my memory at all times with an affirmative experience which refuses to be set aside." Emerson and Thoreau often argued with one another, but this was part of the "adversarial" interaction Emerson sought in his understanding of friendship.

## THE DEVELOPMENT OF THOREAU

### The patronage of Emerson

Thoreau's relationship with Emerson also involved difficulties for both, but the development was ultimately constructive over time, as summarized in Table 4.10. There was an ongoing Hegelian dialectic between Emerson and Thoreau throughout the relationship, and even after Thoreau's death, because each valued independence and nonconformity as their source of power. Emerson's modal relationship with Thoreau gradually elevated in a stepwise manner from 4.8 ("comforting") when they first met to 5.0 ("responsible") by 1839. By 1843, Emerson's modal relationship to Thoreau was at level 5.2 (mutually "helpful"), and this was maintained until Thoreau's death. Likewise, Thoreau's relationship to Emerson began in the emotional plane (4.9, "contented") and increased by steps until it was symmetric with Emerson (5.2, mutually "helpful").

However, these changes in the modal DHR of Emerson and Thoreau are largely the result of varying contributions from stable relationships in the individual planes. For example, the detailed relationships described in Table 4.10 show that the relations in planes 2, 3, and 5 were stable. The major change was the emotional conflict resulting from Thoreau's dissatisfaction with Emerson's treating him like

**Table 4.10.** Detailed Diagnosis of Human Relationships between R. W. Emerson and H. D. Thoreau as They Developed over Time

| | Planes of Relationship | | | | | | |
|---|---|---|---|---|---|---|---|
| Date | 2 | 3 | 4 | 5 | 7 | Modal DHR | Modal Descriptor |
| **A. DEVELOPMENT OF EMERSON'S RELATIONSHIP WITH THOREAU** | | | | | | | |
| 8/37 | — | .8 [Patron] | .7 | .3 [Helpful] | .0 | 4.8 | "Comforting" |
| 8/39 | — | .8 | .7 [Empathy] | .3 | .0 | 5.0 | "Reliable" |
| 5/43 | — | .8 | .7 | .3 | .0 | 5.2 | "Helpful" |
| 1/46 | — | .8 | .7 | .3 | .0 | 5.2 | "Helpful" |
| 1/51 | — | .8 | .7 | .3 | .0 | 5.2 | "Helpful" |
| 1/52 | — | .8 | .2 [Unsupported] | .3 | .0 | 5.2 | "Helpful" |
| 1/62 | — | .8 | .2 | .3 | .0 | 5.2 | "Helpful" |
| **B. DEVELOPMENT OF THOREAU'S RELATIONSHIP WITH EMERSON** | | | | | | | |
| 8/37 | .9 [Flattery] | .8 | .7 [Seeking patron/friend/guide] | .7 | .0 | 4.9 | "Contented" |
| 8/39 | .9 | .8 | .7 | .7 | .0 | 5.0 | "Reliable" |
| 5/43 | .9 | .8 | .7 | .7 | .0 | 5.0 | "Reliable" |
| 1/46 | .9 | .8 | .7 | .7 | .0 | 5.2 | "Helpful" |
| 1/51 | .9 | .8 | .6 [Needing warm friend] | .7 | .1 | 5.2 | "Helpful" |
| 1/52 | .9 | .8 | .2 [Unsupported] | .7 | .1 | 5.2 | "Helpful" |
| 1/62 | .9 | .8 | .2 | .7 | .1 | 5.2 | "Helpful" |

a patron instead of a peer. Emerson and Thoreau each felt emotionally unsupported and hurt by the other's behavior. Nevertheless, each continued to cooperate with the other in "win–win" situations.

The stepwise developments in the relationships between Emerson and Thoreau have been well documented. For example, in August 1839, Emerson wrote to Carlyle that Thoreau "writes our truest verses," which suggests both Emerson's executive judgment and ambition for Henry. As he stated in his address *The American Scholar* in 1837, Emerson hoped to attract young people like Thoreau so that they could transform American culture in an authentic way independent of European influence and traditions. In Thoreau he did indeed find such a voice of the future. Emerson had an essential role in developing the spiritual life and literary career of Thoreau. Emerson guided and encouraged him, such as encouraging him to keep a journal and suggesting that he use his gift for naturalistic observation of nature as a literary form by inviting him to write about the natural history of

Massachusetts for the *Dial* in 1842. He also helped Thoreau to get his works published elsewhere, lent him money at times, and provided him with a place to stay and the leisure for his nature study, contemplation, and writing.

In May 1941, Emerson wrote that Thoreau is "a noble manly youth, full of melodies and inventions. We work together by day in my garden." By April 1843, Hawthorne recorded that the "sturdy and uncompromising" Thoreau had become a tolerated inconvenience for the Emerson family after residing with them for two years (Borst 1992). Emerson was regularly helpful to Thoreau during his residence with the Emersons. Later Thoreau began to return the help to Emerson by overseeing the Concord household and working on the *Dial* whenever Emerson was traveling.

Meanwhile, Thoreau had become more objectively aware of Emerson's limitations. During the first winter on Walden Pond (1845–1846), Thoreau wrote in his journal (Broderick 1981) that "Emerson again is a critic poet philosopher—with talent not so conspicuous—not so adequate to his task—lives a far more intense life—seeks to realize a divine life." Many other contemporaries of Emerson felt that his prose was better than his poetry, which lacked meter (Miller 1957, page 217). Nevertheless, Thoreau also expressed his overall fidelity and veneration of Emerson: "His personal influence on young persons greater than any man's. In his world every man would be a poet—Love would reign—beauty would take place—Man & nature would harmonize."

After Emerson's return from Europe in 1848, each became disappointed in the other. While Emerson was away, Thoreau had effectively replaced him as head of the household. Thoreau loved this role and had deep affection for Emerson's wife Lidian and Emerson's children. Thoreau himself was unmarried and may have felt displaced by Emerson's return. In addition, in October 1848 Robert Lowell published a popular parody called *A Fable for Critics* in which he described Thoreau as an imitator who had "stolen all his apples from Emerson's orchard" and urged him to strike out on his own (Baker 1996). In 1849 Thoreau's first book, *A Week on the Concord & Merrimack Rivers*, was a commercial failure and put Thoreau in debt because he followed Emerson's example of assuming responsibility for the publication costs. Emerson could afford this arrangement because his books sold well and he had independent income from his first wife's estate (Richardson 1995, pages 459–476). Thoreau had no such independent income and no established audience (Myerson 1995, pages 25–39). Shortly after Thoreau's book was published in May 1849, Thoreau recorded in his journal feelings of estrangement and anger toward Emerson, after a casual remark Emerson made that was critical of the book:

> I had a friend, I wrote a book, I asked my friend's criticism, I never got but praise for what was good in it—my friend became estranged from me and then I got blame for all that was bad,—& so I got at last the criticism which I wanted.
> While my friend was my friend he flattered me, and I never heard the truth from him, but when he became my enemy he shot it to me on a poisoned arrow.

Nevertheless, in 1850 when Margaret Fuller died, Thoreau responded loyally to Emerson's request that Thoreau help by going to search for Fuller's remains. Fuller was also Thoreau's friend. It is important to remember that a single statement or the disappointments each felt had not severed their mutually helpful relationship. Emerson and Thoreau still shared the same ideals of transcendental thought, but each was disappointed in the way each was applying those ideals.

Even when they were most friendly around 1842, they often did not communicate on a physical level on even a weekly basis. Thoreau recognized that their communication operated at a deeper spiritual level that was invisible to the physical senses. "We communicate," wrote Thoreau to his friend Emerson, "like the burrows of foxes, in silence and darkness, under ground." The dialectic with all its recurrent conflicts continued between the two great transcendentalists. Despite tensions and disappointments, neither ever broke off their helpful relationship with the other, as Emerson had with Brownson and Newcomb. Emerson enjoyed the dialectic with a true friend, a kind of "beautiful enemy," and at the end of his life, he still thought of Thoreau as having been his best friend. Likewise (Richardson 1995, page 464), Thoreau ends his essay on friendship in *Walden* by saying that "Although friendship between good men is interrupted, their principles remain unaltered. The stalk of the lotus may be broken, but the fibers remain connected."

Nevertheless, the fibers of the Emerson–Thoreau relationship were strained and stretched to a considerable distance. By January 30, 1852, Thoreau wrote in his journal, "I doubt if Emerson could trundle a wheelbarrow through the streets, because it would be out of character. One needs to have a comprehensive character." Thoreau disapproved of Emerson's new worldly preoccupation with social appearances and public opinion following his return in 1848 from visiting Europe. Ultimately, Thoreau shared ideals with Emerson, but Emerson himself was no longer the embodiment of that ideal.

Thoreau's emotional distance from Emerson gave Thoreau the freedom to develop "a comprehensive character" of his own through a contemplative life that was inwardly penetrating and outwardly loving. The transformation of Thoreau's thought established him as the essential Transcendentalist, rather than an imitative disciple. By 1856 Emerson recognized Thoreau's illumination but wished he would be less insistent that his own views were truer than Emerson's own views and behavior. Emerson wrote,

> Must we always talk for victory, and never once for truth, for comfort, and joy? Centrality he has, and penetration, strong understanding, and the higher gifts,—the insight of the real or from the real, and the moral rectitude that belongs to it; but all this and all his resources of wit and invention are lost to me in every experiment, year after year, that I make, to hold intercourse with his mind. Always some weary captious paradox to fight you with, and the time and temper wasted.

The illumination of Thoreau

Henry David Thoreau produced the most elevated creative works of all the American transcendentalists, even surpassing his mentor Emerson. His essay on *Civil Disobedience* was used by Gandhi in India and by Martin Luther King to explain the principle of freedom in human relationships, which ranks as a truly wonderful insight of civilization.

The general chronology of the major public events in the life of Henry David Thoreau is summarized in Table 4.11. Throughout his life, Thoreau was an inde-

**Table 4.11.** Chronology of Major Public Events in the Life of Henry David Thoreau

| Year | Event |
| --- | --- |
| 1817 | Thoreau born in Concord, July 12, third of four siblings |
| 1818–1823 | Family moved to Chelmsford, north of Concord, and then to Boston |
| 1823 | Family returned to Concord; attended Concord Academy |
| 1833–1837 | Attended Harvard College, ranked twenty-third of forty-four |
| 1837 | Meets R. W. Emerson, who resided in Concord; begins journal in October |
| 1838 | Taught school in Concord, wrote poetry on transcendental themes, lectured at Concord Lyceum |
| 1839 | Voyage on Concord and Merrimack rivers with brother John |
| 1840 | Published poem *Sympathy* in *Dial*; proposal of marriage to Ellen Sewall was rejected |
| 1841-1843 | At Emerson's home in Concord |
| 1842 | Older brother John died of lockjaw |
| | Published *Natural History of Massachusetts* and *Metrical Prayer* |
| 1843 | On Staten Island as tutor to Emerson's nephew; edits *Dial* in Emerson's absence |
| 1844 | Worked as pencil-maker for father; consolidated material for first book |
| 1845–1847 | At Walden Pond |
| 1846 | Spent one night in Concord jail in July for refusal to pay taxes for past six years |
| 1847–1848 | At Emerson's home; works as surveyor, tutor, writer, and lecturer |
| 1848 | Published *Ktaadn and The Maine Woods* |
| 1849 | Published *A Week on the Concord and Merrimack Rivers, Resistance to Civil Government* |
| 1850 | Thoreau searched for remains when Margaret Fuller shipwrecked; visited Canada and Cape Cod |
| 1853 | Published *Excursion to Canada* |
| 1854 | Published *Walden, Where I Lived, and What I Lived For* |
| 1855 | Published *Cape Cod* |
| 1859 | Published *Plea in Defense of John Brown* |
| 1860 | Went to Minnesota for health |
| 1862 | Published *Walking*, died at Concord on May 6 |
| 1863 | Posthumous essay *Life without Principle* and posthumous poem *Inspiration* published |

pendent, uncompromising nonconformist. Thoreau was usually quiet, but when he spoke he was blunt and contentious with an ironic biting humor. He said "no" more easily than "yes." His prickly independence could make him difficult to deal with socially. In other words, in temperament he was low in Novelty Seeking, Harm Avoidance, and Reward Dependence, which I have called an "independent" temperament profile. In his early schooldays, he was nicknamed "Judge" by his classmates because he was so solemn (Borst 1992, page 1). Similarly, in adulthood, Emerson described him as "brave" with a "grave aspect" and "terrible eyes" that blazed with an icy gray light (Baker 1996, pages 103–104).

His father had discovered a graphite mine and supported the family by running a pencil-making factory. Henry was a good student and entered Harvard College when he was sixteen years old, which was not an unusual age at the time. In college he was a responsible student and was interested in transcendental ideas. He was so impressed by Emerson's book *Nature*, published in 1836, that he gave it as a graduation present to a classmate. At Harvard College, he could be described as average in cooperativeness, but above average in self-directedness and self-transcendence. In other words, he was a young intellectual with a creative character, which attracted Emerson to write a letter of endorsement to the president of Harvard during his senior year, who honored Thoreau with a small stipend.

Upon graduation, Emerson became his patron and advised him to begin keeping a journal, which he did in October 1937. Thoreau recorded over two million words in his journal over twenty-four years (1837–1861). His daily routine for much of his life consisted of walking through the countryside, observing nature and his relationship to nature, and then recording his observations and thoughts in his journal. The variability in Thoreau's thoughts, as recorded in his journals, is summarized in Table 4.12, which is subdivided according to major circumstances in his life. Before living at Walden Pond, Thoreau's average thoughts in his journals were in the material plane (3.8–3.9), which involved his industriousness and wish for power and influence. His maximum thoughts were in the second stage of self-awareness (5.4–5.5), indicating his fondness for meditation. His minimum thoughts were at the beginning of the first stage of self-awareness (3.4–3.5), indicating a tendency toward envy and aggravation.

When living at Walden Pond, Thoreau's thoughts became much more elevated. However, his thought pattern did not actually change immediately on moving to Walden. Actually his pattern of thoughts did not change until after an illumination experience in July 1846, which produced a substantial rise in his maximum thoughts to 5.9, that is, "resourceful," "self-actualized" and "creative." The change in his thoughts over time in his journals suggest that something momentous happened to Thoreau while he was at Walden Pond.

Thoreau's thoughts can be examined more fully by considering his journals along with his publications and other available information (Broderick 1981; Borst 1992; Myerson 1995). A detailed diagnosis of the frequency of the thoughts (DFT) of

**Table 4.12.** Approximate Chronology of Mean and Range of Henry David Thoreau's Thoughts as Recorded in His Journals (1837–1852) and Grouped According to Residence at the Time

| Journal Period | Mean | Minimum | Maximum |
|---|---|---|---|
| TEACHING IN CONCORD | | | |
| 8/37–1/40 | 3.8 | 3.4 | 5.4 |
| | [Industrious] | [Aggravated] | [Conscientious] |
| AT EMERSON'S HOME | | | |
| 1/41–9/41 | 3.8 | 3.4 | 5.4 |
| 11/41–9/43 | 3.8 | 3.4 | 5.4 |
| AT STATEN ISLAND | | | |
| 9/43–3/45 | 3.9 | 3.5 | 5.5 |
| | [Purposeful] | [Curious] | [Calm] |
| AT WALDEN POND | | | |
| 7/45–6/46 | 3.9 | 3.5 | 5.5 |
| 7/46–9/47 | 4.2 | 3.6 | 5.9 |
| | [Privacy seeking] | [Inferior] | [Creative] |
| AFTER WALDEN POND | | | |
| 48–52 | 4.2 | 3.6 | 5.9 |

Thoreau is described in Table 4.13. In Table 4.13, the distributions of his thoughts are compared before and after his jail experience. Thoreau had refused for six years to pay locally collected taxes because the money would go to a federal government that was supporting slavery and making war on Mexico. In July 1846, while living in his cabin on Walden Pond, Thoreau went to town and was unexpectedly arrested. He was detained in the Concord jail for one night until an unknown person secretly paid the tax without his knowledge. While in jail his thoughts became highly elevated, as described in his essay *Resistance to Civil Government*, which was later called *Civil Disobedience*. After this illumination experience in 1846, the pattern of Thoreau's thinking was permanently transformed.

As shown in Table 4.13, before his illumination, Thoreau's thoughts were usually in the higher half of the material plane (3.5–3.6) or the middle of the emotional plane (4.4–4.6). As a result, his global average thought level was 3.9, which is the average of his average thoughts in the five planes weighted by the frequency of thought in those planes.

Thoreau's maximum thoughts up to July 1846 were at the meditative level of 5.5. However, when he was in jail, he experienced an illumination in which his global

**Table 4.13.** Development of the Thought of Henry David Thoreau Before, During, and After His Illumination by Being Jailed One Night for Refusal to Pay Taxes to the State (in Opposition to Slavery) in July 1846: Diagnosis of the Frequency of Thoughts (DFT) Based on His Journals and All Available Sources including His Description of Illumination in His Essay *Civil Disobedience*

| | Plane of Thought Frequency | | | | | | |
| | 2 | 3 | 4 | 5 | 7 | Global | Descriptor |
|---|---|---|---|---|---|---|---|
| A. DFT BEFORE ILLUMINATION IN JULY 1846 | | | | | | | |
| Average | .4 | .5 | .4 | .3 | .0 | 3.9 | "Purposeful" |
| Maximum | .6 | .6 | .6 | .6 | .0 | 5.5 | "Conscientious" |
| Minimum | .2 | .2 | .3 | .2 | .0 | 3.5 | "Curious" |
| B. DFT DURING ILLUMINATION IN JAIL IN JULY 1846 | | | | | | | |
| Maximum | .7 | .8 | .7 | .9 | .2 | 5.9 | "Self-actualized" |
| C. DFT AFTER ILLUMINATION (TYPICAL OF 1847–1862) | | | | | | | |
| Average | .5 | .7 | .5 | .6 | .0 | 4.2 | "Privacy seeking" |
| Maximum | .7 | .8 | .6 | .9 | .2 | 5.9 | "Self-actualized" |
| Minimum | .4 | .4 | .4 | .3 | .0 | 3.6 | "Argumentative" |

thoughts were at 5.9. He felt deeply that active opposition to what was unjust was the only true (choiceless) action of anyone who was aware of the innate spiritual freedom of all human beings. As described in *Civil Disobedience*, Thoreau said,

> I have paid no poll-tax for six years. I was put into a jail once on this account, for one night; and, as I stood considering the walls of solid stone, two or three feet thick, the door of wood and iron, a foot thick, and the iron grating which strained the light, I could not help being struck with the foolishness of that institution which treated me as if I were mere flesh and blood and bones, to be locked up. . . . I saw that, if there was a wall of stone between me and my townsmen, there was a still more difficult one to climb or break through before they could get to be as free as I was. I did not for a moment feel confined. . . . I felt as if I alone of all my townsmen had paid my tax. . . . In every threat and in every compliment there was a blunder; for they thought that my chief desire was to stand the other side of that stone wall. I could not but smile to see how industriously they locked the door on my meditations, and *they* were really all that was dangerous.

After this awakening, Thoreau's thoughts were substantially lighter. His maximum thoughts in his journals and publications were in the illuminative phase of the third stage of self-awareness (5.8 or 5.9). In addition, his average thoughts were elevated from 3.9 to 4.2, which involved the conflict between seeking recognition and seeking privacy. His minimum thoughts were also slightly elevated from 3.5 (quick to complain) to 3.6 (feelings of superiority or inferiority).

The elevation of Thoreau's thought in his publications after his illumination is shown in Table 4.14. After his illumination, Thoreau began long walks in 1849 and began to study biology systematically, particularly botany. He saw "walking" as a self-aware immersion in the universal unity of being. This was inspiring and satisfying to Thoreau and he felt that well-being was the result of sympathetic reverence for an infinite intelligence immanent in nature.

The mature works of Thoreau have had lasting spiritual impact. They reveal his deepening awareness of the inseparable bonds connecting all humanity and nature. This awareness awakened a deep respect for the freedom inherent in all human beings. Thoreau's resistance to unjust laws was a choiceless expression of his Platonic compassion. His insight corresponded well with the philosophy of Lamartine during the French Revolution of 1848; Lamartine enacted the freedom of all slaves in France. Thoreau's harmonious immersion in nature and his deep respect for individual freedom are timeless in spiritual value.

A substantial part of Thoreau's work was published during his lifetime, although not with much commercial success or personal recognition. The scope and depth of his spiritual transformation became clearer when Emerson and others read his

**Table 4.14.** Development of Henry David Thoreau's Thought as Shown in Creative Works Published from 1840 to 1863, including Average Thought Level of the Work and Thoreau's Title and Publication Date

| Thought Level | Descriptor of Publication | Thoreau's Title |
|---|---|---|
| BEFORE ILLUMINATION | | |
| 4.8 | Poem | *Sympathy* (1840) |
| 4.9 | Poem | *Rumors from an Aeolian Harp* (1842) |
| 5.0 | Poem | *The Inward Morning* (1842) |
| 5.1 | Poem | *Smoke* (1843) |
| AFTER ILLUMINATION | | |
| 5.6 | Essay | *Ktaadn & The Maine Woods* (1848) |
| 5.6 | Book | *A Week on the Concord & Merrimack Rivers* (1849) |
| 5.7 | Essay | *Civil Disobedience* (1849) (originally *Resistance to Civil Government*) |
| 5.7 | Essay | *Excursion to Canada* (1853) |
| 5.7 | Essay | *Where I Lived, and What I Lived For* (1854) |
| 5.6 | Book | *Walden* (1854) |
| 5.6 | Book | *Cape Cod* (1855) |
| 5.6 | Essay | *A Plea for Captain John Brown* (1859) |
| 5.6 | Essay | *Walking* (1862) |
| 5.6 | Essay | *Life without Principle* (1863) |
| 5.6 | Poem | *Inspiration* (1863) |

journals after his death. However, it is remarkable that Emerson minimized the importance of Thoreau's writing in his eulogy of Thoreau and the memoir *Thoreau*, which was published later after Emerson had the opportunity to study Thoreau's journals. In his eulogy and memoir of Thoreau, Emerson chose to depict Thoreau as a peculiar "hermit" and "ascetic" and said little about the importance of his mature writings (Myerson 1995, pages 25–39). Emerson's eulogy is misleading and self-centered, as was remarked by the daughter of Bronson Alcott, Louisa Mae Alcott, who attended the funeral (Myerson 1995, pages 36–39). Emerson's memoir of Thoreau also had the effect of perpetuating a myth that Thoreau had wasted his talents and died without accomplishing anything of lasting value. This had the effect of slowing general public recognition of the importance of Thoreau's mature writing. Essentially, Emerson was continuing his dialectic with Thoreau about the understanding and application of transcendentalism in life. Emerson was helpful to Thoreau mainly when doing so served his own purposes. Emerson was obviously defending his narcissistic self-image as the pre-eminent torchbearer of transcendental truth, when in reality it was Thoreau who had held the torch of truth at its greatest height in America since 1848.

## THE SIGNIFICANCE OF THE TRANSCENDENTALISTS

### The spiritual and cultural interest of the movement

We can how step back and take a broader perspective on the American Transcendentalist Movement from the details of our study of the development of their thoughts and relationships. In the case of the American transcendentalists, it is informative to distinguish the periods of diffusion in which Emerson was preeminent (1833–1846) from the period in which the mature Thoreau (1847–1862) also made important contributions.

The levels of thought inspired in each phase of the movement are indicated in Table 4.15 as the "spiritual interest" of each phase. This is a measurement of how psychologically interesting the movement is to other people in terms of its ability to inspire lightness of thought—in Emerson's own statement of intent on June 2, 1830, to "lead men to improve themselves, to keep the ear and soul open to receive truth." Emerson's illumination in the Jardin des Plantes in Paris marked the debut of the movement, as indicated in Table 4.3 and described in detail in the accompanying descriptions from his journal for July 13, 1833. At its debut, the spiritual interest of the movement is about 5.2, indicating that it was intended "to arouse the intellect," as indicated in Emerson's journal on August 18, 1937 about the function of a scholar. Emerson's illumination was followed by an intense period of diffusion to his disciples between 1834 and 1842. He also wrote his seminal book *Nature* in 1836 and gave his most influential addresses, such

**Table 4.15.** Overview of Spiritual Interest of the American Transcendentalist
Movement in Relation to the Life of Emerson (1803–1882) Based on the Level of
Thought It Inspired in Others at Different Times in the Movement

| Phase of Movement | Description | Spiritual Interest |
|---|---|---|
| Debut (7/13/33) | Illumination of Emerson in *Jardin des Plantes* in Paris, France | 5.2 |
| Emerson's diffusion (1833–1846) | Recruitment of disciples, and creative writing and lectures by Emerson and disciples | 5.1 |
| (7/46) | Illumination of Thoreau in Concord jail | 5.0 |
| Thoreau's diffusion (1847–1862) | Inspired writing by Thoreau on nature and freedom (no new disciples, but Emerson continues to lecture with more humanistic interests after return from Europe in 1848) | 4.8 |
| Popular spread (1863–1882) | After death of Thoreau, works by Emerson are popular and participation is broad but lacking in original fervor and mainly concerned with social aspects of everyday living | 4.1 |
| End | Death of founder and disciples | 3.1 |

as *The American Scholar* (1837), *The Harvard Divinity School Address* (1838),
and *The Method of Nature* (1841) well before 1846. Throughout the period 1833
to 1846, the spiritual interest of the movement remained in the intellectual plane.

In July 1846, Emerson's disciple Thoreau had his own illumination experience.
However, by this time, the movement's overall spiritual interest had slipped into
the emotional plane and was largely regarded as a humanistic movement (4.8).
Thoreau's writings were not of commercial success at the time. Thoreau did not
recruit disciples, but he produced a series of elevated creative works, which have
had enduring appreciation as classics of naturalism and civil disobedience.

After the death of Thoreau in 1862, the American transcendentalist movement
continued through the popular lectures and publications of Emerson throughout
the United States and Europe. It is in this form that the movement is most widely
known, but this phase is mainly concerned with basic emotional issues, such as
social sympathy, and self-reliance, rather than with spiritual awakening. Without
spiritual transformation of others or the recruitment of new disciples, the movement stagnated and then died with the death of its founder in 1882.

However, fortunately, inspired works like those of Emerson and Thoreau can
have a lasting impact beyond the immediate activity of the movement. May 2003
was the bicentennial of Emerson's birth, and his impact on American culture
remains substantial. Indeed, the creations of Thoreau, Emerson, and his other

disciples continue to stimulate interest today throughout the world among individual readers, as well as among historians, philosophers, and students of literary form and method. Hopefully, the psychological method of study described here may be of some benefit in understanding the method and message of the transcendentalists.

## CONCLUSIONS ABOUT THOUGHT AND SOCIAL RELATIONS

In brief, each person has a characteristic range of thought and of human relationships, which can be reliably and precisely measured in a quantitative fashion by the DFT and DHR. The range depends on the depth of self-awareness and understanding of particular emotional conflicts. The state of elevation of our thoughts and relationships depends on various parameters that influence our position within our characteristic range. Changes in the depth of understanding in our subconscious are possible in advanced stages of self-aware consciousness, leading to improvement in our character that are permanent. Our mood and cognitive state can be elevated or lowered in different states of self-aware consciousness, but improvement in self-awareness and character elevate the minimum level to which our thoughts and relationships may fall. This indicates that growth in self-awareness can lead to stable reduction in vulnerability to extreme states of mental disorder. Consequently growth in self-awareness can lead to cure of the underlying causes of mental problems, rather than merely acute relief of the symptoms of the underlying disorder.

The American Transcendentalist Movement has served to familiarize us with the measurement method and its underlying processes as a vivid and well-documented example. In the next chapter, we need to examine the question of what underlying psychophysical mechanisms can explain the structure and dynamics of self-aware consciousness.

## REFERENCES

Baker, C. (1996). *Emerson among the eccentrics: A group portrait.* New York, Viking.
Borst, R. R. (1992). *The Thoreau log: A documentary life of Henry David Thoreau.* New York, GW Hall & Co.
Brands, H. W. (2000). *The first American: The life and times of Benjamin Franklin.* New York, Anchor.
Broderick, J. C., ed. (1981). *Journals of Henry David Thoreau, 1837–1852.* Princeton, New Jersey, Princeton University Press.
Brownson, O. (1957). A dissenting definition. *The American Transcendentalists: Their prose and poetry.* P. Miller, ed. Garden City, New York, Doubleday & Co.: 39–47.
Cassirer, E. (1955). *The philosophy of the enlightenment.* Boston, Massachusetts, Beacon Press.

Emerson, E. W. and W. E. Forbes, Eds. (1914). *Journals of Ralph Waldo Emerson with annotations.* Boston, Massachusetts, Houghton Mifflin Co.

Emerson, R. W. (1841). The method of nature. *The American Transcendentalists: Their prose and poetry.* P. Miller, ed. Garden City, New York, Doubleday & Company: 49–68.

Emerson, R. W. (1880). Historic notes on life and letters in New England. *The American Transcendentalists: Their prose and poetry.* P. Miller, ed. Garden City, New York, Doubleday & Company: 1–20.

Emerson, R. W. (1939). *The letters of Ralph Waldo Emerson.* New York, Columbia University Press.

Emerson, R. W. (1960–82). *Journals and miscellaneous notebooks of Ralph Waldo Emerson.* Cambridge, MA, Harvard University Press.

Emerson, R. W. (1964). *The correspondence of Emerson and Carlyle.* New York, Columbia University Press.

Erikson, E. H. (1964). *Insight and responsibility.* New York, W. W. Norton & Co.

Haskins, D. G. (1887). *Ralph Waldo Emerson, his maternal ancestors.* Boston, Cupples Upham & Co.

Kohut, H. (1984). *How does analysis cure?* Chicago, Illinois, University of Chicago Press.

Locke, J. (1690). An essay concerning human understanding. *Great Books of the Western World.* M. J. Adler, ed. Chicago, Illinois, Brittanica: 85–402.

Miller, P., ed. (1957). *The American Transcendentalists: Their prose and poetry.* Garden City, New York, Doubleday & Company.

Myerson, J., ed. (1995). *The Cambridge companion to Henry David Thoreau.* New York, Cambridge University Press.

Plato (1986). *The dialogues of Plato.* New York, Bantam Books.

Richardson, R. D. J. (1995). *Emerson: The mind on fire.* Berkeley, California, University of California Press.

Rogers, C. R. (1980). *A way of being.* Boston, Massachusetts, Houghton Mifflin.

Sturgis, E. (1957). To R. W. E. *The American Transcendentalists: Their prose and poetry.* P. Miller, ed. Garden City, New York, Doubleday & Co.: 273–275.

Svrakic, D. M. (1990). "The functional dynamics of the narcissistic personality." *American Journal of Psychotherapy* 44: 189–203.

Teilhard de Chardin, P. (1978). *The heart of matter.* New York, Harcourt Brace Jovanovich.

Updike, J. (2003). Big dead white male. *The New Yorker.* August 3: 77–81.

Viereck, P. R. E. (1965). *Conservatism revisited.* New York, Free Press.

Weber, M. (1958). *The Protestant ethic and the spirit of capitalism.* New York, Scribner.

Winnicott, D. (1958). *Collected papers: Through pediatrics to psychoanalysis.* New York, Basic Books.

# 5

# PSYCHOPHYSICAL THEORIES
# OF CONTEMPLATION

## THE PREVALENCE OF CONTEMPLATIVE THOUGHT

Contemplative thinking has beneficial effects of major clinical significance. Contemplation enlarges consciousness and improves character through the nondualistic reconciliation of worries, struggles, and conflicts. In contrast, dualistic thinking blocked the full development of awareness in Emerson and his disciples. Later, Freud denied the reality of his oceanic feelings when visiting the Acropolis, which is a symbol of wisdom and universal order, because of his inability to trust in the goodness of the deepest aspect of himself, that is, his psyche (Freud 1936).

Consequently, Freud split the functions of the unconscious into the perfection-seeking superego and the pleasure-seeking id. The split between the conscious and unconscious prevented Freud from recognizing the human potential for full coherence of all aspects of our being. Freud attributed all moderating intelligence to the ego. This dualistic structure implies perpetual conflict between the soma and the psyche, as well as division between the conscious and unconscious, which can never lead to stable happiness and well-being.

Such dualistic thinking was reinforced by the classic view of cause and effect prevalent in the nineteenth century. Nevertheless, the metacognitive work of psychoanalysis provides a natural foundation for the development of contemplative thinking. Consequently, it was natural that some of Freud's disciples, such as Carl

Jung and Sandor Ferenczi, recognized the possibility and the importance of self-transcendence as the foundation for integrity, oceanic feelings, and creativity (Gay 1998). Later, Erik Erikson described maturation as a progressive increase in social radius leading to integrity and wisdom (Erikson 1963, 1964), which is based on recognition that each individual is like a wave that is an inseparable part of the eternal ocean of life. Likewise, Kohut (1984) and Winnicott (1958) emphasized the unity of the psyche and soma and the importance of developing authenticity. Hence, contemplative thinking, which begins with oceanic feelings, is a natural step in human development, building on the foundation of metacognition or meditation.

Many people attain the third stage of self-aware consciousness in spontaneous peak experiences, even if their usual view of reality assumes mind–body dualism. In fact, most people (59%) report peak experiences of either oceanic feelings or inseparability, as shown in Table 5.1. The observations in Table 5.1 were based on administration of the Temperament and Character Inventory (TCI) to a sample of 632 individuals representative of the population of the St. Louis metropolitan area as part of our St. Louis Health Survey in 1995. The peak experiences tabulated in Table 5.1 are dramatic in their quality, including feelings of boundlessness, ecstatic union, nonduality, and inseparability. Even these intense peak experiences occur in most people sometimes in their life. In addition, 82% of people report that they often lose awareness of the passage of time when absorbed in doing something they enjoy. Hence, contemplative thought is a normal experience, although peak experiences of inseparability occur only infrequently to most people who do have them.

Contemplative thought is a prevalent phenomenon that must be described and understood to have a general theory of self-aware consciousness. In this chapter, we ask two basic questions. "What are the fundamental properties of self-aware thought, particularly in the third stage of self-aware consciousness?" Based on an examination of these observable phenomena, we try to specify testable questions about the psychophysical mechanisms underlying the third stage of self-aware consciousness. Knowledge of the psychophysical mechanisms of contemplative consciousness is essential to shed light on why this stage of thought is so uplifting and serene. Knowledge of the psychophysical mechanisms is also important to demonstrate what facilitates and what blocks the development of third-stage self-awareness. Unfortunately, most past work on the development of self-aware consciousness has been purely descriptive. For example, what psychoanalysts have described as ego defense mechanisms are merely descriptions of thought processes. The psychophysical mechanisms that explain individual differences in ego processes are unknown (Vaillant 1993). In other words, there is no scientific theory to predict who will develop self-transcendence and integrity or to teach practical ways for mental health practitioners to help people develop coherence of personality.

Our second question is, "What are the fundamental assumptions in physics about the relationship of mind and matter that correspond to the different stages of self-

**Table 5.1.** Prevalence of Peak Experiences, including Oceanic Feelings and
Inseparability Based on Self-reports in the TCI in 632 Individuals Representative
of the General Population of St. Louis

| *Prevalence* | | *TCI Question Endorsed* |
|---|---|---|
| OCEANIC FEELINGS | | |
| (1) | 20% | (Boundlessness) |
| | | "Sometimes I have felt like I was part of something with no limits or boundaries in time and space." |
| (2) | 38% | (Ecstatic Union) |
| | | "I have had moments of great joy in which I suddenly had a clear, deep feeling of oneness with all that exists." |
| (1 or 2) | 45% | |
| INSEPARABILITY | | |
| (3) | 23% | (Nonduality) |
| | | "I sometimes feel so connected to nature that everything seems to be part of one living organism." |
| (4) | 26% | (Nonlocality) |
| | | "I often feel so connected to the people around me that it is like there is no separation between us." |
| (3 or 4) | 39% | |
| OCEANIC FEELINGS OR INSEPARABILITY | | |
| (1–4) | 59% | |

Items for oceanic feelings and inseparability are from subscales 1 and 2 of TCI Self-Transcendence.

aware consciousness?" To evaluate these questions, different theories of causality
and consciousness will be compared in terms of the level of thought that they seek
to explain. Certain aspects of thought, such as creative gifts and the Savant syndrome, will also be examined to illustrate its quantum-like properties. Creative gifts
are associated with contemplative thinking in specific domains and provide important clues for understanding the fundamental nature of self-aware consciousness.

## THE STAGES OF UNDERSTANDING CAUSALITY
## AND CONSCIOUSNESS

Most discussion of consciousness in psychology, philosophy, and physics has been
confused because it failed to distinguish between the three stages of self-aware
consciousness. For example, many modern theories of consciousness are based
on dualistic representation in which subject and object, thinker and thought, are
assumed to be separate (Seager 1999). Essentially, such theories apply only to

the first stage of self-aware consciousness because such consciousness assumes classical mechanical determinism, which works fairly well for the ordinary cognition of everyday activities that do not demand much meditative awareness or compassion for others. Unfortunately, theories that are adequate for only the lower range of human thought are sometimes advocated as general models, or the higher range of human thought is claimed to be intractable, inconsequential, or illusory.

The underlying assumptions about causality in the successive stages of self-aware consciousness are summarized in Table 5.2. *There is a close parallel between the stages of self-aware consciousness and the progression in the way physics incorporates understanding of causality and the integration of the mental and physical aspects of nature.* In Table 5.2, the lowest level of understanding is chaos and chance, which represent darkness, disorder, or the absence of self-aware consciousness of information. Self-aware consciousness of order grows toward unity and coherence (i.e., lightness), which is characterized by awareness of our inseparability (nonlocality) and the spontaneity of gifts (noncausality). Between the extremes of chaos and coherence, there are intermediate steps based on local realism (Branning 1997).

Galileo, Descartes, and Newton developed the concepts of classical physics during the seventeenth century. According to classic physics, the whole universe is a purely mechanical system or machine like a clock (Newton 1713). In the classic model of physical reality, nature consists of localized bits of matter. Even living bodies and brains are regarded as simply mechanical systems. Furthermore, the motion of all material elements is completely determined by contact interactions between adjacent elements.

According to the classic view, the subjective aspects of nature, such as human thoughts and feelings, are passive bystanders of mechanical processes. Information content depends passively on the way matter is organized, so that subjective consciousness is an inconsequential epiphenomenon of life. According to classic physics, thought cannot cause any material motion because every such action is

**Table 5.2.** Assumptions about Causality in Different Theories of Physics and Stages of Self-Aware Consciousness

| Stage | Self-Awareness | Causality | Perspective |
|-------|----------------|-----------|-------------|
| 0 | No self-awareness | Chaos chance | Singular |
| 1 | Ordinary cognition | Local | Classic (dualistic and local) |
| 2 | Metacognition | Local | Relativistic (dualistic and universal) |
| 3 | Contemplation | | |
| A | Illumination | Nonlocal | Quantum nonlocality |
| B | Unitive phase | Noncausal | Nondual (nonlocal and noncausal) |

completely determined by purely mechanical forces. That is, thought lacks energy and the capacity to do work. Of course, such complete mechanical determinism contradicts the direct human intuition that each person can willfully cause physical actions, like moving a hand purposefully, and mental activity, like choosing freely to attend to external or internal cues. Such deterministic views have profound implications for human self-awareness and moral values, leading to intense philosophical controversy, as discussed in Chapter 1. In psychology, the claim of William James that our emotions and thoughts are the consequence but not the cause of our actions was quickly dismissed by the systematic findings of William Cannon (1927), as noted in Chapter 1. Nevertheless, the ideas of classic physics still recur even in modern philosophy of the mind, neuroscience, and molecular psychiatry. This persistence of an incomplete model of the nature of physical reality may be partly explained by the fact that people are taught to use the assumptions of classic physics for many practical activities. We grow accustomed to such assumptions and fail to recognize the important ways they contradict the experienced fact that our thoughts can influence our actions.

The relegation of thought processes to the position of a passive bystander also has profound implications for understanding the evolution of learning abilities. If thought has no causal effects, then it is not subject to any selective pressures in evolution. Yet there appears to be close and systematic coordination between the evolution of brain structure and consciousness! The evolution of consciousness, which is considered further in Chapter 7, strongly suggests that consciousness does have causal effects.

The progression from the first to the second stage of awareness of the relationship between matter and mind, as well as between causality and consciousness, was the development of Einstein's theories of special and general relativity. Einstein had been reading the philosophy of Ernst Mach just before he wrote his paper on special relativity, and he credited Mach with influencing his thinking (Goonatilake 2000). According to Einstein's viewpoint, what is true about nature depends on the observer as well as on the observed and the subjective sense of time is an illusion. Nevertheless, Einstein maintained the assumptions of classic physics about local realism. Einstein used Mach's principles to exclude the reality of nonlocality, which is often described as "action at a distance." According to the philosophical view of local realism, nature is composed primarily of physical matter, which can only act through contact with adjacent bits of matter.

However, Einstein also established the equivalence of mass and energy, as expressed in his famous equation $E = mc^2$, where $E$ refers to energy, $m$ to mass, and $c$ to the speed of light. Einstein strongly held to his assumption of local causality, but modern quantum physics has now rigorously demonstrated violations of local realism by the quantum phenomena of nonlocality and noncausality.

Nevertheless, the first stage of self-aware consciousness can still be maintained while using quantum mechanics to describe physical reality, as in the interpretation of Niels Bohr. The quantum theory was based on Max Planck's discovery of the quantum of action and was largely developed in the years 1925–1927, primarily by Heisenberg, Bohr, Dirac, Schroedinger, and Max Born (Gamow 1966; Stapp 2000). The Copenhagen interpretation of quantum physics is at the thought level of rational materialism (i.e., 5.0). According to the Danish physicist Bohr and his followers, reality can be meaningfully described only by assuming the dualistic separation of the observer and the observed. The observer operates according to the laws of classic mechanical determinism and can make probability statements about the behavior based on analysis of information according to quantum mechanics. Although the behavior of the observed is predicted by quantum mechanics, nothing meaningful can be said about particles of matter at the quantum level prior to measurement. In other words, quantum physics deals with bits of information that are diffused as waves and not with localized particles of matter, which are objects that are only inferred by an observer in a state of dualistic consciousness.

Essentially, the Copenhagen interpretation of quantum mechanics does not allow conscious awareness of reality at the quantum level. In fact, according to the Copenhagen interpretation, not only is there nothing to be said but there is no reality before measurement. According to this materialistic view, all that is real and consciously meaningful is what is observed at the classic level of mechanical determinism.

Einstein was not satisfied with Bohr's interpretation. His theories of special and general relativity operate in the second stage of self-aware consciousness, which maintains the dualistic assumption of local causality (i.e., local realism) but extends the perspective of the observer to an infinite number of positions in the universe of space and time. Einstein's new basic step in the special theory of relativity in 1905 was to regard physics as the observation of *relationships* among the various aspects of the universe, rather than the absolute underlying substance of the universe, such as matter or ether (Bohm 1996, page viii). Consequently, what is observed as true depends on the observer. The second stage of self-awareness assumes local causality, as in the first stage of self-awareness. However, the second stage of self-awareness also assumes a universal perspective, as in the third stage of self-awareness. Both the theories of relativity and quantum physics take a global perspective that is universal; that is, both theories are based on the assumption of "undivided wholeness" (Bohm and Hiley 1993, page 176).

The third stage of self-aware consciousness is distinguished from the earlier two stages by conscious awareness of aspects of nonduality. In the illuminative phase, action at a distance is recognized, whereas in the unitive phase, noncausality is also recognized. *Action at a distance* is another term for nonlocal causality. *Noncausality* refers to actions that are not fully explained by antecedent causes, such as spontaneous gifts or free choices. Erwin Schrodinger, who developed the quantum wave equation, was a monistic philosopher whose views of life were close to those of positive philosophers like Spinoza (Schrodinger 1983, 1992).

Schrodinger's theory of matter and mind is typical of the illuminative phase of self-aware consciousness, which transcends the assumptions of local realism.

Based on their understanding of local realism (Einstein, Podolsky et al. 1935), Einstein, Podolsky and Rosen assumed that "if, *without in any way disturbing the system*, we can predict with certainty the value of a physical quantity, then there exists an element of physical reality corresponding to this physical quantity." However, as Bohr pointed out, the use of any macroscopic physical instrument for measurement results in a disturbance of the observed physical system. Consequently, in physics there is a "measurement problem," which has been the topic of controversy since the introduction of quantum physics. The measurement problem is variously described as the problem of Schrodinger's cat, or Wigner's friend, or the collapse of the quantum wave function with measurement, or quantum state reduction (Stapp 2000).

This measurement problem does not occur in contemplation, that is, when the observer is the observed. It may be that only contemplation satisfies Einstein's condition that observation can be made without disturbing the observed system. Furthermore, in contemplation the perspective is nondualistic because the observer is the observed. Consequently, local causality, which was Einstein's most cherished assumption, simply does not apply in contemplation. The third stage of self-aware consciousness begins with the subjective experience of nonlocality, which is usually described as oceanic feelings. *Oceanic feelings* are "a sensation of *eternity*, a feeling of something limitless, unbounded, something 'oceanic'" (Freud 1929, page 767). Freud also described such feeling as the experience of an "indissoluble connection, of belonging inseparably to the external world as a whole" (Freud 1929, page 767).

The experience of nonlocality leads to increasing depth of recognition of phenomena that are unique to quantum physics, such as noncausality and nonlocality. Nonlocality refers to the inseparability of the bits of information. It is the beginning of the recognition that information may be the fundamental basis of reality. Localized particles of matter cannot be the fundamental basis of reality, as shown by rigorous demonstrations of action at a distance. When there is nonlocal causality or action at a distance, a causal influence on one "object" has an instantaneous influence on another remote but "entangled object." Noncausality and nonlocality are the properties that distinguish quantum physics from classic and relativistic models of local physical realism.

According to modern (post-Copenhagen) interpretations of quantum physics, "Classical physics was a deterministic theory about imaginary bits of localized matter, whereas quantum theory is a probabilistic theory about real bits of information" (Stapp 2000, page 2). The post-Copenhagen interpretation of quantum physics corresponds to the third stage of self-aware consciousness, which begins with the direct experience of oceanic feelings or nonlocality. Henry Stapp (2000) has pointed out that this shift in perspective allows the integration of the mental and physical aspects of nature. Work to integrate the subjective and objective aspects of nature was begun in the early 1930s by John von Neumann and Eugene Wigner. The French Nobel Laureate Louis de Broglie and the American David Bohm worked on a way of trying to describe physical particles at the quantum level (Bohm 1980; Albert 1994). In contrast, Henry Stapp has taken the more radical step of regarding the fundamental basis of reality to be information, not localized matter at all.

Frequently people have assumed that the world is primarily composed of separate material particles and that information is a secondary phenomenon derived by the organization of matter. The opposite may be true: information may be the primary basis of the universe, and material objects are secondary phenomena derived by inferences from the organization of information. In 1989, the American physicist John Archibald Wheeler expressed the idea of the primacy of information in the pithy phrase "it from bit" (Davies 1992; Davies 1999).

This revolutionary notion is not really new. It is a partial expression of the Greek concept of *logos* as the complete information from which all the various forms of nature are derived. However, before to the development of the post-Copenhagen quantum theory, concepts suggesting that anything other than matter might be the basis of reality were scientifically obscure. Now the objective and subjective aspects of nature can be integrated and studied in a scientifically rigorous manner in modern quantum theory with a rationally coherent concept of man and nature. According to Henry Stapp (Stapp 2000),

> The basic message of both Copenhagen and post-Copenhagen quantum theory is that the physical world must be understood in terms of INFORMATION. The "bits of matter" that classical physics had assumed the world to be built out of are transmuted into diffused spread-out nonmaterial structures that combine to form a new kind of physical reality that functions as an objective carrier of a growing collection of "bits of information."
>
> Each subjective experience injects one bit of information into this objective store of information, which then specifies, via known mathematical laws, the relative probabilities for various possible future subjective experiences to occur. The physical world thus becomes an evolving structure of information and propensities, rather than an evolving material structure.

According to Stapp, information provides the basis for our understanding of energy and matter. This is not quite the same as saying that information is actual reality, but only that it is what we know about reality. The distinction between what is real and what we can say about what is real is made clear in Roy Frieden's work on the derivation of the laws of physics (Frieden and Sofer 1995). Frieden and his colleagues have used a precise definition of information to derive many of the fundamental laws of physics (Frieden and Cocke 1996; Frieden 1998; Matthews 1999). Frieden and Sofer (1995) make two conjectures:

All things physical are information-theoretic in origin and this is a participatory universe. . . . Observer participancy gives rise to information; and information gives rise to physics.

Matter and consciousness are two realities in themselves, which are capable of mutual interaction.

According to Frieden's dualistic view of information, matter and consciousness are two fundamental realities, and information is what a dualistic observer can say about these two realities.

A nondualistic view of reality can be based on the further conjecture that all things are equivalent to energy. Einstein established the equivalence of energy and mass. Likewise, information can be shown to measure the free energy in a system, or inversely its entropy. Specifically, information (I) is defined as the complement of entropy (S). That is, information $I = 1 - S$. Entropy is also directly proportional to the difference between the energy (E) bound in a system and that energy free (F) to do work. That is, entropy $S \sim (E - F)$. Therefore, information about a system is a measure of the energy in the system that is available to do work. Both mass and information are measures of energy, so energy may be the fundamental basis of reality. If so, this would require that consciousness is also a measure of energy, which would mean that consciousness does work and exerts real effects in the processes of living.

According to Quantum Field Theory, space is a universal field of infinite energy. In other words, space is not really an empty void. Rather space is filled with energy, which is the beginning and end of all physical phenomena in space-time. This concept has been confirmed repeatedly by experimental high-energy physics, which regularly encounters phenomena that can only be explained by quanta emerging from space or returning into space. This movement in space-time indicates a direction of all physical developments to and from its source.

Physics is lacking a general theory of the nature of space and the space energy field. However, a consensus has emerged that a universal field, called a Higgs field, pervades all space (Higgs 1964). The Higgs field has been used to develop a unified field theory incorporating all the fundamental interactions of matter. Experimental support for the field has been indicated in recent particle discoveries, but not all predicted particles have yet been observed.

Such phenomena as noncausality and nonlocality were so contrary to everyday experience that physicists, including Einstein, were forced to undergo a revolution in their thinking during the past century (Bell 1993). Now these phenomena are firmly established experimentally in physics (Bouwmeester, Pan et al. 1997; Tittel, Brendel et al. 1998; Weihs, Jennewein et al. 1998; Zeilinger 2000). Nevertheless, many conservative psychologists, neuroscientists, and philosophers of mind continue to think in terms of classical physics (Rey 1997). In contrast, more liberal leaders in the same fields have begun to consider quantum phenomena in relation to human cognition seriously (Eccles 1989; Penrose 1989; Chalmers 1996; Stapp 1999; Walker 2000). Hence, it is instructive to examine the explanatory power of alternative theories.

## EXPLANATORY LEVEL OF CAUSAL THEORIES

Different theorists of physics and of consciousness have tried to provide explanations for action and thought at various levels of self-aware consciousness. Representative theorists are listed in Table 5.3 for various levels of thought for which the theorists provide explanatory accounts. Please remember that the actual level of thought of the theorists may be higher or lower than the level of thought they seek to explain, so this is not a personal evaluation of the thought of the theorists. For example, someone with a low level of thought may try to explain elevated phenomena. Vice versa, people with high personal levels of thought may sometimes devote their attention to lower phenomena.

What is important to recognize here is that a theory cannot explain phenomena that it ignores or denies are real. For example, the influential modern philosopher Daniel Dennett reduces consciousness to intentionality in his writings (Dennett 1987, 1991, 1993). According to my system of measuring thought, intentionality refers to thought in the plane 3, which is called either the material plane or the plane of intention. Intentionality provides no account whatsoever of phenomenal consciousness (i.e., emotionality and rationality) or meta-cognition. Dennett is well aware of this elimination of higher levels of thought, which he argues do not exist and should be ignored in a scientific understanding of human beings. Dennett makes this strong claim because he assumes that fundamental reality is best described by classical mechanical determinism, that is, local realism. For example, in *Consciousness Explained* (Dennett 1991), he assumes that "a brain is always going to do what it is caused to do by local mechanical disturbances."

If classic determinism were a complete model of reality, Dennett's arguments might be valid. Likewise, if classic determinism were complete, there would be no rational basis for creativity, free will, moral values, or spirituality. The observation of one's thoughts could have no consequence in a person's life. According to modern quantum theory, however, Dennett's assumption is false: the events in a human being's brain can be strongly influenced by self-observation and free conscious choices. As Henry Stapp (Stapp 2000, page 4) comments,

> Consciousness can play the influential role in the determination of our actions that we intuitively feel that it plays, and that religions have normally assumed that it plays. Thus this underlying conflict between religion and science evaporates when one goes over to quantum theory, which makes our minds co-authors of our actions.

**Table 5.3.** Representative Theorists of Physics and Consciousness According to the Level of Action and Thought for which They Provide an Explanatory Account

| Level Explained | Physics | Consciousness |
|---|---|---|
| 0 Connectionism<br>behaviorism<br>(thought < 3.4) | Isaac Newton | David Hume<br>Thomas Hobbes<br>Paul Churchland |
| 1 Intentionality<br>local realism<br>(thought 3.4–3.9) | Isaac Newton | Daniel Dennett<br>Gerald Edelman<br>Eli Robins and Sam Guze<br>Joseph LeDoux |
| Emotionality<br>(thought 4.0–4.9) | | Fred Dretske<br>David Rosenthal |
| Rational materialism<br>(thought 5.0–5.3) | Niels Bohr<br>Stephen Hawking<br>Steven Weinberg | Franz Brentano<br>Ned Block<br>Thomas Nagel<br>John Searle<br>Martin Seligman<br>Wm. Seager |
| 2 Metacognition<br>meditation<br>(thought 5.4–5.7) | Albert Einstein | Aristotle<br>René Descartes<br>Immanuel Kant<br>Sigmund Freud<br>Aaron Beck<br>Antonio Damasio<br>Richard Davidson |
| 3 Nonlocal causality<br>oceanic feelings<br>thought 5.8–7.0) | Erwin Schrodinger<br>David Bohm<br>John S. Bell<br>Roger Penrose<br>John A. Wheeler | Carl Jung<br>Adolf Meyer<br>David Chalmers<br>M. Csikszentmihalyi<br>Charles Alexander |
| Noncausality<br>Contemplation<br>(thought 7.1–7.7) | Henry Stapp<br>Evan H. Walker | G. W. F. Hegel<br>J. Krishnamurti |
| Coherence<br>(thought 7.8–7.9) | Peter Higgs | Plato<br>Augustine<br>M. K. Gandhi |

At a higher level of explanation than Dennett, rational materialists like William Seager (1999, page 142) have tried to steer a narrow course between what they see as the "Charybdis of supernaturalism and the Scylla of a blinkered reductionism." Such materialism risks irrelevance by its failure to recognize the significance of recent progress in cognitive neuroscience and in quantum physics. There has been substantial empirical progress in the neuropsychology of metacognition (Damasio 1994; Gusnard, Akbudak et al. 2001; Gusnard and Raichle 2001), attention (Posner and Fan 2003), and meditative states (Wallace 1970; Cade and Coxhead 1989; Csikszentmihalyi 1991, 1993), which I previously described in Chapter 3. Concepts about physical reality from the seventeenth century are unable to explain the full range of human thought:

> Classical dynamics is 'local' in the sense that all causation is via contact interaction between neighboring bits of matter. But the interaction of subjective experiences with the physical world turns out to be 'nonlocal': what a person decides to do in one place can instantly influence what is true in distant places . . . to the extent that a rationally coherent conception of physical reality is possible, this reality will be informational in character, not material. (Stapp 2000)

The movement of thought in the higher stages of self-aware consciousness has been well documented for more than a century, as was described in Chapter 3. Although many theories are limited to the first stage of self-aware consciousness, progress in experimental demonstration of nonlocality has stimulated work relevant to understanding the higher stages of consciousness. Likewise, work on the neuropsychology and brain imaging has stimulated interest in understanding the brain mechanisms associated with the higher stages of consciousness. It is difficult to regard metacognition as an illusion when the self-observation of internal cues results in substantial measurable variation in the activity of specific brain regions above and below the default state of subconscious activity (Gusnard and Raichle 2001). Furthermore, the activation of specific brain regions is also strongly correlated with individual differences in character development. Fortunately, leading neuroscientists and physicists have recognized the importance of understanding consciousness for the interpretation of physics, as well as the importance of quantum phenomena in understanding consciousness (Bohm 1980, 1996; Penrose 1989; Bohm and Hiley 1993; Stapp 2000; Walker 2000). Hopefully, the ability to quantify self-aware consciousness, as described here, will stimulate further progress in the dialogue between physics and psychology.

## FACILITATING CONTEMPLATIVE EXPERIENCE

It is impossible to understand anything that has not been personally experienced; therefore, it is important to identify practical ways for facilitating the experience of contemplative thinking, particularly for clinicians who want to help their patients mature optimally. In Chapter 3, I described three phases of the silence of mind meditation, which helps people to exercise their mind in ways that move them in a stepwise fashion toward contemplation. Another meditation that is particularly helpful in the development of contemplative thinking is called *union in nature*. It is especially useful to demonstrate the fact that our senses are often partially asleep and that they can be awakened to produce a state of joyful awareness in which there is no real separation between self and nonself. In contemplation, the boundaries between self and nonself (i.e., conscious and unconscious) are relaxed. In the process of meditation on our union in nature, we become aware that our senses were partially asleep and that we actually exist in a participatory union with all that exists.

In the first phase of the union in nature exercise, a person is instructed to awaken each of their five physical senses in the order of their typical biological maturation. That is, they awaken their senses of touch, taste, smell, hearing, and vision one at a time in the stated sequence. When people are stressed or preoccupied, their awareness of sensory experiences is reduced. For example, the average person can usually observe that their sense of smell is reduced (i.e., partially "asleep" or subconscious) when they try to smell a pleasant odor after they have been "stressed out." To "awaken" the physical and intuitive senses, you first make an effort to awaken each of your physical senses. The exercise can be done anywhere, whether in an office, bedroom, or in a garden. You may touch something smooth or with a complex texture, or simply feel the weight of your body on your seat or feet. Then you may taste something like a mint if you are outside in a garden, perhaps a piece of chewing gum or candy, or just your own skin or saliva if nothing else is available. Third, you check to see how easily you can smell the room you are in, or something fragrant in your home or garden. Fourth, you can check your awareness of the sounds around you by listening attentively to your environment and the sounds of your own body. Fifth, you can heighten your vision by looking around you to see what you may have overlooked in your other preoccupations or you may close your eyes and see what image appears in your mind.

The first sequence is then repeated again, but this time an effort is made to keep each sense awake when the next is awakened, until all your senses are fully awake simultaneously. When your senses of touch and taste are both awake, you realize that the external skin and internal mucosa are not barriers but gateways for communication between what is outside and what is inside. Such penetration of the subject–object boundary may lead to the early steps of nonlocal awareness at thought levels of 7.1–7.3, as described in the next section.

When your senses of touch, taste, and smell are all awake, you may experience an emotional communion with all that exists. When you are aware of this communion, there is also the experience of serenity along with an enlightening alertness that is calm, freely mobile in creative discovery, and impartially loving. In this state of union in nature (i.e., thought levels of 7.4–7.5), all of your experience is a participation in the universal unity of all being.

When your senses of touch, taste, smell, and hearing are all awake, there may be an awakening of your awareness that your own intelligence is inseparable from a limitless collective intelligence. Such integrated intelligence combines reason and love in a selfless perspective, which occurs at thought levels 7.6–7.7. When all of your senses are fully awake, there may be the experience of cosmic consciousness at thought levels 7.8–7.9, as described in the next section.

The meditation on union in nature is a moment of pure joy, which you can be practice as often and anywhere you like. It takes about half an hour to do this properly, and optimally should be done the first time with someone with previous experience, particularly if you are tense, preoccupied, or have many fears and blocks limiting your self-awareness. The hope and encouragement of a compassionate therapeutic alliance can help others to awaken their own self-awareness. The exercise can be done as often as is practical. With repetition, there is increasing likelihood of learning to experience and maintain contemplative thinking as a usual or even permanent way of living.

## DESCRIPTION OF CONTEMPLATIVE THOUGHT

The maximal thoughts of the American transcendentalists were in the beginning phase of contemplative thought (that is, thoughts from 5.8–7.0). To give a fuller description of thought in plane 7, the aspects of contemplative thought from 7.1 to 7.9 are summarized in Table 5.4. In this section, I describe thought in five subplanes of plane 7 in terms of both the content of thought and my understanding of the underlying worldview at each level. For each aspect of thought in Table 5.4, the corresponding gift of the spirit that influences thought is described. The described thought is listed along with what I propose as the spiritual mechanism and the quantum phenomenon that may explain the occurrence of such thoughts. Quotations of thoughts at various levels of elevation in plane 7 will be used as illustrations for clarity.

Thought in the sexual subplane 7–2 is characterized by a sense of wonder and awe. More specifically, there is personal humility combined with awe of the boundlessness of the universal unity of being, which leads to an understanding of hope. We understand ourselves as an integral aspect of the universal unity of being, just as all things are, which is both wonderful and humbling. We are branches of the vine of life—dependent creatures, not gods, but inseparably connected to the source of our fulfilling hope. There is wonder and hope because we are an indissoluble part of what is infinite and eternal, so there is no justification for despair or fear of annihilation. At the same time, there is deep humility because there is no basis for anyone to be regarded as superior or inferior to anyone—all are really aspects of the whole and dependent on the whole as the source of sustenance.

**Table 5.4.** Characteristics of Contemplative Thought

| Aspect | Gift | Mechanism | Principle |
|---|---|---|---|
| Sexual | Awe, hope, humility | Being | Nonduality (all is information) |
| Material | Reverence, kindness, charity | Freedom (pleasant) | Noncausality (gifts, spontaneity) |
| Emotional | Calm alertness, mercy | Love (not fear) (no conflict) | Complementarity (serenity) |
| Intellectual | Patience (seeking holiness, choiceless awareness, impartiality) | Truth | Nonlocality (inseparability) |
| Spiritual | Wisdom (peacemaker, single-heartedness, well-being) | Goodness | Fluidity (coherence, all is energy, cosmic feelings) |

In other words, when the level of thought is at 7.1, there is direct awareness of nonlocality, which is the beginning of cosmic consciousness. The term *cosmos* is derived from the Greek *kosmos*, referring to the "universal unity of being," that is, the universe conceived as a whole that is undivided, orderly, harmonious, intelligent, and creative. The conscious awareness of nonlocality involves access to what was previously unconscious, which is experienced as a node in the nonlocal (i.e., collective) unconscious. Such nonlocal consciousness has been variously described as self-remembering (Ouspensky 1938), as being cognition (Maslow 1962), as God consciousness (Maharishi 1969), or as psychedelia (Gowan 1971). All these terms refer to the seventh state of consciousness, which I designate at thought levels from 7.1 to 7.7. This seventh state is distinguished from two earlier phases of contemplation. Specifically, thought at 5.8 is the fifth state of lucid awareness, oceanic feelings, and integrity. Thought at levels 5.9–7.0 refers to creativity, which has been called the sixth state of consciousness (Cade and Coxhead 1989). Thought at 7.1 is the beginning of wisdom (i.e., the awakening of the mind to self-awareness of the light of the spirit of truth). At this elevation of thought there is freedom from dualistic thinking, that is, freedom from what Krishamurti called the "known" (Krishnamurti 1975) or what is called "knowledge of good and evil" in the book of Genesis in the Bible.

A disciple of the transcendentalist Walt Whitman, the Canadian psychiatrist Richard M. Bucke (1837–1902) studied reports of the experience of cosmic consciousness after he had a brief peak experience of nonlocality himself in 1872 during a visit to England. Bucke was a respected superintendent of a large psychiatric hospital in Canada. He was professionally respected for his innovative and compassionate care of the mentally ill. Bucke's experience of cosmic consciousness occurred at the end of an evening he had spent with two friends "reading Wordsworth, Shelley, Keats, Browning, and especially Whitman." On his long ride home, he described the following experience in his book *Cosmic Consciousness*:

> His mind, deeply under the influence of the ideas, images and emotions called up by the reading and the talk of the evening, was calm and peaceful. He was in a state of quiet, almost passive enjoyment. All at once, without warning of any kind, he found himself wrapped around as it were by a flame-colored cloud. For an instant he thought of fire, some sudden conflagration in the great city; the next, he knew that the light was within himself. Directly afterwards came upon him a sense of exultation, of immense joyousness accompanied or immediately followed by an intellectual illumination quite impossible to describe. Into his brain streamed one momentary lightning-flash of the Brahmic Splendor which has ever since lightened his life; upon his heart fell one drop of Brahmic Bliss, leaving thenceforward for always an after-taste of heaven. Among other things he did not come to believe, he saw and knew
>    that the Cosmos is not dead matter but a living Presence,
>    that the soul of man is immortal,
>    that the universe is so built and ordered that without any peradventure all things work together for the good of each and all,
>    that the foundation principle of the world is what we call love and that the happi-ness of everyone is in the long run absolutely certain. (Bucke 1951, pages 9–10)

Bucke's experience was brief and never repeated, but afterwards he felt trans-formed. He was filled with hope and confidence. He felt a consistent consequence of the experience of nonlocality was that those who experienced this later felt a sense of immortality and lost the fear of death and the sense of sin. Bucke's trans-formation is a clear example of Erikson's insight that the development of integ-rity through contemplative thought involves transcendence of despair and the fear of death. Hence the understanding of hope is based on the recognition of our eternal participation in what is wonderful and eternally fresh. This is the initial recogni-tion of the nondual nature of all being. One is all, and all is one. Such recognition of nonduality seems to require letting go of the assumption that the fundamental components of reality are local particles of matter; rather, nondual consciousness leads to the assumptions of the positive philosophy.

The quantum physicist Erwin Schrodinger pointed out that living things must overcome the natural tendency of dead things to fall into disorder (i.e., to in-crease in entropy) (Schrodinger 1992). Schrodinger said that a living thing maintains a high level of orderliness (i.e., a low level of entropy) by "continu-ally sucking orderliness from its environment" (1992, page 73). In other words, illumination (i.e., thought at level 5.8) involves self-awareness that all things participate in the unity of being, which has the natural properties of universal order, life, and love.

Schrodinger also observed that all things are inseparable components of one whole only if the components are universal fields. Fields are simply a way of describing inseparable aspects of the whole. According to Schrodinger's monistic perspective, ultimately there is one universal field of pure consciousness, but this infinite source of energy and information can be rearranged in infinite ways. Hence, rather than concern with individual reproduction and sexuality, our sexual needs can be sublimated to subplane 7–2, giving rise to wonder and hope. Contemplation of the mystery of our finite self in relation to what is infinite may give rise to awe, which is a composite of wonder, humility, and hope. For example, Emerson described such awe during his visit to the Jardin des Plantes in Chapter 4.

As a psychiatrist, Bucke was able to study the similar experiences of others, which he summarized in *Cosmic Consciousnesss* (Bucke 1951). Bucke documented fourteen individuals whom he concluded had even more elevated contemplative thoughts than he had himself. These fourteen included the founders of major religions, such as Gautama Buddha, Jesus Christ, and Mohammed, and others such as Paul, Plotinus, Dante, Francis Bacon, Jacob Boehme, William Blake, Balzac, John of the Cross, and Walt Whitman. Bucke also identified others in whom he thought the illumination was less complete and more transient, such as Emerson, Thoreau, and himself.

Thought in the material subplane 7–3 is characterized by a feeling of kindness and reverence. There is an understanding of charity based on recognition of non-causality. In other words, we recognize that the spontaneity of life is a gift and that all our talents are gifts. What is spontaneous in us is kindness, not fear or mean-spiritedness, which are consequences of the errors of dualistic thinking. Any lack of kindness or lack of reverence for others would be self-defeating resistance to the spontaneous source of all life. In contemplation of the mystery of good and evil, we transcend our fear of evil within our self and others. We are free to act independent of any old habits or traditions if we act spontaneously. In other words, the mechanism underlying noncausality is freedom or spontaneity of action. What we know is a gift, and our spontaneous actions are free. Hence, knowing is acting spontaneously and effortlessly. Krishnamurti also described the equivalence of knowing and acting in freedom, which he described as "choicelessness" (Krishnamurti 1992).

Thought in the material subplane 7–3 is sometimes described as the gift of piety or reverence. Rather than selfish desire or seeking of pleasure, our material desires from plane 3 are sublimated to subplane 7–3. In other words, our intentions become spiritual in their basis. This leads to charity and spontaneous kindness and compassion for others and reverence for the universal unity of being. For example, at thought level 7.2, Augustine said, "Our greatest efforts should be for a most virtuous life." At thought level 7.3, Lamartine said, "To love, pray, and sing: here is all my life."

At thought level 7.2 or 7.3, a person may still be moved to tears when experiencing the suffering of others, so there is not full serenity. In contrast, thought in the emotional subplane 7–4 is peaceful and serene. Serenity is an alertness that is calm, freely mobile, unconditionally loving, and always appropriate for

the person's context and content of thought. Thought at level 7.4 or 7.5 is compassion without any personal suffering. Such compassion and freedom from individual suffering are the result of the sublimation of all emotional conflicts from
plane 4 to the emotional aspects of spirituality. Sublimation of emotions to serene
compassion leads to direct recognition of the dual nature of the self as a localized
individual and as a universal being. Through contemplation of the mystery of love,
we understand that the love is necessarily both impartial and compassionate because of the indivisibility of all things. The universal unity of being is all-loving
and omnipresent because its essence is an eternal sharing of divine being. What
could be a greater gift than to share your whole being in the act of creation? All
life has already received everything and is only growing in awareness of its fundamentally divine nature. Human beings are not sterile machines—they share in
the unconditional and inexhaustible love of all that is, which is divine. The essence of each form of life is the same. Everything develops within the all-encompassing love that is the essence of everything.

The dual nature of a person is comparable to the dual nature of light as a particle and a wave. Krishnamurti stated the quantum principle that "the observer is
the observed" or "you are the world," as we have previously discussed (Bohm
1995). However, this intuition has been stated previously many times. For example,
as quoted by Bucke (1951, page 185), the uneducated shoemaker Jakob Boehme
(1575–1624), said at thought level 7.4,

> If you will observe your own self and the outer world, and what is taking place therein,
> you will find that you . . . are that external world. You are a little world formed out of
> the large one, and your external light is a chaos of the sun and the constellation of stars.
> If this were not so you would not be able to see by means of the light of the sun.

When thought is in the emotional subplane 7–4, we are acting only as inseparable agents on behalf of the harmony of all, so violence and fear have no basis.
Thought at this level is sometimes described as the gift of counsel, as compassion, or as the understanding of love. For example, as quoted by Bucke (1951,
page 89), Gautama Buddha said at thought level 7.4,

> When to a man who understands, the self has become all things, what sorrow, what
> trouble can there be to him who once beheld that unity.

At this sublevel thought is nonviolent, merciful, and loving because all things
are complementary manifestations of the universal unity of being. Serenity is based
on the mechanism of love, whereas all fear is a perturbation of the mechanism of
love. Our concerns about receiving sympathy and appeasement from others in
plane 4 are sublimated to subplane 7–4, so that we seek only to give love and
reconciliation to others without fear for our individual self.

When thought is at the level of 7.4 or 7.5, there is serenity but experience is not consistently joyful. In contrast, thought in the intellectual subplane 7–5 involves patience filled with joy. This is a state of choiceless awareness in which reason and love are integrated efficiently, which is joyful and effortless. Such unconditional awareness is based on recognition of the nonlocal and noncausal nature of all things, which gives rise to an understanding of the mystery of faith. Understanding of nonlocality and noncausality gives rise to patience. Hence thought at this level is sometimes described as the gift of fortitude. For example, at thought level 7.6, Montaigne said in his *Essays* (Montaigne 1998), "I do not bite my nails about the difficulties I meet with. . . . I do nothing without gaiety."

When thought is at level 7.6 or 7.7, intelligence is integrated and joyful, but there may be limited wisdom about the most fruitful direction of action. In contrast, thought in the spiritual subplane 7–7 is characterized by coherence of personality and full cosmic consciousness. Thought at this level has also been called unity consciousness or the eighth state of consciousness (Cade and Coxhead 1989).

States of coherence can also be described as the optimal state of consciousness, "flow," or fluidity (Csikszentmihalyi 1991). However, the full range of contemplative states (i.e., thoughts from 5.8 to 7.9) are regarded as states of flow by Csikszentmihalyi and as cosmic consciousness by Bucke. However, it is useful in my opinion to quantify thought within this wide range, that is, to recognize subplanes within the range of contemplative thought.

In any case, the psychological fluidity of contemplative thought can be viewed as the counterpart of physical coherence in states of superfluidity. In its pure form (i.e., in subplane 7–7), psychological coherence is comprised of wisdom, well-being, and creativity. There are no complaints whatsoever when thought is fully coherent. In other words, at this level of thought a person is a wise truth seeker and a single-hearted peacemaker. Coherent thought is associated with deep understanding of the mystery that all matter and information is derived from a universal field that is a source of boundless energy, as postulated in modern quantum physics. Often such awareness occurs only in transient peak experiences, but there are some individuals in whom the average level of thought is transformed to stable coherence in a state of constant awareness. For example, at thought level 7.8, Gandhi (1997, *Young India*, October 11, 1925) said,

> I do dimly perceive that whilst everything around me is ever-changing, ever-dying, there is underlying all that change a Living Power that is changeless, that holds all together, that creates, dissolves, and re-creates. That informing Power or Spirit is God. And since nothing else I see merely through the senses can or will persist, He alone is.

Furthermore, according to Gandhi's view (*Young India*, 11, 1925;) Gandhi 1997, page 52), the universal source of all energy is pure consciousness and benevolent power:

And is this Power benevolent or malevolent? I see it as purely benevolent. For I can see that in the midst of death life persists, in the midst of untruth truth persists, in the midst of darkness light persists. Hence I gather that God is Life, Truth, Light. He is Love. He is the Supreme Good.

Gandhi provides many examples of coherent thought, which deals with every aspect of life in an integrated manner. For example, at thought level 7.8, Gandhi also said, "When I despair I remember that all throughout history the way of Truth and Love has always triumphed. There may be tyrants and assassins, and for a time they may seem invincible, but in the end they always fall. Think of it—Always." Gandhi's thoughts and actions throughout his life are an inspiring example of nondual consciousness as a stable way of living.

## QUANTUM-LIKE NATURE OF INSIGHT AND GIFTEDNESS

### Insight learning

So far in this chapter, I have suggested that there is a quantum-like nature to self-aware consciousness on the basis of indirect evidence. Theories of physics have developed in ways that are analogous to theories of self-aware consciousness. Likewise, the content of contemplative thought corresponds to the fundamental aspects of quantum phenomena, including nonlocality, noncausality, and coherence. However, the most important evidence for the quantum-like nature of thought are the directly observable features of learning based on insight, that is, intuitive learning and creativity.

A quantum is defined as a discrete and indivisible unit, such as the units of energy in light of varying frequencies. Likewise, the development of insight ("enlightenment") progresses by means of a succession of discrete but inseparable events, which often occur suddenly in the transition from one thought to another. This quantum-like nature is characteristic of both insight and humor. Insight is sudden recognition, which we designate by the expletive "Ah-ha!" The humor of jokes also involves a sudden recognition, which we designate by the expletive "ha-ha!" as discussed in *The Act of Creation* (Koestler 1964). The humor is lost if the joke must be explained analytically, just as the joyful life of art is lost in intellectual criticism. More generally, character development involves a succession of discrete steps in insight, which we have already examined in detail in Chapters 2 and 3, showing that these discrete steps move in a spiral pattern in time. In contrast, to this stepwise hierarchical development of character, the conditioning of habits varies continuously in its strength (Adamec and Stark-Adamec 1983). *Hence, self-aware thoughts, but not habits or procedural skills, have a quantum-like pattern of development.*

Even more striking evidence for the quantum-like nature of insight learning are gifts, as seen in prodigies in art and science, such as Mozart in music or Ramanujan in mathematics (Kanigel 1991). These special abilities are called gifts because they are unpredictable in terms of a person's prior experience and genetic background (Winner 1996; Treffert 2000). In other words, gifts are spontaneous and unpredictable abilities unique to each individual. Such gifts are intuitive in nature in the sense that those with the gift have immediate recognition and understanding the gist of things independent of any reasoning process. They learn more easily, more quickly, and often have a deeper understanding of what they are doing than do other people regardless of their general level of intelligence (Winner 1996). Individuals with severe mental retardation may still have genius in discrete aspects of intelligence, such as music, art, or mathematics. The special abilities that are most common in savant syndrome are extraordinary memory, mathematical ability (including calendar calculating), and artistic and musical talent (Winner 1996; Treffert 2000). These extraordinary gifts are not consistently associated with any individual differences in brain structure or family background (Treffert 2000, pages 264–265). Psychiatrist Darold Treffert attributes the gifts of savants to "ancestral memories," which are inherited somehow like instincts even though there is no consistent family resemblance for gifts (Treffert 2000, page 218). Similarly, Treffert quotes psychiatrist William B. Carpenter, who concluded that the extraordinary abilities of savants must be based on innate intuition (Treffert 2000, page 200):

> In each of the foregoing cases, then, we have a peculiar example of the possession of an extraordinary congenital aptitude for certain forms of mental activity, which showed itself at so early a period as to exclude the notion that it could have been acquired by the experience of the individual. To such congenital gifts we give the name of intuitions: it can scarcely be questioned that like the instincts of the lower animals they are the expressions of constitutional tendencies embodied in the organism of the individuals who manifest them.

Hence, a gift can be accurately described as a quantum of intuition, that is, a specific capacity for insight learning using rational intuition. Gifts also resemble the innate modules of intuition that shape the development of language and other forms of knowledge unique to human beings (Chomsky 1980, pages 1–61). Gifts may be extraordinary forms of rational intuition, but even ordinary learning may depend on intuition generally. Gifts are exceptional only because most people lack the particular intuitive capacity. For example, if most people could not acquire languages as easily as normal human children, then we would regard those who could acquire language as "gifted." Chomsky made the point that ordinary cognition (which is the first stage of self-aware consciousness) differs from behavioral conditioning in that self-aware consciousness has a modular structure that depends on a rich innate endowment. Chomsky noted,

My own suspicion is that a central part of what we call 'learning' is actually better understood as the growth of cognitive structures along an internally directed course under the triggering and partially shaping effect of the environment. . . . Scope and limits of development are intimately related. Innate factors permit the organism to transcend experience, reaching a high level of complexity that does not reflect the limited and degenerate environment.

Chomsky also observed that behaviorists like Skinner and Piaget have assumed that development is uniform across domains and that the intrinsic properties of the initial state are homogeneous and undifferentiated. In contrast, most cognitive scientists now recognize that cognition is modular and dependent on a rich innate endowment. Chomsky has observed that "those who tend toward the assumption of modularity tend also to assume rich innate structure, while those who assume general multipurpose learning mechanisms tend to deny modularity" (Chomsky 1980, page 3).

Furthermore, the human capacity for empathy and development of civilized society depends on the channeling of cognitive development along a common path. For example, he noted (Chomsky 1980, page 4):

Consider again the question whether cognitive functions are both diverse and determined in considerable detail by a rich innate endowment. If the answer is positive, for some organism, that organism is fortunate indeed. It can then live in a rich and complex world of understanding shared with others similarly endowed, extending far beyond limited and varying experience. Were it not for this endowment, individuals would grow into mental amoeboids, unlike one another, each merely reflecting the limited and impoverished environment in which he or she develops, lacking entirely the finely articulated and refined cognitive organs that make possible the rich and creative mental life that is characteristic of all individuals not seriously impaired by individual or social pathology. . . .

In other words, the development of a shared language and other aspects of self-aware consciousness in humans depends on there being a common path of the development of human self-aware consciousness. There are always differences between individuals in the development of psychophysical systems. If this reasoning is valid, then gifted individuals are simply those who are precociously elevated in their development of modular cognitive abilities along that common path of development. Otherwise there would be no coordination between the development of brain processes and the development of self-aware consciousness throughout evolutionary history. Without such coordination, communication in society would be impossible.

## Intuition and uniquely human gifts

The hypothesis that gifts are precocious developments along a common path of consciousness needs to be carefully examined. Experimental studies have shown that algorithmic models of human intelligence, which involve verbatim statements in memory like a computer program, provide an inadequate description of cognitive growth and development (Bjorklund 1997). They do not account well for the facts of cognitive growth, such as how children learn intuitively in play, how children learn languages, how forgetting and reminiscence occur, or how true memories are distinguished from false memories. This has led to the dissociation of intuitive learning of the gist of things from the rational learning of verbatim memories (Reyna and Brainerd 1998). Human intelligence involves intuition as well as reasoning and sensory observation.

Beyond such basic human abilities, creativity and wisdom are aspects of human intelligence that have an intuitive, holistic, integrative mechanism that is distinct from reasoning ability and verbatim memory (Labouvie-Vief 1990; Sternberg 1990). More specifically, only human beings have had the creativity to develop science, art, and spirituality. Each of these achievements seems to require the integrative function of intuitive learning, which is required for self-awareness and creativity.

Howard Gardner has examined evidence for multiple intelligences in his studies of creative individuals, who have different types of gifts (Gardner 1983, 1993). In developing his theory of multiple intelligences, Gardner studied creativity through the lives of Freud (psychology), Einstein (mathematics), Picasso (painting), Stravinsky (music), T. S. Eliot (poetry), Martha Graham (dance), and Gandhi (politics and spirituality). His wife, Ellen Winner, described cognitive abilities in the development of gifted children, some of whom grew to be creative adults and some who did not. These important studies provide an important general overview of the psychological characteristics of gifts, which is summarized in Table 5.5. Winner observed that the characteristics of gifts in children with normal or superior intelligence were similar to those described in Savant Syndrome (Winner 1996). Gifts are innate talents that do not depend on reflection or algorithmic reasoning. Gifted individuals are able to observe their own problem-solving strategies but the process is intuitive and spontaneous. When they are using their gift, they often enter into contemplative thought, which is characterized by flow states. They often experience sudden intense feelings, images, and memories, leading to ecstasy, wonder, and awe, and other spiritually elevated experiences. Such experiences often stimulate their creativity. Use of gifts is intensely satisfying, which leads people to enjoy using their gifts as much as possible. These psychological phenomena are common to people with gifts in different domains, although the talent itself is domain-specific to academic subjects, such as language or mathematics, or art, such as music or visual arts.

Hence, creativity of a prodigious degree is an expression of gifts. Gifts are discrete modules in the range of thought possible in a person's self-aware consciousness. Those who have studied savant syndrome, gifts, and creativity have looked unsuccessfully for explanation in terms of brain structure and genetic inheritance.

**Table 5.5.** Prominent Psychological Characteristics of Gifts and Gifted Individuals Described by Ellen Winner (1996)

1. **Innate** talents and abilities
2. **Nonreflective** understanding, a feeling of something given without effort or merit, or direct awareness unmediated by conceptual schemas
3. **Intuitive** leaps, not algorithms, often using a figural mode of representation
4. **Metacognitive** awareness of own problem-solving strategies
5. **Contemplative** thought is frequent, leading to flow states, creative leaps, and spiritual experiences of ecstasy, wonder, and awe
6. **Attunement** to the environment is participatory, leading to intense sensory awareness without effort

Presumably, there are some features of the brain and inheritance that are necessary for the expression of gifts, but the inconsistency of findings about genetics and anatomical structure suggest that it is necessary to consider nonmechanical explanations. The discrete and spontaneous nature of gifts is suggestive of a quantum or quantum-like mechanism. As described earlier, contemplative and creative thinking have many features that are at least suggestive of the fundamental quantum phenomena of nonlocality and noncausality. However, it would be premature to jump to any conclusions for or against the quantum nature of contemplation, creativity, or gifts. It is first necessary to consider more about the biology of human thought in Chapters 6 and 7. Then alternative biological, psychological, or sociological explanations for creativity, which may account for its quantum-like properties, will be tested in Chapter 8.

Is it possible that self-aware consciousness may sometimes operate at a quantum level despite the fact that it occurs in macroscopic organisms at high temperatures? Most quantum processes in matter are observed only at a microscopic level or at extremely low temperatures. However, psychology involves the study of information processing in thought, not mechanical processes in matter. Therefore, psychology has a major advantage over physics for the study of quantum processes. Quantum physics always invokes consciousness of an observer, but the advantage of psychology over physics is that the observer is the observed, so there is no perturbation in the process of psychological measurement of consciousness.

We need to evaluate the materialist hypothesis that the contemplative reports of nonlocality and noncausality are illusory. Alternatively, we need to evaluate seriously the transcendentalist hypothesis that contemplative thinking is characterized by quantum phenomena, such as nonlocality and noncausality. The possible inadequacy of the materialist hypothesis is what philosopher David Chalmers (1996) has called the "hard problem" in understanding consciousness. To determine whether contemplative thinking really operates at a quantum level, we need to define specific spiritual parameters that can be reliably measured as demanded by Einstein as evidence of reality. Einstein and his colleagues (Einstein, Podolsky et al. 1935) assumed that "if, *without in any way disturbing the system*, we can predict with certainty the value of a physical quantity, then there exists an element of physical reality corresponding to this physical quantity." If spiritual parameters are not illusory, then we need to be able to show that that they can be predicted with certainty.

What is the range of reality?

In the first stage of self-awareness, only matter is recognized as real and consequential. In the second stage, both matter and consciousness of information about matter are recognized as real. In the third stage, energy is recognized to be variously manifest as matter, as consciousness of information about matter and spirit, and as spirit (i.e., pure consciousness, which is noncausal and nonlocal).

What is meant by energy in the third stage of self-awareness? In general, energy is defined as the ability to do work, that is, to have consequences or real effects. If reality is limited to matter, then mind and spirit are subjective phenomena that are inconsequential. If mind, or spirit, or both are real, then they must have measurable consequences about observable phenomena in life that can be predicted. For example, no one can see gravity or love, but they are nevertheless forces that have real effects. We can measure the effects of gravity from mutual attraction of heavy objects, which is the displacement of mass in material relationships. Likewise, we can measure the effects of love in terms of generosity, which is the displacement of selfish desire in human relationships.

More generally, to show that mind and/or spirit have energy, they must be shown to have predictable effects. For example, the observations made in Chapter 3 about the spiral path of self-aware consciousness suggest strong and testable predictions about the levels of energy associated with different types of thought. If the elevation of thought requires an increase in energy, then elevation of thought may involve a reduction in resistance to an energy potential underlying consciousness, which is normally untapped in the subconscious mind or the unconscious spirit. The more elevated the thought, the greater is its level of energy to motivate order and coherence in self-aware consciousness. If the hypothesis that mind and spirit are measurable manifestations of energy is true, then the spiritual level of self-aware consciousness should have the highest frequencies of energy because it is associated with the most elevated levels of thought. More specifically, the third stage of self-aware consciousness should lead to measurable differences in real phenomena, such as shorter reaction times in executive decision tasks and more flexibility and calmness in conflict tasks.

Matter, consciousness of information, and spirit are the manifestations that are usually designated as the body, mind, and spirit of a human being. In other words, the body or soma is characterized by material parameters, the mind is characterized by informational parameters, and the psyche is characterized by spiritual parameters. Mass is an example of a material parameter. Factual knowledge is an example of information. What are some examples of spiritual parameters that have real predictable effects? This is such a vast question that there can be no complete answer, but I will offer some brief preliminary answers to dispel some misconceptions and to begin defining some more specific questions that we still need to examine empirically in the following chapters.

I propose that thoughts are influenced by both the soma and the psyche. I also propose that the functional organization of the soma and the psyche must be compatible because coherence of personality is possible. The functional organization of thought, therefore, provides a model of the functional organization of the central nervous system and of the psyche. The most fundamental spiritual parameters are likely to be energies underlying the three movements in the spiral path of the psyche. The path of the psyche corresponds to steps in the development of self-aware consciousness. As described in Chapter 3, there are three dimensions of movement in self-aware consciousness, which can be measured by the three TCI character dimensions. Each dimension is about equally explained by genetic variability and by variability unique to each individual (Gillespie, Cloninger et al. 2003), thereby providing a model of the influences of the soma and the psyche on human thought. I propose that these dimensions are the mental expression of the spiritual parameters of the transcendentalists.

Transcendentalists have already described specific spiritual parameters that have substantial effects on self-aware consciousness, which is of great practical significance for an adequate psychology and psychiatry. For example, *listening to the psyche* is the transcendentalist parameter for describing the unique human function of contemplative thinking. When the mind of a person becomes aware of itself, that person is listening to his psyche. Listening to the psyche allows a person to grow in awareness, which is pleasant and satisfying. The contribution to thought of the global average level of listening to the psyche can be measured quantitatively by the level of TCI Self-Transcendence. The contribution of listening to the psyche in each plane of thought can be measured by the subscales of Self-Transcendence: sensibility (self-forgetful common sense and fresh experience of sensory responsivity) vs. repression (sensory numbing) (ST1, plane 2), moral idealism vs. practicality (ST4, plane 3), transpersonal awareness vs. individualism or narcissism (ST2, plane 4), faith vs. skepticism (ST5, plane 5), and spiritual awareness (nonlocal intuitiveness) versus local realism (ST3, plane 7). Spiritual awareness, as measured as a subscale of TCI Self-transcendence, involves nonlocal awareness using the intuitive senses in contrast to the dualistic assumptions of local realism. Nonlocal (spiritual) awareness eliminates the intuitive sense of being controlled, so as Self-Transcendence increases to nonlocal awareness the conflict between being controlled or controlling is reconciled. TCI Self-Transcendence provides a reliable quantitative measure of the degree to which the conflict between being controlled externally and being controlling is reconciled by patient contemplative listening to the psyche.

The conflict between being controlled and being controlling is modulated by a brain network including the anterior cingulate and dorsolateral prefrontal cortex, which interact with the posterior inferior parietal cortex, as described in Chapter 3. When we want something external to our self, we are constrained or controlled by external influences, which leads to overactivity of the inferior parietal cortex. Only letting go of our struggles and wants allows full listening to the nondualistic psyche. The variability in Self-Transcendence that is not determined by genetic factors or prior conditioning provides an empirical measure of the variability unique to each individual, thereby providing an objective test of the reality of the quantum nature of individual differences in the human awareness of the judicial monitoring and control of voluntary actions. Sublimation to full listening to the psyche is blocked by not letting go of struggles (i.e., low Self-Transcendence, impatience), fear or arousal (i.e., low Cooperativeness, lack of freedom of will, excessive attachments, wants, desires, or aversions), or narcissism (i.e., low Self-Directedness, inflated ego, lack of enlightenment). Failure to listen to the psyche leads to reduced well being, mood disorders when severely deficient, and anhedonia in extreme cases. On the other hand, increases in listening to the psyche lead to increases in well-being from illumination experiences, as described previously for Bertrand Russell, Ralph Waldo Emerson, Henry Thoreau, and Richard Bucke. Such contemplative experiences have the predictable and lasting effect of transforming the person's worldview and level of well-being as measured by increased coherence of personality and positive emotionality. By listening to our psyche, we lighten our unconscious and nourish our subconscious, thereby improving our character. Such strong effects are natural and predictable effects of a practical nature—they are not unnatural, unpredictable, or magical in any way. Some may choose to describe such transformations as mystical or miraculous, but please recall that a miracle is simply something that we cannot explain or do not understand. Our ability to explain phenomena improves in a stepwise fashion as our finite understanding is deepened by the elevation of our self-aware consciousness. Sometimes when highly elevated beings, like the positive philosophers, talk about communion with the unity of being, the phenomena seem so unlike the confused lives of most people that it sounds fantastic or utopian. On the other hand, it seems fantastic to a positive philosopher that individuals would voluntarily persist in the misery of self-centered living when they could be wise and happy! We all want to be happy and we are all on a common path of increasing wisdom that is made up of modular gifts of insight. To progress in our insight, we need to listen to the lightness of our psyche and work to understand and let go of our personal heavy baggage of fears, struggles, and conflicts. This takes committed work—small step by small step—but the work has predictable and lasting effects, as has been documented in longitudinal studies described in Chapter 6.

Even if people are equally devoted to listening to their psyche, there are marked differences between individuals in their worldview, which is strongly correlated with the average level of a person's thoughts throughout their life. Such differences in worldview are ascribed by transcendentalists to differences in the *level of the psyche*, which has sometimes been called the *magnitude of the psyche* (Augustine 388). Like a person's world view, the level of the psyche is much more stable than momentary fluctuations in thought and affect. Our world view reflects the collective memories of the psyche that determine our initial perspective on experience. The description of a person's world view is therefore an important part of mental status examination. It can be quantified on exactly the same scale used for rating the level of thought, as detailed in the Appendix.

*Freedom of will* is the transcendentalist term for the uniquely human capacity to make choices in behavior flexibly and spontaneously—that is, undetermined by prior conditions and habits. Freedom of will is low when a person's behavior is highly conditioned by conflicts or maladaptive habits, as in individuals who have substance dependence or personality disorders. On the other hand, a person with a high level of free will is expected to have flexibility in legislative functions, such as fluidity of speech, good modulation of the intensity of affect, and adaptive problem solving, which can be reliably rated in a thorough mental status examination. The contributions to thought of individual differences in a person's global average level of freedom of will can be measured quantitatively on the basis of both legislative functions in the mental status examination and the level of TCI Cooperativeness. The component subscales of TCI Cooperativeness measure the effects of free will in each of the five planes of human self-aware consciousness: tolerance vs. prejudice (CO1, plane 2), forgiveness or compassion vs. revengefulness (CO4, plane 3), empathy vs. inconsiderateness (CO2, plane 4), helpful versus unhelpful (CO3, plane 5), and charitable principles vs. self-serving opportunism (CO5, plane 7). Individuals who score highly in the TCI subscale charitable principles are altruistic and kind, whereas those who score low on this subscale regard life in terms of causal determinism: life is merely a "zero sum game" in which each person should take as much as they can at every opportunity. Altruism, in contrast, is based on the recognition of noncausality as a fundamental principle of living systems.

The progressive development of cooperativeness, charity, and altruism requires a mapping of experience in an allocentric space, as is provided by the inferior parietal cortex, rather than in an egocentric space, as provided by the anterior insula (see Chapter 3). Flexibility of voluntary choice is not possible without an allocentric representation, so TCI Cooperativeness provides a quantitative measure of awareness of choice in what we want, that is the qualia of voluntariness or free will. There is no freedom in wanting something external to one's finite individual self, so full freedom involves wanting to give to others, who are understood as part of one's whole and infinite Self. The underdetermination of flexibility of voluntary choice by prior conditions in empirical studies of the awareness of agency can provide an objective test of the reality of the quantum nature of freedom of will.

The freedom of our will atrophies when we yield to fears or selfish desires, but it can increase when we increase in self-awareness and make a commitment to change based on our increased awareness of what would be wholeheartedly satisfying. The importance of cultivating freedom of will is the central message of Krishnamurti's life and writings (Krishnamurti 1975; Jayakar 1986). Increased freedom of will is also associated with predictable changes in the sense of subjective time (Krishnamurti and Bohm 1985). When we are free, we are beyond any self-centered concern about subjective time. More practically, growing freedom of will is essential in the development of flexibility in our executive functions, which is an essential component of the balanced self-government of a coherent person.

One apparent advantage of the transcendentalists' labels for the spiritual parameters is that they suggest a way of psychologically understanding the heterogeneous nature of emotions and making testable predictions about the complex interactions among different parameters in their psychosocial effects. For example, a little reflection easily allows most people to understand that the development of both freedom of will and better listening to the psyche is needed to grow in serenity and in the degree to which we are *following the path of the psyche*. Think about what it means to follow the path of the psyche: the level of a person's reality-testing is strongly related to the degree to which he or she is following the path of the psyche toward wisdom and well-being. A person who is psychotic with hallucinations and delusions is very low in following the path, whereas an individual who has integrated intelligence with pure rational intuition is very high in following the path. The contribution to thought of following the path of the psyche can be measured quantitatively on the basis of the degree of reality testing on mental status examination and by the level of TCI Self-Directedness. When the degree of following the path of the psyche is high, thought and relationships are highly sublimated. The sublimation of thought is measured by the TCI Self-Directedness subscale hopefulness (enlightened second nature) (SD5). The contribution of following the path of the psyche in each plane of thought is indicated by the components of TCI Self-Directedness: responsible vs. controlled and blaming (SD1, plane 2), purposeful vs. capricious or goal-less (SD2, plane 3), self-accepting vs. self-striving (SD4, plane 4), resourceful vs. inept (SD3, plane 5), and hopeful (enlightened second nature, spontaneous agency) vs. compromising and deliberate (SD5, plane 7). A person's ability to adapt realistically can be reduced by low freedom of will, or poor listening to the psyche, low serenity, or a low level of the psyche. When we recognize what is true by listening to the psyche as well as we can, and if we are flexibly adaptive because we are free from conditioning and we are calm and attentive, then we can and will do whatever is appropriate and adaptive. Both listening to the psyche and freedom of will are necessary to follow the path of the psyche to well-being. Such interactions are typical of the nonlinear dynamics that is typical of complex biopsychosocial systems, as we will describe in Chapter 8.

The *serenity of the psyche* is another putative spiritual parameter that is closely related to the degree of coherence of personality, but it is different than following the path of the psyche. The degree of calmness and appropriateness of a person's affect on mental status examination indicate their level of serenity. The serenity of the psyche is very low when the affect is inappropriate for both the content of thought and the person's context. It is mildly low when the affect is appropriate for content but mildly inappropriate for a person's context. Serenity is very high when a person is calm regardless of circumstances. Serenity should be distinguished from well-being, which I rate in terms of the range of affect, rather than its appropriateness. In many people the degree of serenity and well-being will be congruent, so studies of normal individuals often confound these aspects of healthy adaptation (see Table 1.1). The dissociation of these phenomena becomes obvious, however, in thorough mental status examinations of the differential diagnosis and treatment of psychopathological states, which I will describe in detail in another book. A person's serenity is the affective component of the level of understanding of the psyche, which is an indicator of the degree of purity of a person's rational intuition. For example, in Chapter 4, the level of serenity was predictive of the precision of people's ability to recognize and measure the elevation of thought of what they read (see Tables 4.3 and 4.4).

What we read also can be characterized in terms of its *spiritual interest*, which is not the same as the *level of thought* of what is written. A violent movie may contain little dialogue that is self-aware, but seeing the real consequences of such behavior may inspire a person to seek nonviolent *human relationships*. On the other hand, the consequences of violence may be sanitized or even glorified in some movies, so that people are misled to seek happiness by aggression. The spiritual interest of a book or movie can be measured in terms of philosophical (see Chapter 1), psychological (see Chapters 3 and 4), or physiological variables (see Chapters 2 and 6). In Chapter 4, we discussed the spiritual interest of Emerson in reading Montaigne's *Essays* and visiting the Jardin des Plantes in Paris in 1833. More generally, the spiritual interest of something is its interest to the person's psyche. The interest of something to the psyche is another way of describing how coherent or wise the related action would be. Will reading a book uplift or lower a person's thoughts? Will watching a movie be relaxing or inspiring, or will it be disturbing and self-defeating? What will be the consequence of reading the book on the elevation of thought?

Obviously these parameters are of practical significance to psychological function. At least some of the parameters can be reliably measured and make useful predictions, but can a transcendental explanatory model make valid predictions in systematic experiments on self-awareness? The answer to this question requires systematic research to supplement the anecdotal accounts provided by transcendentalists. Gandhi and others have quite reasonably argued that the best evidence for the reality of spirituality is the historical record of the transformed lives of people who learn to listen to their psyche and follow its path to wisdom and well-being. Bucke and others have relied on evidence of transformation in personality to validate reports of spiritual illumination (Bucke 1951). However, Bucke's observations were based only on anecdotal reports of subjective experiences.

As I began to investigate the measurement and effects of transcendental phenomena empirically in 1995, I came to appreciate the central fact that spirituality simply cannot be explained adequately at a lower level. In the course of the development of self-aware consciousness, the second stage cannot explain the third stage—it can only lay the foundation for the next step into the unconscious in a state of calm receptivity. Cognitive-behavioral approaches to radical personality transformation are dualistic and reductive, so they cannot produce wisdom or well-being.

## Is free will an illusion?

The extent to which consciousness has real effects on physical movement has been experimentally examined in ground-breaking neurophysiological studies by Benjamin Libet (Libet 1982; Libet, Wright et al. 1982; Libet, Gleason et al. 1983; Libet, Wright et al. 1983; Libet 1993). Libet observed that there was a consistent sequence of observable phenomena prior to voluntary physical movements (Libet, Gleason et al. 1983). The actual movement of muscle was measured by an electromyogram (EMG). Subjects reported that they were conscious of movement beginning about 90 milliseconds on average prior to the EMG detecting any movement. When subjects made "spontaneous, capricious" movements, they reported awareness of wanting to move (W) prior to movement on the EMG by an average of about 350 milliseconds and by a minimum of about 150 milliseconds. When asked to plan the movements thoughtfully, they reported awareness of wanting to move (W) prior to movement on the EMG by about 800 milliseconds on average. Electroencephalograms (EEGs) showed preparatory cortical activity before any movement on the EMG by about 1050 +/– 175 milliseconds when movements were preplanned and by about 575 +/– 150 milliseconds when movements were capricious (Libet, Wright et al. 1982). The cortical activity prior to any conscious awareness of wanting to move was measured as a readiness potential, which consists of a succession of an initial slow-rising brain wave from about 1500 ms to about 400 milliseconds before movement and a later wave with a rapidly rising negative slope from about 400 milliseconds to approximately the time of movement. The readiness potential may consist mainly of the negative slope component when movements are not preplanned. Libet concluded that "cerebral initiation of a spontaneous, freely voluntary act can begin unconsciously, that is, before there is any (at least recallable) subjective awareness that a decision to act has already been initiated cerebrally." In other experiments, Libet concluded that it takes about 500 milliseconds for the sensation evoked by any given external stimulus to reach conscious awareness, but that the time of the sensation is subjectively "back-referred" to the time of the stimulus, so that there does not seem subjectively to be a half-second lag in our awareness of the world (Libet 1993; Pockett 2002). Both the studies of sensory stimulation of brain and brain activity prior to motor activity suggest that conscious awareness of sensori-motor events occurs after preparatory brain activity has already begun. Such data have been used to support the belief that consciousness is an inconsequential epiphenomenon of complex sequences of unconscious brain activity (Wegner 2002). We become consciously aware of wanting to move *after* the brain has already initiated its preparations for action, so how could consciousness represent anything but an illusion of agency and voluntary choice? This question has been called the "deep problem" in the concept of will, which is defined as voluntary agency or the capacity to choose what action to perform or withhold (Spence, Hunter et al. 2002; Hunter, Farrow et al. 2003).

Libet's findings describe replicable phenomena that must be explained by any adequate theory of consciousness and mind–body relationships, but the interpretation of the results has been highly controversial, as evidenced by the acrimonious debates in an entire issue of the journal *Consciousness and Cognition* in June 2002 (e.g., Pockett 2002). In my opinion, the controversy over interpretation of Libet's replicable results has occurred because both Libet and other interpreters have assumed that self-aware consciousness is a dichotomous variable that is either fully present or totally absent. In fact, the movement of self-aware consciousness has multiple stages that are modulated by multiple quantitative variables, as shown in Chapter 3, so treating consciousness as a dichotomous variable is inadequate, as evidenced by the controversy about the interpretation of the results. The interpretation of the findings becomes more clear once it is realized that the subject's self-reports indicate variably incomplete degrees of self-aware consciousness. Measures of individual differences in self-aware consciousness are needed in order to describe and interpret the timing of the five stages of development of self-aware consciousness in human thought. The onset of the readiness potential was usually substantially earlier than the awareness of wanting to move, but the difference varied from 1010 milliseconds to only 15 milliseconds (Libet, Gleason et al. 1983). Libet himself has begun to recognize the need to take personality into account in understanding such individual differences. For example, individual differences in Self-Trancendence (measured as tendency toward repression rather than sensory responsivity) are correlated moderately with length of sensory stimulation needed to elicit awareness of sensation (Shevrin, Ghannam et al. 2002). Less transcendent (i.e., more hysterical and repressive) subjects take longer to become aware of sensory stimulation.

More generally, measures of individual differences in personality are needed to interpret each stage in the development of self-aware consciousness. The five steps in human thought are summarized in Table 5.6 along with the TCI character measures of the underlying aspects of agency (i.e., following the path of the psyche

**Table 5.6.** Five Stages of Human Thought and Underlying Dynamic Processes Measured by TCI Character Subscales of Self-Directedness (SD), Cooperativeness (CO), and Self-Transcendence (ST)

| Step in Self-aware Consciousness | *TCI Measures of Functional Processes* | | |
|---|---|---|---|
| | *Agency (SD)* | *Flexibility (CO)* | *Understanding (ST)* |
| (1) Intuition | Responsible *vs.* controlled | Tolerant *vs.* prejudiced | Sensible *vs.* repressive |
| (2) Reasoning | Purposeful *vs.* aimless | Forgiving *vs.* revengeful | Idealistic *vs.* practical |
| (3) Emotion | Accepting *vs.* approval-seeking | Empathic *vs.* inconsiderate | Transpersonal *vs.* individual |
| (4) Intention | Resourceful *vs.* inept | Helpful *vs.* unhelpful | Faithful *vs.* skeptical |
| (5) Action | Hopeful sublimation *vs.* compromising deliberation | Charitable principles *vs.* self-serving opportunism | Spiritual awareness *vs.* local realism |

or TCI Self-Directedness), flexibility (i.e., freedom of will or TCI Cooperativeness), and understanding (i.e., listening to the psyche or TCI Self-Transcendence), as described in the prior section. The character subscales quantify differences in the degree of elevation of thought in each plane. For example, in plane 2, Harm Avoidance is progressively elevated from feeling controlled (low SD1), prejudiced (low CO1), repressive and empty (low ST1) to feeling responsible (high SD1), tolerant (high CO1), sensible and self-respecting (high ST1).

As described in Chapter 3, the first step in self-aware consciousness is the initial perspective, which is always intuitive. The first step corresponds to the onset of preparatory activity in the brain, as measured by Libet with the cortical "readiness potential." The degree of preparatory activity is also indicated by the amplitude of the P300 evoked potential in other experimental paradigms (Vedeniapin, Anokhin et al. 2001). The time course of cortical event-related potentials allows the dissociation of the early intuitive recognition of stimuli from later decision making (Van Rullen and Thorpe 2001). Intuitions are only immediately conscious in the third stage of self-awareness, which are contemplative states of flow or choiceless awareness. The second step in consciousness involves labeling and reasoning, which varies from purposeful planning to capricious wants and aversions. The longer the objective deliberation in the second stage, the slower will be the reaction time of the subjects because of reduced spontaneity of agency. The second step defines our wants when our actions are purposeful, as in Libet's experiments in which subjects were asked to plan their movements thoughtfully. The labels and plans of the second stage elicit emotional responses in the third stage, which are modulated by the emotion-related aspects of the character dimensions (accepting, empathic, transpersonal vs. striving, inconsiderate, individualistic). The third stage defines our wants when our actions are capricious, as in Libet's experiments in which subjects were asked to act "spontaneously" and "capriciously." The fourth step involves the actual intention to act, which corresponds to Libet's subjects awareness of movement beginning before it is actually measurable by the EMG. The final step is the overt action, measured by Libet as physical movement in the EMG.

The impression that self-aware consciousness occurs after the initiation of preparatory activity in the brain is, in my opinion, a misleading artifact of treating consciousness as a dichotomous variable that is either fully present or totally absent. TCI Self-Directedness is moderately correlated with the P300, which may measure initial brain preparatory activity for action (Fuster 1984; Fuster 1997). For example, the amplitude of the P300 is positively correlated with TCI Self-Directedness in parietal leads about 0.4 (Vedeniapin, Anokhin et al. 2001). In addition, TCI Self-Directedness is positively correlated ($r = 0.6$) with total reaction times in tests of executive function requiring a simple motor response like a finger movement (Gusnard, Ollinger et al. 2001; Gusnard, Ollinger et al. 2003). When actions are capricious, the readiness potential consists mainly of the negative slope component. Similarly, Contingent Negative Variation (CNV) in parietal leads is correlated with TCI Cooperativeness and Self-Transcendence, but not Self-Directedness (Cloninger 2000). The parietal cortex is the region in which allocentric mapping of relationships occurs, which is necessary for cooperative behavior, as previously described.

Available data show that individual differences in TCI character scales will help to understand the stages of self-aware consciousness more rigorously than has been possible when consciousness is treated as a dichotomous variable. Much more work is needed about the higher stages of consciousness in which agency becomes increasingly spontaneous and free of emotional conflicts and intellectual deliberations. Little can be gained by assuming that consciousness is dichotomous and that everyone is equally aware.

In fact, there is substantial evidence that there are substantial differences between individuals in their self-efficacy and that self-efficacy can be enhanced voluntarily regardless of prior conditioning and biological predisposition. Self-efficacy is the confidence that one can change and that one wants to change, which is a combination of basic confidence and awareness of flexibility in choice of what one wants. Self-efficacy corresponds to what is also called initiative, which is the beginning of the first stage of self-aware consciousness (see Chapter 6). Self-efficacy requires awareness of both personal agency (i.e., the will to be responsible and purposefully self-directed, rather than controlled by external circumstances) plus awareness of flexibility (i.e., the freedom to forgive oneself and change bad habits rather than continuing self-defeating behavior) in the intuitive and reasoning steps of thought (see Table 5.6). In other words, individuals with self-efficacy should score average or higher on the TCI character subscales that modulate Harm Avoidance and Novelty Seeking (i.e., planes 2 and 3 in Table 5.6). Substantial evidence shows that individuals with substance dependence can give up substance dependence without treatment if they have awareness of their self-efficacy. Success in quitting substance abuse can be predicted from a person's level of self-efficacy, not his or her degree of physiological dependence on a substance of abuse, such as heroin (Robins, Helzer et al. 1995) or tobacco (DiClemente, Prochasta et al. 1985; Kavanagh, Pierce et al. 1993; Hill, Schoenbach et al. 1994; Kenford, Fiore et al. 1994).

Some people lack awareness of their self-efficacy because they lack the sense of responsibility (measured by the SD1 subscale) and sensibility (measured by the ST1 subscale). Such patients are usually described as having conversion disorders or as being hysterical and repressive (Shevrin, Ghannam et al. 2002). Patients with conversion disorders, such as nonepileptic seizures or "psychogenic" tremors, exhibit behaviors that appear to be voluntary but do not have explicit self-awareness of voluntary agency or motivation for their actions. They do have an intuitive awareness of what they are doing, which they can recall and describe vaguely (Cloninger 1986). Their recall and descriptions lack contextual understanding as in children without full self-object differentiation, so they are often inconsistent historians. In the absence of explicit self-awareness, individuals with conversion disorders regard their actions as involuntary. The interpretation of their motivation is highly vulnerable to suggestions from others. EEG studies of individuals with conversion disorders have observed movement-related cortical readiness potentials that appear normal (Toro and Torres 1986; Terada, Ikeda et al. 1995). Such readiness potentials do not indicate awareness of agency because patients with tics regard their movements as voluntary but frequently have a cortical readiness potential that is absent or brief (Karp, Porter et al. 1996). Differences between individuals in their awareness of agency are correlated with individual differences in the activation of the prefrontal cortex and parietal cortex (Spence, Crimlisk et al. 2000; Frith and Frith 2003), which are also highly correlated with TCI Self-Directedness (Gusnard, Akbudak et al. 2001; Gusnard, Ollinger et al. 2003). Hysterical features are also correlated with sensory numbing and slower awareness of sensory stimulation (Shevrin, Ghannam et al. 2002).

A person can also voluntarily increase his or her awareness of self-efficacy. Most people can do this without treatment once they recognize that they have developed a maladaptive habit. For example 95% of cigarette smokers who quit do so on their own without any treatment (Surgeon-General 1989). Among bulimics seeking treatment, the pretreatment level of TCI Self-Directedness is the best predictor of success with cognitive behavioral therapy (Bulik, Sullivan et al. 1998). Regardless of the initial level of character development, antidepressant medications and/or cognitive behavioral therapy increase the post-treatment levels of Self-Directedness, thereby establishing an upward spiral of increasing character development in ongoing therapy (Tome, Cloninger et al. 1997; Bulik, Sullivan et al. 1998; Anderson, Joyce et al. 2002; Joyce, Mulder et al. 2003).

If free will is an illusion, it is an illusion that can be quantitatively measured, has substantial variance unique to each individual, is subject to voluntary change by each individual, and has real life consequences! Actually, the lack of awareness of freedom of will is what appears to be an illusion based on the misleading impression produced by the assumption that consciousness is a dichotomous variable that is fully present or completely absent. Most work on the development of self-efficacy has been carried out with individuals with personality disorders or little development of the character traits of Self-Directedness and Cooperativeness. In order to be more certain of the psychophysical reality of higher stages of self-awareness in which Self-Transcendence is elevated, I concluded that it was necessary to identify the psychophysiological characteristics of thought in different stages of self-aware consciousness. I thought that it was necessary to understand more about the experimental manipulation and psychophysiology of self-aware consciousness before the alternative hypotheses of materialists, idealists, and transcendentalists regarding contemplative thinking could be adequately tested.

For the study of well-being to be a rigorous science, we must know whether there are reliably measurable physiological changes characteristic of different stages of self-aware consciousness. Such characteristic physiological changes appear to be likely since the level of self-aware consciousness can be quantified by reliable individual differences in TCI character scales and by objective changes in mental status. Also character can be developed voluntarily in many, but not all, people. If there are predictable changes in psychophysiology, these changes may help to explain the variables that facilitate or obstruct the development of creative gifts and contemplative thinking. Could specific changes in self-aware consciousness produce specific physiological effects that predicted improvements in character and long-term psychosocial outcomes? To answer this question, we next examine the psychophysiology of thought in different stages of self-aware consciousness.

## REFERENCES

Adamec, R. E. and C. Stark-Adamec (1983). "Limbic kindling and animal behavior— Implications for human psychopathology associated with complex partial seizures." *Biological Psychiatry* 18: 269–293.

Albert, D. Z. (1994). "Bohm's alternative to quantum mechanics." *Scientific American* 269 (May): 60–67.

Anderson, C. B., P. R. Joyce, et al. (2002). "The effect of cognitive-behavioral therapy for bulimia nervosa on temperament and character as measured by the Temperament and Character Inventory." *Comprehensive Psychiatry* 43: 182–188.

Augustine (388). The magnitude of the soul. *Writings of Saint Augustine*. New York, Cima Publishing Co.: 51–59.

Bell, J. S. (1993). *Speakable and unspeakable in quantum mechanics*. Cambridge, England, Cambridge University Press.

Bjorklund, D. F. (1997). "In search of a metatheory for cognitive development (or, Piaget is dead and I don't feel so good myself)." *Child Development* 68: 144–148.

Bohm, D. (1980). *Wholeness and the implicate order*. London, Routledge.

Bohm, D. (1995). Interview about Krishnamurti. *Krishnamurti: 100 Years*. E. Blau, ed. New York, Stewart, Tabori & Chang.

Bohm, D. (1996). *The special theory of relativity*. London, Routledge.

Bohm, D. and B. J. Hiley (1993). *The undivided universe: An ontological interpretation of quantum theory*. London, Routledge.

Bouwmeester, D., J. W. Pan, et al. (1997). "Experimental quantum teleportation." *Nature* 390: 575–579.

Branning, D. (1997). "Does nature violate local realism?" *American Scientist* 85: 160–167.

Bucke, R. M. (1951). *Cosmic consciousness: A study in the evolution of the human mind*. New York, Dutton.

Bulik, C. M., P. F. Sullivan, et al. (1998). "Predictors of 1-year treatment outcome in Bulimea Nervosa." *Comprehensive Psychiatry* 39: 206–214.

Cade, C. M. and N. Coxhead (1989). *The awakened mind: Biofeedback and the development of higher states of awareness*. Shaftesbury, Dorset, England, Element Books.

Cannon, W. B. (1927). "The James-Lange theory of emotions: A critical examination and an alternative theory." *American Journal of Psychology* 39: 106–129.

Chalmers, D. J. (1996). *The conscious mind: In search of a fundamental theory.* New York, Oxford University Press.

Chomsky, N. (1980). "Rules and representations." *Behavior and Brain Sciences* 3: 1–61.

Cloninger, C. R. (1986). "A unified biosocial theory of personality and its role in the development of anxiety states." *Psychiatric Developments* 3: 167–226.

Cloninger, C. R. (2000). "Biology of personality dimensions." *Current Opinions in Psychiatry* 13: 611–616.

Csikszentmihalyi, M. (1991). *Flow: The psychology of optimal experience.* New York, HarperCollins.

Csikszentmihalyi, M. (1993). *The evolving self.* New York, HarperCollins.

Damasio, A. R. (1994). *Descartes' error: Emotion, reason, and the human brain.* New York, GP Putnam.

Davies, P. (1992). *The new physics.* Cambridge, England, Cambridge University Press.

Davies, P. (1999). "Bit before it?" *New Scientist* 161: 3.

Dennett, D. (1987). *The intentional stance.* Cambridge, Massachusetts, MIT Press.

Dennett, D. (1991). *Consciousness explained.* Boston, Massachusetts, Little, Brown, and Co.

Dennett, D. (1993). "The message is: There is no medium." *Philosophy and Phenomenological Research* 53: 919–931.

DiClemente, C. C., J. O. Prochasta, et al. (1985). "Self-efficacy and the stages of self-change of smoking." *Cognitive Therapy and Research* 9: 181–200.

Eccles, J. (1989). *Evolution and the brain: Creation of the Self.* London, Routledge.

Einstein, A., B. Podolsky, et al. (1935). "Can quantum mechanical description of physical reality be considered complete?" *Physical Review* 47: 777–780.

Erikson, E. H. (1963). *Childhood and society.* New York, W. W. Norton & Co.

Erikson, E. H. (1964). *Insight and responsibility.* New York, W. W. Norton & Co.

Freud, S. (1929). *Civilization and its discontents.* New York, Jonathan Cape & Harrison Smith.

Freud, S. (1936). A disturbance of memory on the Acropolis. *The standard edition of the complete psychological works of Sigmund Freud.* J. Strachey and A. Freud, eds. London, Hogarth Press. 22: 238–248.

Frieden, B. R. (1998). *Physics from Fisher information: A unification.* Cambridge, England, Cambridge University Press.

Frieden, B. R. and W. J. Cocke (1996). "Foundation for Fisher-information-based derivations of physical laws." *Physical Review* E54: 257–260.

Frieden, B. R. and B. H. Sofer (1995). "Lagrangians of physics and the game of Fisher-information transfer." *Physical Review* E52: 2274–2286.

Frith, U. and C. D. Frith (2003). "Development and neurophysiology of mentalizing." *Philosophical Transactions of the Royal Society of London-Series B: Biological Sciences* 358(1431): 459–473.

Fuster, J. M. (1984). "Behavioral electrophysiology of the prefrontal cortex." *Trends in Neurosciences* 7: 408–414.

Fuster, J. M. (1997). *The Prefrontal Cortex: Anatomy, physiology, and neuropsychology of the frontal lobes.* New York, Lippincott-Raven.

Gamow, G. (1966). *Thirty years that shook physics: The story of quantum theory.* New York, Dover Publications.

Gandhi, M. (1997). *All men are brothers: Autobiographical reflections.* New York, Continuum.

Gardner, H. (1983). *Frames of mind: the theory of multiple intelligences*. New York, Basic Books.

Gardner, H. (1993). *Creating minds: An anatomy of creativity seen through the lives of Freud, Einstein, Picasso, Stravinsky, Eliot, Graham, and Gandhi*. New York, Basic Books.

Gay, P. (1998). *Freud: A life for our time*. New York, Norton.

Gillespie, N. A., C. R. Cloninger, et al. (2003). "The genetic and environmental relationship between Cloninger's dimensions of temperament and character." *Personality and Individual Differences* 35: 1931–1946.

Goonatilake, S. (2000). "Many paths to enlightenment." *Nature* 405: 399.

Gowan, J. C. (1971). *Development of the psychedelic individual*. Buffalo, New York, Creative Education Foundation.

Gusnard, D. A., E. Akbudak, et al. (2001). "Medial prefrontal cortex and self-referential mental activity: relation to a default mode of brain function." *Proceedings of the National Academy of Sciences USA* 98: 4259–4265.

Gusnard, D. A., J. M. Ollinger, et al. (2003). "Persistence and brain circuitry." *Proceedings of the National Academy of Sciences USA* 100(6): 3479–3484.

Gusnard, D. A., J. M. Ollinger, et al. (2001). "Personality differences in functional brain imaging." *Society of Neuroscience Abstracts* 27(80): 11.

Gusnard, D. A. and M. E. Raichle (2001). "Searching for a baseline: Functional imaging and the resting human brain." *Nature Reviews Neuroscience* 2: 685–694.

Higgs, P. W. (1964). "Broken symmetries and the masses of guage bosons." *Physical Review Letters* 13: 508–509.

Hill, H. A., V. J. Schoenbach, et al. (1994). "A longitudinal analysis of predictgors of quitting smoking among participants in a self-help intervention trial." *Addictive Behaviors* 19: 159–173.

Hunter, M. D., T. F. Farrow, et al. (2003). "Approaching an ecologically valid functional anatomy of spontaneous "willed" action." *NeuroImage* 20: 1264–1269.

Jayakar, P. (1986). *J. Krishnamurti: A biography*. London, Penguin Books.

Joyce, P. R., R. T. Mulder, et al. (2003). "Borderline personality disorder in major depression: differential drug response and six-month outcome." *Comprehensive Psychiatry* 44: 35–43.

Kanigel, R. (1991). *The man who knew infinity: A life of the genius Ramanugen*. New York, Charles Scribner & Sons.

Karp, B. I., S. Porter, et al. (1996). "Simple moltor tics may be preceded by a premotor potential." *Journal of Neurology, Neurosurgery and Psychiatry* 61: 103–106.

Kavanagh, D. J., J. Pierce, et al. (1993). "Self-efficacy and social support as predictors of smoking after a quit attempt." *Psychiatry & Health* 8: 231–242.

Kenford, S. L., M. C. Fiore, et al. (1994). "Predicting smoking cessation: who will quit with and without the nicotine patch." *Journal of the American Medical Association* 271: 589–594.

Koestler, A. (1964). *The act of creation*. New York, Macmillan.

Kohut, H. (1984). *How does analysis cure?* Chicago, Illinois, University of Chicago Press.

Krishnamurti, J. (1975). *The first and last freedom*. San Francisco, California, HarperCollins.

Krishnamurti, J. (1992). *Complete collected works of J. Krishnamurti*. Ojai, California, Krishnamurti Foundation of America.

Krishnamurti, J. and D. Bohm (1985). *The ending of time*. San Francisco, California, HarperCollins.

Labouvie-Vief, G. (1990). Wisdom as integrated thought: Historical and developmental perspectives. *Wisdom: Its nature, origins and development*. R. J. Sternberg, ed. New York, Cambridge University Press: 52–86.

Libet, B. (1982). "Brain stimulation in the study of neuronal functions for conscious sensory experiences." *Human Neurobiology* 1(4): 235–242.

Libet, B. (1993). *Neurophysiology of consciousness: Selected papers and new essays by Benjamin Libet*. Boston, Birkhauser.

Libet, B., C. A. Gleason, et al. (1983). "Time of conscious intention to act in relation to onset of cerebral activity (readiness-potential): The unconscious initiation of a freely voluntary act." *Brain* 106(3): 623–642.

Libet, B., E. W. J. Wright, et al. (1982). "Readiness-potentials preceding unrestricted "spontaneous" vs. pre-planned voluntary acts." *Electroencephalography & Clinical Neurophysiology* 54(3): 322–335.

Libet, B., E. W. J. Wright, et al. (1983). "Preparation- or intention-to-act, in relation to pre-event potentials recorded at the vertex." *Electroencephalography & Clinical Neurophysiology* 56(4): 367–372.

Maharishi, M. Y. (1969). *Commentary on the Bhagavad Gita*. Baltimore, Penguin Books.

Maslow, A. (1962). *Toward a psychology of being*. Princeton, New Jersey, D. Van Nostrand.

Matthews, R. (1999). "I is the Law." *New Scientist* 161: 24–28.

Montaigne (1998). *The complete essays of Montaigne*. Stanford, California, Stanford University Press.

Newton, I. (1713). *Principia Mathematica*. London, Mothe-Cajori.

Ouspensky, P. D. (1938). *A new model of the universe*. London, Kegan Paul.

Penrose, R. (1989). *The Emperor's new mind: Concerning computers, mind, and the laws of physics*. New York, Oxford University Press.

Pockett, S. (2002). "On subjective back-referral and how long it takes to become conscious of a stimulus: A reinterpretation of Libet's data." *Consciousness & Cognition* 11: 144–161.

Posner, M. I. and J. Fan (2003). Attention as an organ system. *Neurobiology of perception and communication: From synapse to society*. J. Pomerantz, ed. Cambridge, England, Cambridge University Press.

Rey, G. (1997). *Contemporary philosophy of mind*. Oxford, England, Blackwell Publishers.

Reyna, V. F. and C. J. Brainerd (1998). "Fuzzy-trace theory and false memory: New frontiers." *Journal of Experimental Child Psychology* 71: 194–209.

Robins, L. N., J. E. Helzer, et al. (1995). "Narcotic use in southeast Asia and afterward. An interview study of 898 Vietnam returnees." *Archives of General Psychiatry* 32: 955–961.

Schrodinger, E. (1983). *My view of the world*. Woodbridge, Connecticut, Ox Bow Press.

Schrodinger, E. (1992). *What is life? Mind and matter; Autobiographical sketches*. Cambridge, England, Cambridge University Press.

Seager, W. (1999). *Theories of consciousness: An introduction and assessment*. London, Routledge.

Shevrin, H., J. H. Ghannam, et al. (2002). "A neural correlate of consciousness related to repression." *Consciousness & Cognition* 11(2): 334–341.

Spence, S. A., H. L. Crimlisk, et al. (2000). "Discrete neurophyusiological correlates in prefrontal cortex during hysterical and feigned disorder of movfement." *Lancet* 355: 1243–1244.

Spence, S. A., M. D. Hunter, et al. (2002). "Neuroscience and the will." *Current Opinion in Psychiatry* 15: 519–526.

Stapp, H. (1999). "Attention, intention, and will in quantum physics." *Journal of Conscious Studies: The Volitional Brain* 6: 143–164.

Stapp, H. (2000). *Societal ramifications of the new scientific conception of human beings*. Future Visions Conference, State of the World Summit, New York.

Sternberg, R. J. (1990). Wisdom and its relations to intelligence and creativity. *Wisdom: Its nature, origins, and development.* R. J. Sternberg, ed. New York, Cambridge University Press: 142–159.

Surgeon-General, U.S. (1989). *Reducing the health consequences of smoking: 25 years of progress.* Washington, DC, US Department of Health & Human Services.

Terada, K., A. Ikeda, et al. (1995). "Presence of Bereitschaftspotential preceding psychogenic myoclonus: clinical application of jerk-locked back averaging." *Journal of Neurology, Neurosurgery and Psychiatry* 58: 745–747.

Tittel, W., J. Brendel, et al. (1998). "Violation of Bell inequalities by photons more than 10 km apart." *Physical Review Letters* 81: 3563–3566.

Tome, M. B., C. R. Cloninger, et al. (1997). "Serotonergic autoreceptor blockade in the reduction of antidepressant latency: personality and response to paroxetine and pindolol." *Journal of Affective Disorders* 44: 101–109.

Toro, C. and F. Torres (1986). "Electrophysiological correlates of a paroxysmal movement disorder." *Annals of Neurology* 20: 731–734.

Treffert, D. A. (2000). Extraordinary People: Understanding savant syndrome. New York, Ballantine Books.

Vaillant, G. E. (1993). *The wisdom of the ego.* Cambridge, Massachusetts, Harvard University Press.

Van Rullen, R. and S. J. Thorpe (2001). "The time course of visual processing: From early perception to decision-making." *Journal of Cognitive Neuroscience* 13(4): 454–461.

Vedeniapin, A. B., A. A. Anokhin, et al. (2001). "Visual P300 and the self-directedness scale of the temperament-character inventory." *Psychiatry Research* 101: 145–156.

Walker, E. H. (2000). *The physics of consciousness: Quantum minds and the meaning of life.* Cambridge, Massachusetts, Perseus Books.

Wallace, R. K. (1970). "Physiological effects of transcendental meditation." *Science* 167: 1751–1754.

Wegner, D. M. (2002). *The illusion of conscious will.* Cambridge, MA, The MIT Press.

Weihs, G., T. Jennewein, et al. (1998). "Violation of Bell's inequality under strict Einstein locality conditions." *Physical Review Letters* 81: 5039–5043.

Winner, E. (1996). *Gifted children: Myths and realities.* New York, Basic Books.

Winnicott, D. (1958). *Collected papers: Through pediatrics to psychoanalysis.* New York, Basic Books.

Zeilinger, A. (2000). "Quantum teleportation." *Scientific American* 282: 50–59.

# 6

# PSYCHOPHYSIOLOGY OF AWARENESS

## THE BIOPSYCHOSOCIAL APPROACH

Both physiological and psychosocial studies show that mental health depends on the development of self-aware consciousness. The substantial evidence supporting this broad assertion is carefully critiqued in this chapter. The extensive information available from these two approaches has been poorly integrated, nevertheless, because of the tradition of dualistic thinking that separates the mind and the body. The biomedical approach focuses on the brain using somatic therapies such as psychoactive drugs. In contrast, the psychosocial approaches focus on the mind using psychotherapy. Although there is talk about integration of biomedical and psychosocial paradigms, these approaches are really applied by experts from separate ideological camps (Wilson 1993; Michels 1999; Eisenberg 2000). The goals and values of members of the two camps are often antagonistic, rather than complementary and mutually respectful: biomedical experts often think psychosocial experts ignore the real causes of illness, and vice versa. As a result, mental health professionals are not usually trained in any tasks that involve the integration of biomedical and psychosocial skills (Luhrmann 2001).

There are approaches to personality assessment and the psychobiology of learning that are intended to bridge these camps to form a general biopsychosocial paradigm (Cloninger, Svrakic et al. 1993; Kandel 1993; Eisenberg 2000), as described in Chapter 2. However, the history of psychiatry can be viewed as re-current cycles in which there has been alternating dominance by biomedical and psychosocial paradigms with little effort to form an integrative biopsychosocial paradigm. For example, Emil Kraepelin's biomedical approach to categorical diagnosis dominated psychiatry internationally around 1900. Adolf Meyer developed an integrative psychobiology to correct excesses of reductive biomedical or psychosocial approaches. Meyer emphasized the interdependent functions of the soma and the psyche in a social context, and he compared reductive efforts to "make mind out of matter" with futile urges to "square a circle" (Lief 1948, page 625). His integrative approach to the body, mind, and spirit of the whole person was widely respected for its recognition of the dignity of each person and its practical common sense. However, Meyer's holistic approach gave way to the dominance of Freud's psychoanalytic movement in the United States after Meyer retired in 1941. The successful growth of psychopharmacology and neuroscience in the 1960s pushed the biomedical approach and categorical diagnosis back into prominence, as indicated by the dominance of the neo-Kraepelinian approach in the official diagnostic systems of the world since 1980.

During the latter half of the twentieth century, some people attempted to reju-venate the biopsychosocial approach (Engel 1977), but it has never been domi-nant despite its greater generality. The reason for the persistent mind–body dualism, in my opinion, has been the lack of recognition that the brain and mind are in-separable aspects of a self-aware unity. Psychosocial models describe personal-ity in terms of subjective thoughts and feelings motivating voluntary behavior. There are steps in personality development, and these are described in units of "cognitive chunks," that is, transitions between cognitive steps that are discrete. In contrast, biomedical models describe mental phenomena in terms of transitions in the state of the brain (or defects in the brain), which are used to define specific categories of disease. However, there has been little or no work to investigate the relationship between the discrete units of thought ("cognitive chunks") and the discrete states of the brain. The research tools for linking the states of thought and brain function simply were not available until recently. Now functional brain imaging techniques have been developed that are sensitive enough to measure differences between individuals in real time.

Furthermore, dualistic concepts of temperament and character are not adequate to account for the path of self-aware consciousness that underlies the movement of thought and personality development, as discussed in Chapter 2. In Chapters 3–5, I explored the clinical and theoretical requirements of a nondualistic approach to understanding self-aware consciousness. I found that an adequate description of the movement of self-aware consciousness must recognize the spiral path of the psyche as an essential element in the unity of a human being. Separate biomedical and psy-chosocial approaches, even if combined eclectically, provide a degenerate paradigm for a science of well-being, as described later in this chapter.

In this chapter, I present empirical data about synchrony between discrete conscious thought and brain states based on psychophysiological studies, particularly quantitative electroencephalograms (EEGs), functional magnetic resonance imaging (fMRI), and positron emission tomography (PET). The psychophysiology of awareness shows that a nonreductive and nondualistic approach that integrates biomedical and psychosocial perspectives is not just an alternative but is in fact essential to describe human thought with precision. All dualistic approaches ignore the empirical fact that the flow of human consciousness along its spiral path involves synchronous movement of "cognitive chunks" (i.e., discrete units of thought) and brain microstates in which there are sudden transitory connections among changing sets of neural networks distributed throughout the whole brain. In other words, the flow of consciousness in each individual illustrates the universal principle of unity of being.

The psychophysiology of consciousness shows that neither mindless nor brainless approaches provide an adequate basis for describing and treating mental disorders. In saying this, I mean more than that both approaches are essential in delivering effective care for patients. It is already well recognized that we need to attend to the psychosocial needs of patients with severe disorders like schizophrenia, just as we need to attend to the biomedical treatment of patients with personality disorders. I mean that somatic and psychological therapies are truly interdependent and cannot be precisely described, understood, or applied effectively in most people most of the time without integration. In treatment, reciprocal interactions of the soma and the psyche in all thoughts require integrated interventions for the development of well-being. In research, biomedical assumptions must be tested by their ability to predict psychosocial development, and psychosocial assumptions must be tested by their ability to predict neurobiological phenomena.

The fundamental goal of nonreductive psychobiology is to understand how brain activity is organized in its functional relationship to thoughts, feelings, and behavior. This goal is really shared by both biomedical and psychosocial camps, but each camp has delayed effort to integrate its work with what the other camp has learned. This was justified in Freud's time because the tools for studying brain function were too crude to account for observable clinical phenomena. However, recently it has become possible to measure changes in brain function coincident with changes in thought using quantitative EEG, fMRI, PET, and magnetoencephalography (MEG).

Unfortunately, the measurement of thought in such biomedical studies has usually been crude or ignored. On the other hand, psychosocial measurements have been rigorous in longitudinal psychosocial studies, but the associated physiology has been crude or ignored. Nevertheless, both psychosocial and biomedical approaches have made important contributions to our understanding the stepwise nature of self-aware consciousness. However, each approach provides strengths that are needed to complement the other, as I will show.

## TESTING THE STEPWISE NATURE OF DEVELOPMENT

Erik Erikson's model of psychosocial development will be used to document the empirical evidence for adult development of self-aware consciousness because George Vaillant has shown that its stages can be coded reliably in a way that is independent of gender, social class, education, and general intelligence (Vaillant 1993). Erikson extended Freud's model of psychosexual development to a more general model of the stages of psychosocial development (Erikson 1963). In turn, Erikson's model has been carefully tested and modified in longitudinal studies by George Vaillant and colleagues (Vaillant and Milofsky 1980; Vaillant 1993). Erikson described maturation as a spiral of development in which there is an increasing social radius, which is similar to the spiral of self-aware consciousness I described in Chapter 3 based on both psychological and physiological evidence. Erikson's model, as modified by Vaillant, is depicted in Figure 6.1 along with my estimate of the level of thought of each stage.

According to Erikson, the capacity for basic trust of others is the first major developmental stage of psychosocial development. The development of trust rather than mistrust of others corresponds to what Freud called the oral stage. Infants do not develop normally without being touched, held, and hugged by a stable caretaker. Variability of thought at this level is measured by the TCI Harm Avoidance subscale "anticipatory worry and pessimism versus optimism." Thought at level 2.6 is the minimum level of thought characterized by basic trust of others. However, at thought level 2.6, people still feel pessimistic, dependent and helpless and frequently want others to take care of them. Thought level lower than 2.6 is characterized by increasing degrees of Harm Avoidance, that is, mistrust and fear (thought at 2.4), or even lowering of thought to hate (2.2) or total distrust (2.0).

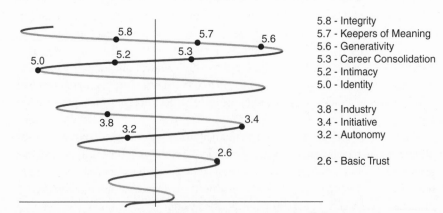

Figure 6.1. Stages of psychological development according to the modified model of Erikson. (From Erikson 1963; Vaillant and Milofsky 1980.)

Erikson called the second major developmental step in his model "autonomy versus shame," which corresponds to Freud's anal stage. Around age two years, children need to master control of their anger and their ability to assert themselves to some degree. The minimum level of thought that involves a sense of autonomy is level 3.2, but at this level people are still selfish and greedy with little restraint on Novelty Seeking. Variability in thought at this level is measured by the TCI Novelty Seeking subscale "extravagance versus reserve." People whose thought is at the level of 3.2 may experience guilt as a result of their extravagance anal greed. Thought below level 3.2 is associated with vulnerability to shame, as described in the Appendix on measurement of thought, which is in agreement with Erikson.

Erikson's third major developmental level is called "initiative versus guilt." Initiative is usually called "self-efficacy" in social psychology, as described in Chapter 5. The development of initiative corresponds to Freud's phallic phase in which children around four to six years of age imitate their parents to show off. The minimum level of thought involving initiative is 3.4, which is the level at which individuals have control of rage but still remain competitive and envious. This level of thought is dominated by novelty-seeking and concrete operations, as described by Piaget. The conformist stage (Loevinger 1976) is nearby at thought level 3.5.

Erikson's fourth major developmental level is called "industry versus inferiority." Industry corresponds to Freud's latency phase. Children between four and ten years of age often experience satisfaction from working with and alongside adults. The consolidation of the concrete operational ability for "conservation" of number and mass usually occurs by the ages of five to seven years. The minimum level of thought associated with conservation and industriousness is 3.8, which involves power-seeking behavior. Variability in thought at this level is measured by TCI Novelty Seeking subscale "exploratory excitability versus stoic rigidity." Thought below 3.8 is associated with feelings of inferiority, which may be compensated by assertiveness and proud claims of superiority. Thought at 3.6 involves the conflict between superiority and inferiority (i.e., secondary narcissism). The difference in thought level between industry (3.8) and inferiority (3.6) illustrates that Erikson's model describes major developmental stages approximately but does not provide a complete description of the movement of thought.

The fifth stage in Erikson's model is "identity versus identity diffusion." Vaillant rated this stage as having been attained when a person was self-reliant and independent of their family of origin. At this level of thought individuals are well-developed in the TCI Persistence scale "work hardened versus spoiled." This level of development also corresponds to what I have called self-directedness at thought level of 5.0. This level of thought marks the onset of the self-sufficient intellect, which Jane Loevinger calls the "self-aware" stage.

The sixth stage of "intimacy versus isolation" involves achievement and cooperativeness. Vaillant rated this stage as having been attained when a person was able to maintain an interdependent intimate relationship, such as a marriage, for a decade. Vaillant considered career consolidation to be a development dependent on having already established a capacity for intimacy. Similarly, I assign a minimum thought level of 5.2 for intimacy and 5.3 for career consolidation.

Vaillant describes the development of the capacity for intimacy as the gateway to adulthood. In approximate agreement, the second stage of self-aware consciousness involves thought beyond 5.3. Thought at level 5.4 is what Jane Loevinger called the "conscientious" stage. TCI Persistence is well-developed at this level of thought. Still more elevated thought at level 5.6 is characteristic of the seventh stage in Erikson's model, which is "generativity versus stagnation." Generativity involves the capacity to care for the well-being of others, to be a productive leader and community builder. Variability in generativity is measured by the TCI Persistence subscale "eagerness of effort versus laziness." Such generative capacity is shown by responsibility for guiding the growth of others. The generative level of thought also corresponds to the capacity for mindfulness. In my experience, this level of thought is what Loevinger called the "individualistic" stage, but at this point there is some tension remaining between generativity and individuality. The disagreements between Erikson and Loevinger reflect the fact that most people only partially understand that individual freedom and generativity are actually not in conflict (if only we are fully self-aware).

Vaillant also distinguished generativity from a slightly higher level of development he called "keepers of the meaning." Keeping the meaning is thought at level 5.7, which I call *self-transcendence* or *transpersonal awareness* and which Loevinger called *autonomy*. For example, Viktor Frankl, the developer of psychotherapy based on the "will to meaning," emphasized the importance of self-transcendence (Frankl 1959). Likewise, Vaillant described this level as developing concern for a social radius that extends beyond one's immediate community. Vaillant suggested that at this level there is development of wisdom. According to Erikson, however, at this level of thought people may still experience despair, which is not resolved until the development of "integrity" at thought level 5.8 to 7.1, which is characterized by emergence of faith and hope. Loevinger called this level (i.e., thought at level 5.8 or higher) the "integrated" stage. The experience of illumination at 5.8 is the foundation of integrity because a person realizes the boundless nature of life, thereby transcending despair about the mysteries of life and death.

Entry into the third stage of self-awareness (at level 5.8) might be considered to be the beginning of wisdom, but it is certainly not the attainment of full coherence of personality. At thought level of 5.8, individuals are still perfectionistic, as measured by the TCI Persistence subscale for perfectionism. Accordingly, I place wisdom at a level in plane 7 of thought, which is not well described by Erikson, Vaillant, or Loevinger. As described in Chapter 5, thought at 5.8 brings a radical transformation of personality, which is really a *metanoia*, or rebirth into the eternal life of the spirit. Erikson's recognition that despair was the lack of integrity or illumination shows that he recognized that death was a mystery, which can only be understood through contemplation.

Erikson's model is consistent with the positive philosophy as far as he went. Hence, Vaillant correctly describes Erikson as Platonic in his perspective and language (1993). Vaillant and Milofsky (1980) examined Erikson's model of the life cycle in two forty-year prospective studies. These were 392 men from high-crime core-city neighborhoods and ninety-four Harvard University graduates. They found that the stages of the life cycle are typically passed sequentially. Failure to master one stage usually precludes mastery of subsequent stages, suggesting the model of a spiral staircase in which each step must be passed before reaching a higher step. Forty years later, 83% of the college graduates had achieved the second stage of self-aware consciousness in their daily life (i.e., the stage of generativity). However, there were large individual differences in the age at which individuals achieved the successive stages of psychosocial development, as shown in Figure 6.2.

Later, Vaillant expanded his studies by the addition of a prospective study of women with high IQ who had been identified by Terman in studies at Stanford University (Vaillant 1993). The psychosocial stages reached by men and women in the three prospective studies are summarized in Table 6.1. Forty percent or more reached the stage of generativity in each sample, excluding individuals with alcoholism or IQ less than 80.

Vaillant found that a warm childhood environment was weakly associated with higher development. However, the same stages were observed regardless of gender, social class, education, or intelligence level, as shown in Table 6.2. The independence from demographic variables is important because some ways of measuring personality and its development are biased by education and intelligence (Kohlberg 1973; Loevinger 1976) or have only weak sensitivity to the stepwise nature of development (Heatherton and Weinberger 1994).

Hence, psychoanalytic research has made the valuable contribution of demonstrating the stepwise nature of personality development. The nature of this progression is not a simple linear staircase, however, as suggested by Vaillant's imagery. Personality development, like thought, involves a nonlinear sequence of changes in which people can move forward and then regress for a while before moving forward again. Even in Vaillant's data, some people do well in career consolidation before establishing intimacy. For example, a person could be a generative leader of the community, yet have problems with intimacy as a result of poor control of sexual impulses. Consequently, a simple linear staircase model of personality development is inadequate even descriptively.

Furthermore, at an etiological level, personality development involves multiple dimensions of temperament as well as of character, which each have unique genetic determinants that influence the path of development. As discussed in Chapter 2, there are strong nonlinear relationships between antecedent temperament

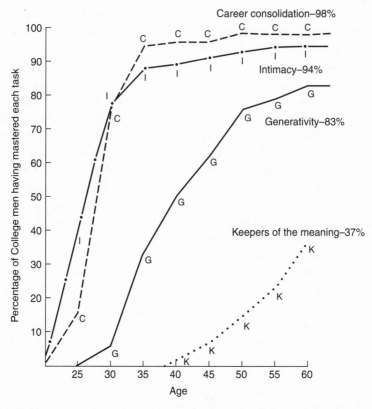

Figure 6.2. Ages of mastery of selected psychosocial tasks (Reprinted by permission from the publisher from *The wisdom of the ego* by George E. Vaillant, page 167, Cambridge, Massachusetts: Harvard University Press, Copyright © 1993 by the President and Fellows of Harvard College.)

dimensions and the level of character development that is attained. Hence the assumption of linearity is not adequate from either a descriptive or an etiological perspective.

Finally, the interpretation of the stages of personality development as ego development is doubtful. It is doubtful because the concepts of ego defense and ego development do not inform any predictions about who does or does not develop to a higher stage of development. Essentially, the stages of development documented by Erikson are purely descriptive—they describe but do not explain the psychobiology of development. What is worse is that the descriptions suggest explanations that are not justified by predictions about the individual differences in development. For example, the motivation for kindness is assumed to be a defense against the spontaneous urge to be bad. The assumption that defending oneself against the unconscious is a mature adaptation is based on fear of the unconscious, which unfortunately limits a person to permanent internal conflict.

**Table 6.1.** Psychosocial Stages Reached by Members of Three
Samples, Excluding Men with IQ Less Than 80 or Alcoholism

| Highest Stage Reached | College Men (n = 186) | Terman Women (n = 40) | Core City Men (n = 212) |
|---|---|---|---|
| Industry | 3% | 0% | 7% |
| Identity | 5% | 10% | 4% |
| Intimacy | 3% | 22% | 15% |
| Career consolidated | 34% | 25% | 33% |
| Generativity | 55% | 43% | 41% |

*Source*: Adapted from Vaillant 1993.

Such profound conflict and confusion actually form an obstacle to the third stage
of self-aware consciousness. The third stage of self-aware consciousness is the
portion of the path of the psyche that leads to wisdom and well-being. The very
existence of wisdom and well-being contradict the assumptions of psychoanalysis. Hence, ego defense mechanisms are descriptive of some aspects of behavior
but do not provide an adequate account of the major motivating forces underlying the path of development of self-aware consciousness.

In summary, longitudinal studies have shown clearly that character develops
in a discontinuous (stepwise) manner. Furthermore, these steps in development
correspond to increases in the level of self-aware consciousness, which leads to
increased coherence and well-being. However, the psychoanalytic models are
purely descriptive and do not provide an adequate explanation of the psychophysical basis of development.

## THE PSYCHOPHYSIOLOGY OF THE STEPS IN THOUGHT

*Personality* is the crystallization of one's usual pattern of thinking. What are
described as personality traits are merely the average pattern of thought, which

**Table 6.2.** Independence of Psychosocial Developmental Stage from
Parental Social Class, Intelligence, and Education

| Background Variable | College Men (n = 187) | Terman Women (n = 85) | Core City Men (n = 277) |
|---|---|---|---|
| Social class | .06 | .05 | .04 |
| IQ | .00 | .01 | .09 |
| Years of education | — | .15 | .12 |
| Warm childhood | .24* | .10 | .17* |

* $p < .001$.

*Source*: Adapted from Vaillant 1993.

nevertheless has a dynamic range that is described as states superimposed on traits in dualistic models such as Axis 1 (clinical states or disorders) and Axis 2 (personality traits) in *DSM-IV*. The spiral path of personality development was observed for character using the TCI (Cloninger, Svrakic et al. 1997) and for Erikson's stages of the life cycle (Figure 6.1). Likewise, thought has a spiral path as described in Chapter 3, which supports the relationship of personality to thought.

Furthermore, if personality develops in a truly stepwise manner, thought and any associated brain mechanisms should also be stepwise in nature. This hypothesis can now be systematically investigated by direct tests using EEG and other techniques such as fMRI and MEG, as mentioned earlier. Many studies have shown changes in EEG patterns during various input conditions, such as listening to music (Petsche, Lindner et al. 1988) or during stressful verbal activity (Berkhout, Walter et al. 1969). Changes are also induced in the EEG by performing different mental tasks known to induce changes in the EEG that vary according to location and wave frequency. For example, verbal and spatial cognitive tasks produce left and right hemispheric activation, respectively, even when matched for task difficulty (Davidson, Chapman et al. 1990). Visual imagery and relaxation of attention produce alpha activity (Barrett and Ehrlichman 1982; Ray and Cole 1985), whereas effortful emotional and cognitive tasks induce beta activity (Ray and Cole 1985). Alpha activity is blocked (after a 200-millisecond delay) by exposure to visual stimuli, by exposure to words that evoke visual imagery, or by suddenly increased attention as a central component of the orienting response (Lehmann and Koenig 1997). Moreover, changes in EEG do not depend on external stimulation or motor output in response to stimulation. For example, different types of stimulus-free and response-free covert thoughts induced different EEG characteristics when thoughts were restricted to a predefined list or catalogue (Ehrlichman and Wiener 1980). However, little was known until recently about the EEG correlates of spontaneous thought in the absence of input or output restrictions.

Studies of spontaneous thought have shown that thought and its associated brain wave activity has a discontinuous stepwise movement. Three of the fundamental characteristics of thought are that it is very fast, sequential, and recursively state-dependent (Newell 1992; Lehmann and Koenig 1997). There is only one conscious thought at one moment in time, but complete thoughts and acts occur within a fraction of a second. In addition, thinking is state dependent in that the same input has different salience and meaning depending on the current state of self-aware consciousness of the person. Furthermore, the state dependency of information processing is recursive: the result of initial information processing may result in changes in the momentary state of consciousness (e.g., changing valence, arousal, or need to control conflict), leading to different responses to future stimulation. Even the potentials evoked to specific stimuli depend on the prestimulus state of the brain or what the person is thinking just before being stimulated (Lehmann, Michel et al. 1994; Lutz, Lachaux et al. 2002). The information processing strategies and accessible memories depend on the preparatory functional state of the brain (Koenig, Prichep et al. 2002; Lutz, Lachaux et al. 2002). In clinical cognitive terms, the labels we give to events initiate a concatenated chain of responses that are at least partially automatic. Consequently, self-report of thoughts can help to specify the preparatory brain state, reducing variability in response to internal and external events (Lutz, Lachaux et al. 2002).

The state defined by analysis of the spectrum of temporal frequencies of the brain's electrical field can be segmented into time series (Barlow 1985) that are generally much longer than the expected duration of single thoughts (Newell 1992). Consequently, these time series define what are called "macrostates" of cognition. Also, the same EEG frequency may be generated from different sources that differ in function and location. However, the sequences of momentary spatial distributions (i.e., the topography) of the electrical field of the brain change more quickly and more often. The duration of discrete epochs in the changing spatial distribution of the brain electrical field is in the millisecond range, which corresponds to the duration of single thoughts.

The topography of the brain electrical field is a characteristic of the whole brain that depends on transient connections in changing sets of many underlying distributed brain networks operating in parallel. The spatial resolution of EEG is not as fine as that of MRI or PET, but it has been improved substantially by recent refinements. Good spatial resolution of brain activity has been achieved by recording EEGs from many electrodes, by registering EEG data with anatomical images, and by correcting the distortion caused by volume conduction of EEG signals through the skull and scalp (Givens, Smith et al. 1999). Statistical methods have also been developed to measure the interdependencies that occur within subsecond epochs between the instantaneous functional networks that form between different brain regions during higher cognitive processes, such as language, attention, working memory, and self-aware consciousness.

*Self-aware consciousness* is a discontinuous sequence of discrete thoughts changing in synchrony with transient connections in changing sets of brain networks. The spatiotemporal changes in brain states have the dynamics of a scale-free system (Lehmann and Koenig 1997), which follow a power–law distribution, as described in Chapter 8. Momentary configurations of the topography of the brain electric field are manifestations of the momentary global functional state of the brain. Field configurations tend to persist in a quasi-stable condition for only a fraction of a second (Lehmann, Grass et al. 1995; Lehmann, Strik et al. 1998; Givens, Smith et al. 1999). These quasi-stable field configurations are the result of transient connections of a particular set of distributed brain networks and are called "brain microstates." These microstates influence the processing of information and accessible memories that allow a person to integrate new information adaptively with prior knowledge and self-awareness of the internal and external milieu.

Dietrich Lehmann and his associates (Lehmann, Grass et al. 1995; Lehmann, Strik et al. 1998) have shown that changes in the topography of the electrical activity of the brain are strongly discontinuous, changing in discrete steps lasting a fraction of a second coincident with transitions between conscious thoughts. The initial observation was that the alpha activity during resting occurred in brief time segments of the electrical field configuration that had a stable topography. These segments of brain topographical activity were called "microstates" because they were discrete and brief. These observations led to the development of formal methods to parse the ongoing series of brain electric field maps into time epochs characterized by quasi-stable field configurations. The duration of the microstates is usually between 80 and 120 milliseconds (Koenig, Prichep et al. 2002). The segmentation into microstates of spontaneous brain field series at rest filtered for alpha activity is shown in Figure 6.3 (Lehmann and Koenig 1997). Note the persistence of the map configuration for several frames and the quick changes in topography.

The relationship of brain microstates to the changing content of thought was demonstrated by asking subjects to report their spontaneous thoughts under conditions of relaxation, drowsiness, and sleep onset (Lehmann, Grass et al. 1995). It had been previously well established that these relaxed conditions provide a rich repertoire of very different EEG patterns varying in arousal and thought content, but little was known about the associations between EEG spectral patterns and thought content. Correlation coefficients between spontaneous conscious thoughts and EEG power spectral profiles were investigated in twenty normal volunteers. The subjects were prompted with a gentle buzz sound fifteen times at about seven-minute intervals in each of two sessions at the individual subject's usual bedtime to give brief reports of "what just went through your mind" just before the prompt. The reports of thoughts were audio-taped and later transcribed for coding by two independent raters on twenty-three descriptive scales with strong interrater reliability. The scales referred to quality of recall, different sensory modalities, time orientation, emotional characteristics, involvement of ego, involvement of reality, perception of one's body and its orientation, and level of alertness or vigilance. The sixteen seconds of EEG recorded immediately preceding each of the prompts were spectral analyzed. Four channels of EEG data were continuously recorded in the left and right temporal-parietal and parietal-central areas. Canonical correlation coefficients were computed for the ratings of thoughts and the EEG spectral values to identify pairs of thoughts and brain microstates. Four of the possible twenty-three pairs of variables were highly significant, with correlation coefficients ranging from .78 to .62. The four pairs of canonical variables showed distinctive features in the EEG spectra and styles of thought, as summarized in Table 6.3. The results showed lawful correspondence between the brain microstates and the thoughts of all subjects. Among other things, the results demonstrated the reliability of introspective reports in a setting of relaxation, isolation, and trust.

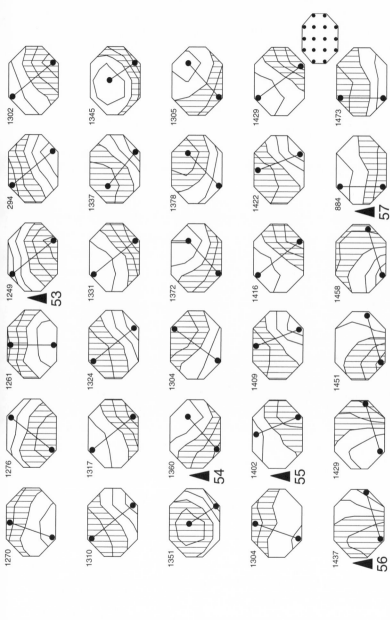

Figure 6.3. Segmentation into microstates of an alpha brain field series during resting. The illustrated momentary potential distribution maps white (positive) and hatched (negative), equipotential lines at 10 mV) at successive times of maximal global field power were assessed by locations of their extreme values (dots connected by line). The spatial window was one electrode distance (sagittal and transverse). Note the persistence of map configuration (disregarding polarity) for several frames and the quick changes. Arrowheads indicate determined microstate borders. Total time covered by the map sequence is 1.6 seconds (Reprinted from Lehmann D, et al., *Electroencephalography and Clinical Neurophysiology*, 67: 271–288, "EEG alpha map series," copyright © 1987, with permission from Elsevier.)

**Table 6.3.** Psychophysical Descriptors of Four Discrete Microstates of Thought Defined by Pairs of Quantitative Features of the EEG and Coincident Spontaneous Thoughts Identified by Canonical Correlations

| Thought Level and Content | EEG Feature |
| --- | --- |
| 5.8 Oceanic feelings (sudden unfamiliar ideas, not goal oriented, passive and sleepy, low recall quality, remote to local reality] | Delta and theta |
| 5.6 Mindfulness (visual imagery, good recall quality, restful, emotions neutral or positive) | Alpha-Blocking and Right theta |
| 3.8 Industry (waking cognition, sounds in present, no free association) | Beta and fast alpha |
| 3.4 Initiative (future oriented, based in local reality, emotionally neutral) | Beta and fast alpha Absence of slow alpha |

*Source*: Adapted from Lehmann, Grass et al. 1995.

The four pairs of psychophysiological variables were identified using the variables about the EEG and thought content identified by Lehmann and his associates. In addition, to provide continuity with our prior discussion of personality development, I used the original detailed ratings to measure the level of thought and its associated descriptor using the Diagnosis of the Frequency of Thought (DFT) method described in Chapter 3. For example, some of the prominent features of the indivisible schema of "initiative" (i.e., thoughts at level 3.4) were being future oriented, reality based, and emotionally neutral. Such thoughts were paired with beta and fast alpha activity along with the absence of slow alpha activity. In contrast, some of the prominent features of "mindfulness" (thought at 5.6) were clear internal visual imagery with good recall quality in a restful state that was emotionally neutral or positive. Such thoughts were paired with blocking of alpha activity and right-sided theta activity. Each level of thought was associated with distinct cognitive variables and a synchronous brain microstate.

The observation that spontaneous visual imagery and abstract thought were associated with distinct brain microstates occurring within the two seconds before being prompted to report their thoughts was later replicated (Lehmann, Strik et al. 1998). The two-second EEG period before the prompts was segmented into microstates. Thoughts involving visual imagery were correlated with brain microstates in which the spatial localization of the alpha source differed from that associated with abstract thoughts without visual imagery. Most important, *only* the last microstate just before the prompt was correlated with the change in the localization of the alpha response predicted by the content of the person's thought.

Topographical configurations of brain electrical activity provide a sensitive indicator of transitions in what Lehmann and associates called the "atoms of thought" in view of their discrete nature. Different spatial landscapes of the distribution of the electrical potential are generated by different active populations of neurons, so the different frequencies of thought occur synchronously with transitory connections of different sets of neural networks distributed throughout the whole brain, bound by will as the strong force binds particles in atoms.

In addition, schizophrenic patients have been observed to have a brain microstate associated with mistrust and ignoring of information (Lehmann 1998; Koenig, Lehmann et al. 1999), as is characteristic of thoughts rated at level 2.4 using the DFT. The duration of this microstate was inversely correlated with the severity of paranoid thinking in the patients. The schizophrenics had other brain microstates that were entirely normal. This suggests that schizophrenic symptoms do not result from continuously biased brain functions but rather from recurrent brain states lacking in self-awareness interspersed between normally self-aware brain states. In psychoanalytic terms, such distortions of memory associated with a deviant brain microstate at a thought level below that associated with basic trust (2.6) can be described as a "psychotic defense," such as delusional projection or distortion.

It is also important to note that transitions of thoughts are also associated with sudden spontaneous changes of the distribution of energy levels in the global electromagnetic field of the brain. In other words, there are spontaneous changes in the distribution of activity throughout the whole brain in the subsecond range that cannot be predicted from the antecedent microstates but covary freely with changes in voluntary thought (Koenig, Prichep et al. 2002). The global field power is the integral of the local energies throughout the whole brain, and the local energies are the squared amplitudes of electrical activity at each local point. The unpredictable variability in global field power indicated that the sequences of brain microstates are at least partially spontaneously self-organized in that they are underdetermined by initial conditions (i.e., external stimuli and prestimulus conditions).

Likewise, there is variability in the global coherence between individuals and within individuals over time, which can be measured as the inverse of global dimensional complexity of the brain (Lehmann and Koenig 1997). There are also age-related changes in the distribution of brain microstates in normative samples of subjects ranging from six to eighty years of age. Using spectral analysis, slow delta (1–4 Hz) and theta (4–7 Hz) waves tend to decrease gradually throughout life, whereas the faster alpha (8–12 Hz) and beta (13–30) waves increase linearly from age six until about age thirty, when they begin to decrease again. Using topographical EEG mapping, asymmetrical microstates diminish with increasing age in normative samples, whereas symmetrical microstates increase (Koenig, Prichep et al. 2002). In contrast, patients with dementia show an increase in asymmetrical microstates involving both abstract thoughts and visual imagery as the dementia progresses in severity, whereas symmetrical microstates decrease with the progression of dementia. However, longitudinal studies of healthy subjects across the lifespan in which thoughts and brain microstates are rated prospectively have not been carried out because the technology has only recently been developed.

In summary, the relationships that have been observed between thoughts and brain microstates are summarized in Table 6.4 along with the general characteristics of cognition. Each of these ten characteristics needs to be considered carefully because most people have been unaware of these properties. As is often the case, in the absence of knowledge, we often make many false assumptions implicitly about thought and the relationships of brain and mind. Thoughts and their associated brain microstates are discrete and usually very brief. The psychophysical building blocks of cognition must be discrete microstates with an average duration of less than one second. Changes in thoughts and associated brain microstates are synchronous and sequential. However, the sequence of development is nonlinear in that there are recurring mind-brain states that do not overlap in time. Microstates may remain stable for less than a second but may repeat several times within a second (Koenig, Prichep et al. 2002). Moreover, the changes are singular and global (i.e., approximately nonlocal) and at least partially spontaneously self-organized in nature (i.e., non-causal), involving overall changes in the field of the brain associated with transient connections of different neural networks. The nonlinear sequential pattern is consistent with parallel processing because each microstate depends on the activity of large multifocal neural networks with distributed parallel processing (Mesulam 1990). Hence, I propose that the global energy level of the brain at rest, which is

**Table 6.4.** Characteristics of Human Thought and Brain Microstates

1. Thoughts and brain microstates are discrete and brief, with average durations of around 100 milliseconds.
2. There are synchronous changes in thought and brain microstates as a nonlinear sequence of recurring brain–mind states that do not overlap in time.
3. Different thoughts are strongly associated with characteristic brain microstates with predictable properties.
4. The same thought generates the same brain microstate, whether spontaneous or experimentally induced.
5. Responses to input depend on the prestimulus brain microstate and momentary thought of the person.
6. The state dependency is recursive, initiating chains of subsequent thoughts that are partially automatic (and partially spontaneously self-organized; see 9).
7. The development of thought with age is associated with corresponding developmental changes in brain microstates.
8. The changes in the topography of the brain field potential are sudden, reversible, and global (i.e., involving the whole brain).
9. The changes in the global field potential of the brain are sudden, reversible, and partially noncausal (i.e., depend on spontaneously self-organized thoughts).
10. Self-aware consciousness is singular but can develop in its coherence (i.e. the scope and stability of self-awareness).

characteristic of its sustained ongoing activity independent of specific thoughts and tasks, corresponds to the average level of conscious thought, which in turn corresponds to the energy potential of subconscious thought (i.e., the portion of the total energy potential of consciousness available to self-aware thinking). This proposal predicts that individual differences in the average DFT co-vary with individual differences in the brain's global energy level. The highest global energy level in most healthy adults, measured electrophysiologically, usually appears during deep (stage IV) slow wave sleep in which high amplitude delta waves are prominent. Furthermore, this level can be experimentally changed, as is discussed in the next section. Specifically, contemplation, but not lower levels of self-awareness, may transform the average level of thought predictably, as is described in the next section. According to my proposal, therefore, contemplation elevates the global energy level of the brain because it elevates the level of the subconscious by lightening the unconscious in a stepwise manner.

In other words, the brain can be viewed as a system that goes through a nonlinear sequence of discrete, global states as a function of time, like a sequence of waves in the ocean spanning an irregular landscape. Moreover, these thought waves vary in their frequency as measured in the DFT described in earlier chapters. It is appropriate to describe the waves of thought and brain microstates as different aspects of the singular phenomenon of self-aware consciousness and to describe the global field power as an indicator of the level of subconscious understanding. It is striking that self-aware consciousness seems to display properties like those expected of quantum phenomena: discreteness, nonlocality, noncausality, and wave-particle dualism. The psychological and physiological significance of the occurrence of quantum-like phenomena will be examined further by considering the psychophysiology of the stages of consciousness.

## THE GLOBAL BRAIN ENERGY STATE

The studies of brain EEG mapping have demonstrated the important finding that specific changes in thoughts are associated with transitory changes in the brain's global field power. The spontaneous, ongoing electrical activity of the brain is measured in the EEG. Many people have assumed that the brain's activity would vary unpredictably if it were not constrained by the demands of carrying out specific tasks. In contrast, recent findings with fMRI suggest a very different pattern: the sustained spontaneous activity of the brain may generate globally coherent processes by itself (i.e., independent of any goal-directed tasks). In other words, the spontaneous (baseline) activity of the brain at rest may support sustained functions that are crucial to the brain's global coherence.

A brief summary of the brain's energy budget may be helpful to evaluate the fluctuations in the brain's field power. In the average adult human, the brain represents about 2% of the weight of the body. Despite the brain's relatively small size, it accounts for about 20% of the oxygen and calories consumed by the body. Hence it has been clearly established that the metabolic activity of the brain is about ten times greater than the activity of the rest of the body. Furthermore, it is well known that this high rate of metabolism varies only slightly despite wide variations in mental and motor activity (Raichle and Gusnard 2002).

It has been suggested that the global coherence of the distribution of energy in the brain's electromagnetic field may be maintained by a continuous, high-level but balanced input of both excitatory and inhibitory activity (Salinas and Sejnowski 2001; Raichle and Gusnard 2002). This balance between excitatory and inhibitory inputs can maintain the brain at a quasi-stable equilibrium that is highly responsive to context-dependent changes from internal or external stimuli. Most of the energy consumption of the brain is required for the propagation of action potentials and for restoring postsynaptic ion fluxes after receptors have been stimulated by neurotransmitters. Recent work has emphasized the role of glutamate signaling in the brain because greater than 90% of synapses release glutamate (Attwell and Laughlin 2001). It has been suggested that most energy use in the brain is the result of excitatory glutamate signaling even in the resting state.

In fMRI and PET studies, it has been possible to measure the global energy activity of the brain, as well as variation in energy consumption coincident with specific tasks and also spontaneously (i.e., independent of any tasks). For example, the relationship between blood flow and oxygen consumption is measured quantitatively in PET studies as the oxygen extraction fraction (OEF). The OEF is the ratio between oxygen delivery (i.e., blood flow) and oxygen consumption. The OEF has been found to be globally uniform throughout the brain in a resting state, such as restful alertness, when averaged across groups of subjects (Raichle, MacLeod et al. 2001). This global spatial uniformity exists despite considerable variation in the ongoing oxygen consumption and blood flow within gray matter and a 4-fold difference between gray and white matter in both oxygen consumption and blood flow.

This global coherence of the distribution of energy in the brain is measurably changed in the normal brain only when specific mental or motor tasks are carried out. Moreover, deactivations consistently appear within the same configuration of areas when subjects engage in a wide variety of goal-directed behaviors (Gusnard and Raichle 2001). When specific mental or motor tasks are carried out, there are quantitative and qualitative changes in metabolic activity compared with the resting state of global coherence. The signal used to map activations in the brain with PET or fMRI is based on local changes in blood flow. Increased neuronal activity in a region of the brain is associated with an increase in blood flow. Surprisingly, however, oxygen consumption increases less than blood flow and glucose utilization (which increase in proportion to one another). Consequently, the oxygen content of hemoglobin in blood increases in proportion to blood flow and neuronal activity. The change in oxygenation of hemoglobin is the practical basis for variation in the magnetic resonance signal intensity. That is, magnetic resonance signal intensity reflects the increases in blood flow and oxygenation of blood in proportion to regional neuronal activity.

The major relevance of recent work on brain energy metabolism to understanding self-aware consciousness is that most brain energy utilization involves spontaneous activity independent of any goal-directed tasks. In fact, goal-directed activity actually decreases the level and the coherence of the distribution of energy in portions of the brain. This suggests the intriguing possibility that global coherence is the spontaneous characteristic of the brain and is only disturbed by goal-directed activities characteristic of the lower stages of self-aware consciousness, including meditation. As I review in the next few sections, global coherence of the electrical activity of the brain increases in the restful alertness of the second and third stages of self-aware consciousness. In addition, global coherence depends on orchestration of both hemispheres by the frontal poles, which is associated with efficiency in carrying out multiple tasks simultaneously (Burgess, Veitch et al. 2000) and creativity (Alexander and Langer 1990). Accordingly, studies of brain psychophysiology in different stages of consciousness provide an important way of understanding the functional significance of variability in the global field power of the brain.

## PSYCHOPHYSIOLOGY OF THE STAGES OF CONSCIOUSNESS

The discrete psychophysical nature of thought suggests that each stage of self-aware consciousness may be distinguished by a specific EEG pattern generated by different connections of neural networks. Fortunately, psychophysiological studies have been conducted for a wide range of states of consciousness.

To understand the psychophysiology of different levels of consciousness, it is helpful to review key aspects of autonomic nervous system activity in relation to the five planes of thought. Some key points are summarized in Table 6.5 based on the functional neuroanatomy of personality (Cloninger, 2002). Thought in planes 2 and 3 activate defensive responses characterized by sympathetic hyperarousal. Sympathetic hyperactivity is also called the fight-or-flight response and is associated with anxiety and physiological effects characterized as preparing a person for "fight-or-flight." These changes include elevation of blood pressure, generally lower amplitude and increased rate of breathing, with increased oxygen consumption, pupillary dilatation, muscle vasodilation, and increased blood flow to muscles. There is decreased sensitivity to aversive stimulation and decreased skin resistance. In the EEG, there is much fast activity at a frequency of thirteen to thirty per second, which is called *beta activity*.

**Table 6.5.** Temperamental Aspects of the Planes of Thought and Their
Neuroanatomical Correlates

| Thought Plane | Temperament Aspect | Limbic Network | Attention Network | EEG–EMG Correlate |
|---|---|---|---|---|
| 2 | Harm avoidance | Septal | Valence | Startle |
| 3 | Novelty seeking | Amygdaloid | Arousal | Defense |
| 4 | Security seeking | Thalamocortical | Conflict control | Relax |
| 5 | Persistence | Striatal | Reward | PREE |
| 7 | — | — | Coherence | |

Defense reflex, fight-or-flight response (sympathetic hyperarousal—beta rhythm on EEG);
relaxation response, decreased sympathetic activity and increased parasympathetic activity
(alpha rhythm on EEG, as in hypnagogic states); PREE, partial reinforcement extinction
effect; coherence, synchrony in homologous regions of two cerebral hemispheres.

In contrast, when a person is relaxed or at rest, there is a decrease in sympathetic activity and an increase in parasympathetic activity. This is sometimes called the *relaxation response* (Benson 1976) and is associated with changes that are generally opposite to those of the fight or flight response: decreased blood pressure, decreased rate of breathing and oxygen consumption, increased skin resistance. On the EEG, there is a decrease in Beta activity with a shift to slower activity in the range of 4–13 Hz, which is called *alpha activity*. Deep diaphragmatic breathing and closing of eyes often induce the relaxation response. In ordinary waking consciousness (i.e., the first stage of self-aware consciousness), the function of the autonomic nervous system is involuntary. However, in advanced stages of self-awareness, individuals can consciously influence functions that are normally autonomic, such as heart rate and breathing rate (Wallace & Benson, 1972; Alexander et al., 1990).

The EEG correlates of different levels of consciousness that have been documented in systematic research are summarized in Table 6.6. Five levels of consciousness have been well documented in systematic studies, designating deep sleep as level 0. The levels of consciousness can be readily distinguished by characteristic spectral frequencies in quantitative EEGs, as shown in Table 6.6. The initial levels of consciousness are distinguished by a single EEG frequency in quantitative EEG studies of the brain macrostate. Deep sleep is characterized by delta rhythms, which are produced by increased activity of a system in the brain stem that synchronizes cortical activity. Dreaming is characterized by theta rhythms, which are generated in subcortical limbic areas, such as the septohippocampal system (Robinson 2000). The septohippocampal system encodes information for long-term storage by processes, such as condensation, that distinguish dream content from waking cognition (Freud 1900). The hypnogogic state between sleep and waking, characterized by relaxed inattention to external or internal stimuli, is associated with alpha activity, which is generated in the thalamic cortical activating system (Cade and Coxhead 1989; Robinson 2000).

**Table 6.6.** EEG Correlates of Specific States of Self-Aware Consciousness

| *Level of Consciousness* | *EEG Correlate* |
| --- | --- |
| 0  Deep sleep | Delta rhythm (1–4 Hz) |
| 1  Dreaming | Theta rhythm (4–7 Hz) |
| 2  Hypnagogic state, hypnopompic state (drowsy-relaxed) | Alpha rhythm (adults 8–13 Hz; children 4–7 Hz) |
| 3  Awake cognition (first stage of self-awareness) | Beta rhythm (13–30 Hz) (variable levels of sympathetic activity) |
| 4  Meditation (second stage of self-awareness) | Slow alpha and theta (decreased sympathetic activity: little or no fight-or-flight response) |
| 5  Contemplation (third stage of self-awareness) | Slow alpha and theta plus beta (16–18 Hz) and delta (1–4 Hz) (bilateral symmetry & coherence) |

*Source*: Adapted from Wallace 1970; Cade and Coxhead 1989; Alexander, Davies et al. 1990.

Waking cognition in the first stage of self-awareness is associated with varying levels of the fight-or-flight response, which produces beta rhythms associated with sympathetic arousal of the cerebral cortex. A combined study using PET and quantitative EEG in nine young adults showed greater activity of the brain attention network regulating control of conflict when ordinary cognition was compared with the restful state of meditation (Lou, Kjaer et al. 1999). Specifically, compared with meditation, ordinary wakeful consciousness involved greater signs of activity in the conflict control network of attention, including increased activity in the lateral prefrontal cortex, anterior cingulate gyri, and basal ganglia.

In contrast, higher stages of self-aware consciousness have been characterized by coherent patterns of multiple wave frequencies. Both second and third stages of self-aware consciousness combine pleasant calmness with increasing breadth and depth of conscious awareness. Consequently the background of activity is a slowing of alpha activity from the usual frequency of 9–12 cycles per second (Hz) down to 7–9 Hz. The slow alpha activity is also regular and high in amplitude, particularly in the frontal and central regions of the brain (Wallace and Benson 1972). In the second stage of self-aware consciousness, the slow alpha background is occasionally blocked by long trains of low-voltage theta activity in the frontal area (Wallace 1970; Wallace and Benson 1972; Cade and Coxhead 1989; Alexander, Davies et al. 1990). This meditative state is similar to the transitional period between wakefulness and sleep, except that such transition to sleep is usually brief and followed by sleep spindles, delta waves, and loss of consciousness. In contrast, restful alertness is maintained for prolonged periods during meditation. In addition, when repeated trials of stimulation by auditory clicks are carried out in individuals in the state of mindfulness, there is no habituation of the alpha-blocking response that is usually seen in states of simple relaxation or drowsiness (Wallace 1970). Consequently, mindful meditation is considered a distinct state of consciousness.

Not everyone who practices meditation enters into the second stage of self-aware consciousness. In a study of fifteen healthy college students who had practiced the yoga called transcendental meditation (TM) for six months to three years, only four of fifteen subjects had the EEG characteristics of mindfulness (Wallace 1970). In addition, when the EEG is monitored continuously for prolonged periods, individuals differ in their ability to maintain a mindful state while resuming other everyday activities (Cade and Coxhead 1989). For some individuals, the mindful state is their usual level of consciousness, whereas for others it is the maximum part of their range of thought. It is important to distinguish between meditation as a procedure and the actual state of consciousness experienced during and after meditation.

The second stage of self-aware consciousness is what I refer to as a *mindful meditative state*. Mindfulness is also called the "fourth state" of consciousness, as shown in Table 6.6. Using topographical EEG mapping, mindfulness may correspond to the brain microstate associated with thought level 5.6 described in Table 6.4. However, additional EEG mapping studies are needed to compare brain microstates associated with mindfulness with those associated with the transition to or from sleep. Mindful meditation is associated with increased metabolic activity of specific brain regions, including the lateral and orbital prefrontal cortex, cingulate cortex, and thalamus (Lazar, Bush et al. 2000; Newberg, Alavi et al. 2001). The activity of the dorsolateral prefrontal cortex and the superior parietal lobe were negatively correlated during meditation, which may reflect the altered sense of space that is often experienced in mindfulness. The increased frontal regional blood flow may reflect internally focused attention (i.e., mindfulness), whereas the global increase in cortical activity may reflect the increased thalamic activity during meditation (Newberg, Alavi et al. 2001).

In the third stage of self-aware consciousness, there is greater coherence of the EEG pattern in homologous regions of both hemispheres than in other stages of awareness. Slow alpha activity is interspersed by occasional trains of slow theta and delta activity (Cade and Coxhead 1989; Alexander, Davies et al. 1990). However, unlike sleep, subjects in contemplation maintain calm alertness for prolonged periods. They can carry on everyday life activities, such as work and conversations. However, when the thought level is 5.8 or higher, there is an experience of nonlocality (i.e., nonseparation of self and others) associated with increased frontal activity in the EEG (Lehmann, Faber et al. 2001). At the same time, individuals experience oceanic feelings, which are described as "blissful." The blissful state is synchronous with increased theta synchronization in the frontal poles, as well as enhanced theta connectivity between prefrontal and posterior association cortex (Aftanas and Golocheikine 2001). Quantitative ratings of internalized attention are correlated with both slow alpha and theta synchronization (as in the second stage of self-awareness), whereas subjective scores for blissfulness are correlated with frontal theta activity (Aftanas and Golocheikine 2001). In addition, if the thought level is 5.9 or higher, the cognitive state is often described as highly creative (Cade and Coxhead 1989; Alexander, Davies et al. 1990). Consequently, contemplation may be regarded as a distinct "fifth" state of consciousness, as shown in Table 6.6.

The emergence of theta and delta activity in the higher stages of consciousness provides a concrete demonstration of what is meant by an increase in the breadth and depth of self-awareness. In the second stage of self-awareness, the mind becomes aware of its own subconscious, which is coincident with the emergence of theta activity generated by the limbic cortical activating system. In the third stage of self-awareness, the mind becomes aware of its own unconscious, which is coincident with the emergence of delta activity generated by the brainstem cortical activating system.

Essentially, the greater energy level of higher stages of consciousness may allow awareness of an increasing depth of brain processes that activate the cerebral cortex with decreasing wave frequencies. That is, it takes a higher DFT level to activate conscious awareness of deeper brain processes. Specifically, the relaxation of thought in the first stage of self-aware consciousness (below level 5.4) activates only the alpha generator in the thalamic activating system. Thought in the second stage of self-aware consciousness (levels from 5.4 to 5.7) can activate the limbic cortical activating system. In the third stage of self-aware consciousness (i.e., levels of 5.8 and higher), thought can activate the brain-stem cortical activating system.

Available information suggests the possibility that the memories of the body, mind, and psyche are unconscious to varying degrees depending on the depth of a person's self-aware consciousness. If this hypothesis is true, then meditation and contemplation should result in objective changes in the coherence of both psychosomatic and psychosocial functions of our being. Distinctions between what is voluntary versus involuntary may diminish with increasing depth of self-awareness until we are in a constant state of nearly full awareness.

In fact, changes in biopsychosocial functions to test this hypothesis have been evaluated in detail in several independent studies of behavioral conditioning, relaxation, meditation, and contemplation. Independent studies are available about a wide variety of techniques for facilitating the development of self-aware consciousness (Wallace 1970; Cade and Coxhead 1989; Alexander and Langer 1990; Lou, Kjaer et al. 1999; Khare and Nigam 2000; Lehmann, Faber et al. 2001; Newberg, Alavi et al. 2001).

## PSYCHOSOMATIC EFFECTS OF MEDITATION

### Short-term studies

Meditative and contemplative states have profound acute effects on body physiology in addition to their EEG correlates. Several systematic studies have been carried out using different meditation techniques, including yoga of TM or Zen mindfulness (Wallace and Benson 1972; Alexander, Davies et al. 1990) or biofeedback-assisted mindfulness (Cade and Coxhead 1989).

Well-designed systematic studies have characterized the relaxation response, which induces a "wakeful, hypometabolic state" (Wallace and Benson 1972). Other descriptions of the state are "restful alertness" and "effortless noncontrol," which indicate letting go of the struggles that lead to sympathetic hyperarousal (Alexander, Davies et al. 1990). Wallace and Benson (1972) carried out detailed physiological monitoring of thirty-six adults who had practiced TM for mostly two or three years (range, one month to nine years). The TM technique is described as

> An effortless procedure for allowing the excitations of the mind to settle down until the least excited state of mind is reached. This is a state of inner wakefulness with no object of thought or perception, just pure consciousness. . . . (Maharishi 1976, page 123)

According to Maharishi (1986, page 40), pure consciousness is a form of mindfulness, which is the mind becoming aware of itself:

> Consciousness in its pure state, fully open to itself alone, experiences itself as this self-interacting reality of nature . . . consciousness knows itself to be the knower, the known, and the process of gaining knowledge—all three values simultaneously in one.

Consequently, this approach to mindfulness may elevate thought to either the second stage of self-awareness (meditation) or the third stage (contemplation). Progression to the third stage of self-awareness is marked by the experience of oceanic feelings, which is associated with near suspension of breathing, or by creativity, which is associated with increased frontal EEG coherence (Alexander, Davies et al. 1990).

As a practical procedure, the meditator sits in a comfortable position with eyes closed. He perceives a particular sound or thought that he has been taught. Without attempting to concentrate specifically on this cue, he effortlessly allows his mind to experience it freely, so that his mind may rise to a "finer and more creative level in an easy and natural manner" (Wallace and Benson 1972). The effortless letting go of struggle and control is called "transcending" by its practitioners.

Subjects meditated for twenty to thirty minutes and were also observed for equal periods of time before and after meditation. Regardless of the duration of prior experience with meditation, five to ten minutes of meditation induced a "wakeful, hypometabolic" state comparable to that observed in experts in meditation with many years of experience. The physiological signs of this state of slowed metabolism included rapid reductions in oxygen consumption, rate and volume of respiration, and heart rate within five to ten minutes of meditation. All of the measured physiological parameters returned to the premeditation level within a few minutes after the subjects stopped meditating. The ratio of carbon dioxide elimination to oxygen consumption remained unchanged before, during, or after meditation, indicating that the factor that influenced both was the general rate of metabolism. In addition, there was a substantial reduction in blood lactate, indicating a shift toward oxidative metabolism in muscle, rather than anaerobic metabolism. There was also a rapid 4-fold increase in skin resistance. Meditation did not change arterial blood pressure.

These acute physiological signs indicated that meditation combined calm wakefulness with a general slowing of the body's metabolic rate. The observed signs were very different from what is observed in other states of relaxation, such as sleep or hypnosis (Wallace and Benson 1972). Oxygen consumption and metabolic rate are reduced in sleep only after several hours, whereas they are reduced in meditation within the first five to ten minutes. In contrast, there is no systematic change on oxygen consumption in hypnosis. Any physiological changes that do occur in a hypnotized person have no relationship to the hypnotic state and merely reflect the particular state of activity suggested to the person (Wallace and Benson 1972).

These results showed that meditation takes about five minutes to have substantial central effects on general body physiology. Furthermore, the physiological changes associated with meditation are closely synchronous with the changes in thought level, beginning with onset of meditation and returning to baseline after cessation of meditation. In other words, the physiology of the body depends on a person's level of thought during a meditation session.

Subsequent work has replicated and extended the findings of Wallace and Benson about the physiological effects of TM (Alexander and Langer 1990). The subjective experience of transcending is highly correlated with heightened EEG coherence across cortical regions and frequency bands, suggesting an increase in long-range spatial ordering and functional integration of the cortex (Badawi, Wallace et al. 1984). Increased alpha coherence occurred during TM but not in randomly assigned controls at rest following muscular relaxation (Dillbeck and Bronson 1981; Gaylord, Orme-Johnson et al. 1989). In comparison to simple relaxation, the heightened alertness during TM has been supported by increased cortical blood flow and marked increase in plasma arginine vasopressin (which is associated with improved learning and memory) (Alexander, Davies et al.

1990). The enhanced calmness of TM is distinguished from simple relaxation by greater decreases in plasma cortisol and greater increases in serotonergic turnover (Alexander, Davies et al. 1990). Mindfulness training can also increase left prefrontal activity (Davidson, Kabat-Zinn et al. 2003).

Furthermore, other studies have shown that people can learn to maintain meditative thinking indefinitely. In other words, the way a person usually thinks can be mindful. For example, Cade and Coxhead (1989) used continuous monitoring of EEG and skin resistance with biofeedback during a variety of meditation and contemplation techniques. They found that a substantial fraction of people who had meditated for many years did not produce the EEG state characteristic of mindfulness. With biofeedback, though, most people quickly learned the level of mindful thinking that produced high skin resistance and high-amplitude alpha interspersed with trains of theta activity in the quantitative EEG. About a third of those who were mindful also learned the level of contemplative thinking that also produced delta activity in the EEG in a wakeful state. Moreover, some people were able to maintain the fourth state (i.e., mindfulness) or the fifth state of consciousness (i.e., contemplation) when tested by requiring that they keep their eyes open, carry on conversations, do mental arithmetic, and other attention-demanding tasks and activities of daily living.

By comparison, remember that without such mental exercises, Jane Loevinger found that less than 0.5% of individuals ever achieve the stage of integration or integrity that is based on contemplative levels of thought (Alexander, Davies et al. 1990). Hence, meditative and contemplative exercises are helpful in raising the maximum level of thought. The experience of elevated maximum thoughts in peak experiences, meditation, or contemplation lays the foundation for such thinking to become the usual way of thinking, but it does not guarantee such long-term outcomes. Moreover, the assessment of long-term outcomes requires careful methodological consideration.

I suggest that it is the level of thought induced by an experience that appears to be crucial in determining biopsychosocial outcomes. Inspiring conversations in a hopeful, compassionate alliance may elevate thought and stimulate a person to maintain such ways of elevated thinking. Brief experiences of elevated thought from visiting a garden or reading the elevated thoughts of positive philosophers can transform a person's thoughts. For example, in Chapter 4, reading Montaigne's essays and visiting a botanical garden inspired Emerson greatly. As described in Chapters 3 and 5, the reading and discussion of poetry were inspirational to Russell and to Bucke and transformed their world views.

For example, much systematic outcome data have been collected on the "Mozart effect" (Rauscher, Shaw et al. 1993; Campbell 1995, 1997; Chabris 1999; Bodner, Muftuler et al. 2001; Thompson, Schellenberg et al. 2001). Listening to some forms of music, and not others, produces an elevation of thought that may have long-term biopsychosocial consequences, although the effects may be explained in terms of the effects of the music on enjoyment and calm alertness. Music by gifted composers, such as Bach, Mozart, or Schubert, has the effect of elevating thought, often to the second level of self-aware consciousness in which we are in a calm wakeful state simply enjoying the order, beauty, and fluidity of the music without judging it critically. Regular exposure to such inspired and inspiring music has been shown in systematic prospective studies to produce increased scores on tests of intelligence and visuo-motor coordination, to reduce distractibility and unproductive hyperactivity, and to enhance well-being (Campbell 1997). Such results are obtained in people of average health, as well as in individuals with disorders such as attention deficit disorder or forms of mental retardation such as Down syndrome. Such effects of music may provide a simple means to elevate thought and enhance well-being but need to be evaluated with quantitative measurement of the level of thought as a mediating variable. The measurement of thought is needed to understand variability in the magnitude and presence of the effect in different groups of subjects (Chabris 1999; Twomey and Esgate 2002).

I think it is important to emphasize that withdrawal from everyday life does not facilitate the development of wisdom and well-being. An ascetic monk who contemplates his navel all day may be in retreat from the challenges that would help him to become more integrated. What is useful is to learn to elevate thought throughout the full range of our activities of daily living. Initially we may need to do this under special conditions of calm and quiet, but then we need to learn to maintain elevated thoughts in the full range of daily activities. Progress in the stability of elevated thinking proceeds by means of many small and discrete steps, as we grow patiently in self-awareness and understanding along the path of the psyche.

## Long-term studies

The ability to measure the thoughts and brain states characteristic of meditation and contemplation provides the much-needed basis for improved studies of treatment to enhance coherence and well-being. With measurement of the level of thought, it is possible to assess the characteristics of people and procedures that produce the intended results. Treatment can be designed in ways that are outcome based and data driven while respecting the freedom and flexibility of both therapists and subjects to act spontaneously and naturally, as long as they are effective. The ability to measure acute brain states also provides a way of testing objectively what acute changes are prospectively predictive of long-term benefit.

Without such measurement of mind–brain states, it is difficult to interpret results in samples of treated individuals or practitioners because of selection and reporting biases. For example, enduring physiological changes have been observed in people identified as regular practitioners of TM. Regular practice with TM is associated with lower respiratory and heart rates, lower plasma lactate levels, and decreased fluctuation in spontaneous galvanic skin responses outside of meditation as compared to nonmeditating controls at rest (Dillbeck and Orme-Johnson 1987; Alexander, Davies et al. 1990). Long-term psychophysiological studies suggest greater autonomic stability, efficiency of endocrine responses, and EEG coherence in regular TM practitioners compared to nonmeditating controls (Alexander, Davies et al. 1990).

The interpretation of such associations is ambiguous. Acute studies show that physiology changes when the level of thought changes. We do not know to what extent the results depend on selection of individuals who are compliant with meditation for a long time (versus those who drop out). We do not know to what extent the benefits depend on maintaining mindful thinking on average or by transiently elevating thoughts under particular unusual conditions that would otherwise be stressful. Nevertheless, the results of long-term studies may be regarded as consistent with systematic short-term studies if it is the case that regular practitioners are learning to generalize their mindful thinking to everyday life. Therefore, we need to examine available data about the psychosocial outcomes associated with various ways of elevating the levels of thought.

## Psychosocial effects of elevating thought

Reports of illumination experiences consistently describe a permanent and radical transformation of thought patterns that strongly influence personal goals and values, as described in Chapters 3 and 4 for Bertrand Russell and the American transcendentalists Emerson and Thoreau. Scientific experiments in which meditation and contemplation are intentionally practiced support such reports (Cade and Coxhead 1989; Alexander, Davies et al. 1990). The most rigorous and extensive program of research has studied the effects of TM. Prospective longitudinal studies with matched controls have been carried out on the psychosocial effects of TM in children, young adult college graduates, convicted felons, and adults over sixty years of age.

A prospective study of the long-term effects of TM compared sixty-eight practitioners of TM with sixty-eight matched controls who were all engaged in some type of self-development, stress management, or exercise to maintain mental or physical health. Development was rated by an expert using Loevinger's test of ego development without knowledge of which subjects were TM practitioners. All 136 young adults were college graduates. Most of the subjects at the time of college graduation were tested as being at or near the "conscientious" stage of development according to Loevinger's classification, which corresponds to a capacity for thought at level 5.4. When followed-up more than a decade later, the proportion of the controls at the autonomous level was 1%, which was the same as when they graduated from college. Loevinger's autonomous level is what I call the level of self-transcendence (maximum thought level 5.7). In contrast, the proportion of TM practitioners who were self-transcendent had increased from 9%

to 38% (Alexander, Davies et al. 1990). In addition, more of the TM practitioners demonstrated principled moral reasoning in other blindly rated tests.

Enhanced psychosocial outcomes were also shown to be dependent on psychophysiological variables. Specifically, higher alpha EEG coherence in the frontal and central regions of the EEGs of adolescents and adults practicing TM was correlated with improved psychosocial development, including greater fluid intelligence, principled moral reasoning, concept formation, and creativity (Dillbeck and Bronson 1981; Alexander, Davies et al. 1990). Frontal EEG coherence is the principal psychophysiological marker of creativity, which is characteristic of contemplative thought at DFT level 5.9. Hence elevation of thought to the third level of self-aware consciousness, as indicated by frontal EEG coherence, has a greater impact on subsequent psychosocial status than does meditation in the second stage of self-awareness. Meditation provides pleasant and relaxing experiences that provide the foundation for transformation of personality in the third stage of self-awareness. These important results illustrate the advantages of a biopsychosocial paradigm, as will be discussed in the next section.

Some studies of the elevation of thought in children raise interesting questions. TM for children is designed to promote shifting to active thinking mind from immediate desires and concrete perceptions (Alexander, Davies et al. 1990). In a prospective six-month study of the effects of elevating the thought of the children, thirty-seven preschoolers (age four to five years old) were compared with twenty-nine demographically matched controls in another school where TM was not practiced. There were greater increases in tests of general intelligence, cognitive reflectivity, cognitive flexibility, conception of conservation of number and mass, field independence, and measures of sustained attention and vigilance. The study involves comparison of rather small numbers of children sampled from different locations, so no definite conclusions can be drawn. Similar reports have been made about the benefits of exposure to elevated music, so additional work is needed to compare different types of intervention that are appropriate for children. It is unclear whether any degree of elevation of thought is beneficial, or whether improvement depends on transitions between the major stages of self-aware consciousness.

In a study of ninety prisoners in a maximum security prison who were taught TM, Charles Alexander observed that one year of practicing TM led to greater improvement in Loevinger's self-development scale compared with wait-list controls, dropouts, and those not interested in learning TM (Alexander, Davies et al. 1990). On average the prisoners improved from the conformist level to the self-aware level in their self-reports. The differences in self-report were supported by the additional finding of recidivism being one third lower in the TM group than in the controls after three and one-half years. An independent study replicated the lowering of recidivism in prisoners practicing TM compared with others in a six-year follow up.

These results in individuals of varying age, education, and maturity suggest that the benefits of elevation of thought may be substantial. However, there are many possible confounding biases in the studies of children, prisoners, and the elderly. Only studies of young adults have used an integrated biopsychosocial model in which psychosocial outcomes could be studied prospectively in relation to intervening changes in psychophysical effects of meditation. The findings in young adults show that the acute physiological effects of transcendental contemplation are predictive of long-term psychosocial outcome. The acute effects of elevating thought to levels below contemplation may possibly be helpful but have much less of a transforming effect on personality than does contemplation. Consequently, the observed results in other groups that did not integrate biomedical and psychosocial observations are ambiguous because their experimental designs were inadequate for any rigorous interpretation. Further work is needed to clarify whether the differences between the effects of meditation and contemplation are quantitative or qualitative.

## DEGENERACY OF REDUCTIVE PARADIGMS

A paradigm is scientifically degenerate if it does not provide a way to test and modify its basic assumptions or if it cannot make predictions that go beyond observed data. In other words, any experimental paradigm is "inadequate" or "degenerate" if it begins with fixed assumptions that cannot be modified in the light of progressively accumulated experience. In contrast, an experimental design is "adequate" or "regenerative" if it can be refined progressively in a stepwise fashion informed by the accumulation of additional experience. Such progress involves a nonlinear sequence of creative intuitive leaps in understanding, as discussed in Chapter 1 (Godel 1961). Such a sequence corresponds to the pattern of awakening of self-aware consciousness. Also, such progressive modification and refinement of initial assumptions is characteristic of the nonlinear optimization process that occurs in complex adaptive systems, such as character development (Cloninger, Svrakic et al. 1997).

The term *degenerate* was initially used as I am defining it in a critical analysis of research on the inheritance of IQ (Urbach 1974). Much research about IQ has neglected the substantial contributions from cultural inheritance and gene–environment correlation, thereby making inflated estimates of the heritability of IQ test scores (Cloninger, Rice et al. 1979; Ehrlich and Feldman 2003). The contributions of genetic inheritance, cultural inheritance, and gene–environment correlation were approximately equal to one another when all available family data were considered (Cloninger, Rice et al. 1979). Studies limited to monozygotic and dizygotic twins do not contain enough information to distinguish cultural and genetic inheritance (Cloninger, Rice et al. 1979), yet nearly all behavioral geneticists and evolutionary psychologists begin by assuming that cultural inheritance and gene–environment correlation can be neglected. As a result of oversimplified assumptions and confusion about the true interpretation of heritability statistics, their conclusions are actually predetermined by initial untested assumptions, which cannot be investigated within their experimental design. Such a self-deceiving combination of fixed and oversimplified assumptions with inadequate experimental designs may be accurately described as degenerate because it is not progressively self-organizing like self-aware consciousness.

Degenerate paradigms can be as seductively misleading as erotic material, which stimulates curiosity and other basic urges but does not lead to increases in wisdom or well-being. For example, psychoanalysis is another well-known example of a degenerate paradigm, which may contain many truths about behavior but cannot be rigorously falsified (Popper 1934). Much like the "just-so" stories of evolutionary psychology (Ehrlich and Feldman 2003), psychoanalytic descriptions provide insightful explanations of any behavior in retrospect but cannot make unambiguous predictions about future development in a reliable manner.

What has not been widely recognized is that *any* reductive or dualistic paradigm of human behavior is degenerate, despite this being pointed out by integrative thinkers about the psychosocial aspects of medicine and biology (Beck 1996; Eisenberg 1998; Gabbard 2000; Sapolsky 2003). For example, the degeneracy of separate biomedical and psychosocial paradigms is the reason that these two conflicting approaches vacillate in their dominance of the field. Whenever one is dominant, its inadequacy becomes obvious to all but its most entrenched advocates. Slowly interest in the inadequate paradigm declines (i.e., it degenerates) and another paradigm rises to replace it. However, if the replacement paradigm is also degenerate, it also declines, and the cycle continues until an adequate paradigm emerges.

Let me give examples of the degeneracy of current research strategies. Rather than selecting examples in which conclusions are simply predetermined by initial assumptions, I have chosen some examples of valuable contributions being made in designs that could easily be made adequate. I have chosen as examples the studies I have already been citing as having made some valuable contributions to a rigorous science of well-being, even though I think there are fundamental limitations to their experimental designs.

First, consider the current state of psychotherapy research. Many insightful and talented clinicians are striving to do replicable research to demonstrate the efficacy of various forms of psychotherapy. The standard of the field is to develop manuals that detail what is supposed to be done under any circumstance. The problem of compliance with such manuals is severe because a complete manual would anticipate every response of the ideal therapist, who is assumed to be the manual writer's own ideal self. However, we are all different and it is impossible to anticipate the boundless possibilities in interpersonal relationships. Consequently, manuals are heterogeneous composites of wisdom, superstition, and error whose assumptions cannot be falsified without a valid external criterion of the critical targets toward which intervention is directed. The manuals may be almost irrelevant if what is important is the level of self-awareness of the therapist, the level of the therapist's relationship with the patient, and the therapist's flexibility in using innovative procedures to elevate the patient's thought, such as how to teach meditation and contemplation. Even the addition of biomedical tests, such as brain imaging or EEG mapping, cannot rehabilitate the psychosocial paradigm unless the psychophysical parameters measured correspond to a valid model of thought and its development. In other words, an adequate (nondegenerate) model of well-being requires a unified model of mind–brain states and human relationships.

Second, recent important biomedical work on the neurophysiology of brain microstates has degenerated because of the absence of an independently validated model of the levels of thought and its development. Once the seminal observation was made that brain microstates exist, the practical problem remained about how to estimate the number of classes of brain microstates. The biomedical researchers wanted to base their conclusions only on observations about the brain. However, such hope is unrealistic in science because all models require extra-statistical information and can be tested only using criteria established in another domain. The need for information from another domain was shown by what happened in efforts to estimate the number of brain microstates. Multivariate methods including canonical correlation analysis were used to estimate the number of significant pairs of mind–brain states, producing four such significant states. However, the number of significant pairs depends on the way the thoughts and brain states are measured. Later, when cluster analysis techniques were applied to the classification of brain states, arbitrary assumptions were required about the number of classes. All brain microstates were statistically forced into four classes. In my opinion, however, the assumption that there are only four brain microstates is unlikely because of what is already known about the richness of human thought and its stepwise development. Perhaps I am wrong in my doubt about this assumption. Nevertheless, the point is that the assumption of four classes was ultimately an arbitrary statistical assumption in the absence of a nonbrain criterion about the relevant variability in human thoughts. The inability of the biomedical paradigm to test its critical assumptions about psychosocial variables occurs because of the absence of a unified model of thoughts and brain states, each of which can be progressively refined. The assumptions about brain microstates need to be tested with observations about thought using something like the DFT, just as the assumptions about thought need to be tested with observations about brain states. Furthermore, assumptions about social relationships need to be tested with observations about the relationships of thoughts of one individual with the brain states of the other individual, and vice versa because relationships can be asymmetric. Remember that a person's psychosomatic response to another person is a bioassay of the interpersonal relationship, which can also be measured using the Diagnosis of Human Relationships (DHR) as in Chapter 4. The way another person relates to us elicits distinct psychosomatic responses, which may remain outside of self-awareness, as in the subliminal effects of some advertising, or, if sufficiently aware, may be consciously experienced and used therapeutically. Direct measurement of thoughts and psychophysical states in social relationships can help to elucidate these important human phenomena. The combined measurement of brain microstates, DFT, and DHR form the basis of an integrated biopsychosocial paradigm.

It should be noticed that nothing I have suggested is really incompatible with the hopes and intentions of either the biomedical or the psychosocial approaches. The biomedical investigators really want to understand the functional organization of brain states and systems in relation to thought and its development. The psychosocial investigators already regard the curative parameters in psychotherapy to be self-understanding, the helping relationship, and procedures for the patient to maintain the gains made in therapy (Luborsky 1989). However, the paradigms being used to achieve these goals are degenerate because of the unnecessary and maladaptive division between the biomedical and psychosocial domains.

I suggest that the only possible reconciliation of the degeneracy of contemporary psychological medicine is the study of mind–brain states as a unified psychobiology. I have begun to describe such a unified psychobiology in this chapter in terms of the synchronous measurement of thought and brain microstates. The quantum-like matrix of thought described in Chapter 3 can be combined with a full matrix of brain microstates. The combination of matrices for thought and brain microstates is possible because they are descriptively compatible and each provides criteria for testing the assumptions of the other domain of measured variables.

For example, in an integrated biopsychosocial paradigm we can measure both biomedical and psychosocial parameters about the patient, about the therapist, and about their interpersonal relationship and interactions. We can investigate which of these variables influence the development of various levels of thought in the patient acutely, and to what degree they do so. We can also investigate what variables predict the long-term maintenance of more adaptive levels of thought. The levels of thought can be objectively tested using measurable psychophysical variables. Then the variables describing the patient, the therapist, and their relationship can be refined iteratively.

Advances in the measurement of both thought and brain states, as described here, now allow a truly integrated biopsychosocial approach to training, research, and clinical practice. However, this possibility is not sufficient to bring about a constructive application of the available potential. We also must grow in awareness about our own problems, struggles, and fears, which create obstacles to our letting go of old degenerate habits of thought and clinical practice.

## REFERENCES

Aftanas, L. I. and S. A. Golocheikine (2001). "Human anterior and frontal midline theta and lower alpha reflect emotionally positive state and internalized attention: High-resolution EEG investigation of meditation." *Neuroscience Letters* 310: 57–60.

Alexander, C. N., J. L. Davies, et al. (1990). Growth of higher stages of consciousness: Maharishi's Vedic psychology of human development. *Higher stages of human development*. C. N. Alexander and E. J. Langer, eds. New York, Oxford University Press: 286–341.

Alexander, C. N. and E. J. Langer (1990). *Higher stages of human development*. New York, Oxford University Press.

Attwell, D. and S. B. Laughlin (2001). "An energy budget for signaling in the grey matter of the brain." *Journal of Cerebral Blood Flow and Metabolism* 21: 1133–1145.

Badawi, K., R. K. Wallace, et al. (1984). "Electrophysiologic characteristics of respiratory suspension periods occurring during the practice of Transcendental Meditation program." *Psychosomatic Medicine* 46: 267–276.

Barlow, J. S. (1985). "Methods of analysis of nonstationary EEGs, with emphasis on segmentation techniques: A comparative review." *Journal of Clinical Neurophysiology* 2: 267–304.

Barrett, J. and H. Ehrlichman (1982). "Bilateral hemispheric alpha activity during visual imagery." *Neuropsychologia* 20: 703–708.

Beck, A. T. (1996). Beyond belief: A theory of modes, personality, and psychopathology. *Frontiers of cognitive therapy*. P. M. Salkovskis, ed. New York, Guilford Press: 1–25.

Benson, H. (1976). *The relaxation response*. New York, Avon.

Berkhout, J., D. O. Walter, et al. (1969). "Alteration of the human electroencephalogram induced by stressful verbal activity." *Electroencephalography & Clinical Neurophysiology* 27: 457–469.

Bodner, M., L. T. Muftuler, et al. (2001). "FMRI study relevant to the Mozart effect: Brain areas involved in spatial-temporal reasoning." *Neurological Research* 23: 683–690.

Burgess, P. W., E. Veitch, et al. (2000). "The cognitive and neuroanatomical correlates of multitasking." *Neuropsychologia* 38: 848–863.

Cade, C. M. and N. Coxhead (1989). *The awakened mind: Biofeedback and the development of higher states of awareness*. Shaftesbury, Dorset, England, Element Books.

Campbell, D. (1995). *The Mozart effect for children*. New York, William Morrow.

Campbell, D. (1997). *The Mozart effect: Tapping the power of music to heal the body, strengthen the mind, and unlock the creative spirit*. New York, Harper Collins.

Chabris, C. F. (1999). "Prelude or requiem for the 'Mozart effect'?" *Nature* 400: 826–827.

Cloninger, C. R., J. Rice, et al. (1979). "Multifactorial inheritance with cultural transmission and assortative mating. II. A general model of combined polygenic and cultural inheritance." *American Journal of Human Genetics* 31: 176–198.

Cloninger, C. R., D. M. Svrakic, et al. (1993). "A psychobiological model of temperament and character." *Archives of General Psychiatry* 50: 975–990.

Cloninger, C. R., N. M. Svrakic, et al. (1997). "Role of personality self-organization in development of mental disorder and disorder." *Development and Psychopathology* 9: 881–906.

Davidson, R. J., J. P. Chapman, et al. (1990). "Asymmetric brain electrical activity discriminates between psychometrically-matched verbal and spatial cognitive tasks." *Psychophysiology* 27: 528–543.

Davidson, R. J., J. Kabat-Zinn, et al. (2003). "Alterations in brain and immune function by mindfulness meditation." *Psychosomatic Medicine* 65: 564–570.

Dillbeck, M. C. and E. C. Bronson (1981). "Short-term longitudinal effects of the transcendental meditation technique on EEG power and coherence." *International Journal of Neuroscience* 14: 147–151.

Dillbeck, M. C. and D. W. Orme-Johnson (1987). "Physiological differences between Transcendental Meditation and rest." *American Psychologist* 42: 879–881.

Ehrlich, P. and M. Feldman (2003). "Genes and cultures: What creates our behavioral phenome?" *Current Anthropology* 44: 87–107.

Ehrlichman, H. and M. S. Wiener (1980). "EEG asymmetry during covert mental activity." *Psychophysiology* 17: 228–235.

Eisenberg, L. (1998). "Nature, niche and nurture: The role of social experience in transforming genotype into phenotype." *Academic Psychiatry* 22: 213–222.

Eisenberg, L. (2000). "Is psychiatry more mindful or brainier than it was a decade ago?" *British Journal of Psychiatry* 176: 1–5.

Engel, G. L. (1977). "The need for a new medical model: A challenge for biomedicine." *Science* 196: 127–135.

Erikson, E. H. (1963). *Childhood and society.* New York, WW Norton & Co.

Frankl, V. E. (1959). *Man's search for meaning: An introduction to logotherapy.* New York, Simon & Schuster.

Freud, S. (1900). *The interpretation of dreams.* New York, MacMillan Company.

Gabbard, G. O. (2000). Psychoanalysis. *Comprehensive textbook of psychiatry.* B. J. Sadock and V. A. Sadock, eds. Philadelphia, Pennsylvania, Lippincott Williams & Wilkins: 563–606.

Gaylord, C., D. W. Orme-Johnson, et al. (1989). "The effects of transcendental meditation and progressive muscle relaxation on EEG coherence, stress reactivity and mental health in black adults." *International Journal of Neuroscience* 46: 77–86.

Givens, A., M. E. Smith, et al. (1999). "Electroencephalographic imaging of higher brain function." *Philosophical Transactions of the Royal Society of London–Series B: Biological Sciences* 354: 1125–1133.

Godel, K. (1961). The modern development of the foundations of mathematics in the light of philosophy. *Collected works.* New York, Oxford University Press.

Gusnard, D. A. and M. E. Raichle (2001). "Searching for a baseline: Functional imaging and the resting human brain." *Nature Reviews Neuroscience* 2: 685–694.

Heatherton, T. F. and J. L. Weinberger (1994). *Can personality change?* Washington, D.C., American Psychological Association.

Kandel, E. (1993). "A new intellectual framework for psychiatry." *American Journal of Psychiatry* 155: 457–469.

Khare, K. C. and S. K. Nigam (2000). "A study of electroencephalogram in meditators." *Indian Journal of Physiology and Pharmacology* 44: 173–178.

Koenig, T., D. Lehmann, et al. (1999). "A deviant EEG brain microstate in acute neuroleptic-naive schizophrenics at rest." *European Archives of Psychiatry and Clinical Neuroscience* 249: 205–211.

Koenig, T., L. Prichep, et al. (2002). "Millisecond by millisecond, year by year: Normative EEG microstates and developmental stages." *NeuroImage* 16: 41–48.

Kohlberg, L. (1973). Continuities in childhood and adult moral development revisited. *Life-span developmental psychology: Personality and socialization.* P. B. Baltes and K. W. Schaie, eds. New York, Academic Press.

Lazar, S. W., G. Bush, et al. (2000). "Functional brain mapping of the relaxation response and meditation." *NeuroReport* 11: 1581–1585.

Lehmann, D. (1998). "Deviant microstates ('atoms of thought') in brain electric field sequences of acute schizophrenics." *European Psychiatry* 13(Supplement 4): 197s–198s.

Lehmann, D., P. L. Faber, et al. (2001). "Brain sources of EEG gamma frequency during

266    *Feeling Good*

volitionally meditation-induced, altered states of consciousness, and experience of the self." *Psychiatry Research* 108: 111–121.

Lehmann, D., P. Grass, et al. (1995). "Spontaneous conscious covert cognition states and brain electric spectral states in canonical correlations." *International Journal of Psychophysiology* 19: 41–52.

Lehmann, D. and T. Koenig (1997). "Spatio-temporal dynamics of alpha brain electric fields and cognitive modes." *International Journal of Psychophysiology* 26: 99–112.

Lehmann, D., C. M. Michel, et al. (1994). "Event-related potential maps depend on pre-stimulus brain electric microstate map." *International Journal of Neuroscience* 74: 239–248.

Lehmann, D., W. K. Strik, et al. (1998). "Brain electric microstates and momentary conscious mind states as building blocks of spontaneous thinking: I. Visual imagery and abstract thoughts." *International Journal of Psychophysiology* 29.

Lief, A., Ed. (1948). *The commonsense psychiatry of Dr. Adolf Meyer: Fifty-two selected papers edited, with biographical narrative.* New York, McGraw-Hill Book Company.

Loevinger, J. (1976). *Ego development.* San Francisco, Jossey-Bass.

Lou, H. C., T. W. Kjaer, et al. (1999). "A $^{15}$O-H$_2$O PET study of meditation and the resting state of normal consciousness." *Human Brain Mapping* 7: 98–105.

Luborsky, L. (1989). *Principles of psychoanalytic psychotherapy: A manual for supportive-expressive treatment.* New York, Basic Books.

Luhrmann, T. M. (2001). *Of two minds: An anthropologist looks at American psychiatry.* New York, WW Norton.

Lutz, A., J.-P. Lachaux, et al. (2002). "Guiding the study of brain dynamics by using first-person data: Synchrony patterns correlate with ongoing conscious states during a simple visual task." *Proceedings of the National Academy of Sciences USA* 99: 1586–1591.

Maharishi, M. Y. (1976). *Creating an ideal society: A global undertaking.* Rheinweiler, West Germany, MERU Press.

Mesulam, M. (1990). "Large-scale neurocognitive networks and distributed processing of attention, language and memory." *Annals of Neurology* 28: 597–613.

Michels, R. (1999). "Looking back: The history of psychiatry in the 21st century." *Archives of General Psychiatry* 56: 1153–1154.

Newberg, A., A. Alavi, et al. (2001). "The measurement of regional cerebral blood flow during the complex cognitive task of meditation: A preliminary SPECT study." *Psychiatry Research* 106: 113–122.

Newell, A. (1992). "Precis of unified theories of cognition." *Behavior and Brain Sciences* 15: 425–492.

Petsche, H., K. Lindner, et al. (1988). "The EEG—An adequate method to concretize brain processes elicited by music." *Music Perception* 6: 133–159.

Popper, K. R. (1934). *The logic of scientific discovery.* London, Hutchinson.

Raichle, M. E. and D. A. Gusnard (2002). "Appraising the brain's energy budget." *Proceedings of the National Academy of Sciences USA* 99: 10237–10239.

Raichle, M. E., A. M. MacLeod, et al. (2001). "A default mode of brain function." *Proceedings of the National Academy of Sciences USA* 98: 676–682.

Rauscher, F. H., G. L. Shaw, et al. (1993). "Music and spatial task performance." *Nature* 365: 611.

Ray, W. J. and H. W. Cole (1985). "EEG alpha activity reflects attentional demands, and beta activity reflects emotional and cognitive processes." *Science* 228: 750–752.

Robinson, D. L. (2000). "The technical, neurological, and psychological significance of alpha, delta, and theta waves confounded in EEG evoked potentials: A study of peak amplitudes." *Personality and Individual Differences* 28: 673–693.

Salinas, E. and T. J. Sejnowski (2001). "Correlated neuronal activity and the flow of neural information." *Nature Reviews Neuroscience* 2: 539–550.

Sapolsky, R. M. (2003). "Gene therapy for psychiatric disorders." *American Journal of Psychiatry* 160: 208–220.

Thompson, W. F., E. G. Schellenberg, et al. (2001). "Arousal, mood, and the Mozart effect." *Psychological Science* 12: 248–251.

Twomey, A. and A. Esgate (2002). "The Mozart effect may only be demonstrable in nonmusicians." *Perceptual and Motor Skills* 95: 1013–1026.

Urbach, P. (1974). "Progress and degeneration in the IQ debate." *British Journal of Philosophy of Science* 25: 99–135, 235–259.

Vaillant, G. E. (1993). *The wisdom of the ego*. Cambridge, Massachusetts, Harvard University Press.

Vaillant, G. E. and E. Milofsky (1980). "Natural history of male psychological health: IX. Empirical evidence for Erikson's model of the life cycle." *American Journal of Psychiatry* 137: 1348–1359.

Wallace, R. K. (1970). "Physiological effects of transcendental meditation." *Science* 167: 1751–1754.

Wallace, R. K. and H. Benson (1972). "The physiology of meditation." *Scientific American* 226: 84–90.

Wilson, M. (1993). "DSM-III and the transformation of psychiatry: A history." *American Journal of Psychiatry* 150: 399–410.

# 7

# THE EPIGENETIC REVOLUTION

## THE SIGNIFICANCE FOR PSYCHOBIOLOGY

At the beginning of the twentieth century, the field of physics was shocked by the recognition of quantum phenomena. Many familiar notions of classic physics had to be abandoned after the discovery of discrete units of energy and the related quantum phenomena of nonlocality and noncausality (Gamow 1966). Now at the beginning of the twenty-first century, the broad field of biology is being shocked by the recognition of the importance of epigenetic phenomena. Epigenetics has been brought to the forefront of attention in biology in the twenty-first century as a result of sequencing the genomes of human beings and more than thirty other organisms (Koonin, Aravind et al. 2000). As a result, "epigenetics" and the "genomic revolution" have become frequent buzzwords (Koonin, Aravind et al. 2000; Lederberg 2001), but their awesome significance is less often appreciated.

Epigenetics is the study of the mechanisms regulating the expression of genes in living organisms (Lewin 1998; Shapiro 1999; Von Sternberg 2002). One of the most surprising findings about the human genome is that less than 5% of the DNA sequences actually code for proteins (Bernardi 1995; Von Sternberg 2000; Makalowski 2001). The same is true of most eukaryotic organisms, such as plants and animals. Most of the eukaryotic genome is comprised of repetitive elements, which neo-Darwinists had long dismissed as "junk DNA." However, there is rapidly accumulating evidence that repetitive elements have important epigenetic roles that influence development, inheritance, and possibly evolution (Shapiro 1999; Chiaromonte, Yang et al. 2001; Von Sternberg 2002).

The "genomic revolution" is particularly crucial for psychological medicine because of the complex regulation of psychological phenomena, such as brain microstates and the related development of personality and psychopathology (Darvasi 2003; Dennis 2003). In fact, what we have observed in prior chapters about personality development holds important clues for understanding the epigenetic processes at the foundation of the development, inheritance, and evolution of complex biopsychosocial processes in general, as we will see in this chapter. The synchronous development of human thought and brain microstates described in Chapter 6 is an example of the transient connections that occur among changing sets of different elements in a complex adaptive system as it organizes itself in response to its environment. In other words, the brain is a complex adaptive system that is composed of cells that are highly differentiated (i.e., specialized) for learning and memory.

Of course, nearly all the cells of the body become specialized to form different organs during development, which begins with undifferentiated stem cells produced by the fertilized egg. Hence, all the cells of an individual normally have the same genome. Nevertheless, the cells become specialized by differential expression of genes through complex adaptive processes. The self-organization of different configurations of specialized cells is called *epigenesis* or *ontogeny*. *Ontogeny* or *epigenesis* refers to the entire process of self-organized development of an organism from the undifferentiated stem cells produced by the fertilized egg.

Genetic factors play an important role in development, interacting with one another and with environmental influences during epigenesis. A wide variety of regulatory processes within the cell influence the expression of genes, including qualitative changes in what is expressed and quantitative changes in the rate and amount of expression. As a result of differences in prior environmental events that induce quasi-stable regulatory states, specialized cells can be in different functional states even though they have the same genome and similar environmental conditions. These alternative quasi-stable functional states are called "epigenetic states" (Rakyan, Preis et al. 2001; Jablonka and Lamb 2002; Thieffry and Sanchez 2002).

Different epigenetic states of cellular tissue are distinguished by distinct patterns of expression of genes, as measured by expression arrays of transcribed messenger RNA or proteins (Enard, Khaitovich et al. 2002; Draghici, Khatri et al. 2003). Changes in epigenetic states are discrete events in which successive quasi-stable states are punctuated by brief periods of rapid change. Qualitative shifts in observed expression patterns indicate a discontinuous change in epigenetic states.

Changes between epigenetic states are adaptive in the sense that they are non-linear self-organizing responses of complex dynamic systems (Zerba, Ferrell et al.

2000). Epigenetic states provide a mechanism of adaptation that can be relatively stable but also rapidly acquired or reversed (Lewin 1998), like short- or moderate-term memory (Cunliffe 2003). In contrast, the transcriptome (i.e., the set of classic genes or DNA sequences that are transcribed to messenger RNA) is more stable, like long-term memories (Von Sternberg 2000). However, like genetic factors, epigenetic changes can be inherited because they involve changes in chromatin and other cytoskeletal structures that can be transmitted from one generation to the next in sperm and egg cells.

In other words, epigenetics suggests that some acquired characteristics can be inherited, but this remains highly controversial. The inheritance of acquired characteristics from one generation to the next is certainly not a frequent event in practice. However, the empirically documented phenomena of epigenetics are forcing all fields of biology to reexamine the oversimplified assumptions of classic Mendelian inheritance that were developed before the advent of molecular biology. The dualistic distinction of classical physics between cause and effect was shown by quantum physics to be an approximation that does not apply well under certain conditions. Likewise, the dualistic distinction of classic Mendelian inheritance between genotype and phenotype is an approximation that does not account well for the development, inheritance, or evolution of complex dynamic phenotypes, such as human personality and other aspects of mental health. *Evolution is partly a creatively adaptive process, not only the result of chance and random drift as assumed in neo-Darwinian models.*

It is crucial for students of mental health to understand the nature of "epigenetic states" because brain microstates are changing connections between a succession of neurons that are in different epigenetic states. Changes in the functional activity of a neuron depend on changes in the regulation of a wide variety of processes that modify gene expression within the neuron (i.e., which modify the epigenetic state of the neuron). Hence, the self-organization of brain microstates in personality development corresponds to the changing configuration of epigenetic states in the brain. In fact, the capacity for learning and memory of cells depends on the quasi-stability of epigenetic states.

Most definitions of an epigenetic state require that they be heritable. Then, *epigenetics* is defined as the study of heritable changes in gene expression that occur without a change in DNA sequence (Wolffe and Matzke 1999). Such inheritance is a broad term, however, including mitosis, which is cell duplication within an individual. When discussing epigenetics, it is important to specify the conditions under which acquired epigenetic states may be heritable from one generation to the next, or if that occurs at all. In this chapter, "epigenetics" refers broadly to all the mechanisms that regulate gene expression and does not imply that these regulatory effects are heritable from parent to offspring.

The term *epigenetics* was originally coined in 1940 by Conrad Waddington (1905–1975) to provide a basis for a unified theory of life by integrating the study of genetics and development ("epigenesis"). Waddington had studied embryology before taking up the study of genetics, so he was interested in integrating these approaches (Van Spreybroeck 2002). The interest in epigenetics has increased rapidly because accumulating data about the regulation of gene expression have revealed the inadequacies of both Mendelian and Lamarckian models of development, inheritance, and evolution, particularly for complex biopsychosocial systems relevant to mental health.


## EARLY THEORIES OF DEVELOPMENT AND EVOLUTION


### The paradigms of Lamarck and Mendel

The two early theories of evolution developed by Lamarck and Mendel are two extreme paradigms, neither of which is adequate to explain the complex behaviors that are influenced by human thought. Neither genetic nor environmental factors alone can account for the complex patterns observed in most aspects of growth and development (Stewart 1998). Nevertheless, it is useful to specify the assumptions of these paradigms and to examine the conditions for which they are adequate to delineate them from the vast range of conditions in which a nonreductive theory of life is needed.

Mendel described the effects of selection on single genes that had such strong and simple effects on the phenotypes he observed that the effects of other genes and environmental influences could be neglected. Such genes were assumed to be discrete units that caused the appearance of the phenotype, with no need to consider regulatory activity of other genetic or environmental factors in development. The inheritance of phenotypes that follow simple Mendelian patterns may involve either qualitative effects (like a color or pattern) or quantitative effects (like height).

Mendel's results were rediscovered at the beginning of the twentieth century. Ronald Fisher was the first to show that quantitative phenotypes could be explained according to basic Mendelian principles (Fisher 1918). In the simplest situation with a quantitative phenotype, the effects of pairs of genes at each locus can be summed up, that is, they are additive. For example, consider the situation where there are two alternative forms of the gene at a locus and one of these is active (an "active allele") but the other is inactive (a "null allele"). Then the grade of the phenotype will depend only on whether a person has zero, one, or two copies of the active allele. If there are two or more loci that make independent contributions to the grade of the phenotype, then we can measure the phenotype by simply counting the number of active alleles at all the loci. Such additive effects of alleles at multiple loci are also described as linear. Genetic models that assume genes are separate units permit simple counting methods. Such counting methods are sometimes called "bean-bag genetics" (Crow 2001).

The basic assumptions of classic Mendelian inheritance define the "central dogma" in neo-Darwinism theories of inheritance and evolution (Lenski and Mittler 1993; Crow 2001; Von Sternberg 2002). According to neo-Darwinism, DNA sequences define the genotype, which is the active, antecedent cause of the phenotype. Genes are discrete units that act and evolve in an independent manner at the DNA level. According to neo-Darwinism, other cellular structures, including the chromatin matrix of chromosomes, are passive and do not influence the development of the phenotype.

In contrast, interactions with the environment that influence gene expression or interactions between the two alleles (e.g., dominance or recessive inheritance) are deviations from linearity. However, such nonlinearity can often be easily accommodated (Morton 1982; Crow 2001). Linear forms of cultural inheritance can also be easily accommodated (Cloninger, Rice et al. 1979; Rao, Morton et al. 1979). The neo-Darwinian model of inheritance is not wrong, just as the Newtonian model of classic physics is not wrong. Both theories are simply approximations that apply only under limited conditions. It is important, therefore, to know when their simplifying assumptions are adequate and when they are inadequate. The main requirement for neo-Darwinian models is that epigenetic inheritance must be negligible, such as when only one gene influences the phenotype to a major degree. A corollary of this major requirement is the assumption that genes that code for proteins operate and evolve as discrete units, rather than being assembled by complex epigenetic processes.

However, the Cartesian-Mendelian assumptions of neo-Darwinism are frequently inadequate. The comparison of the genomes of different eukaryotic animals has shown that genes that code for proteins do not evolve as a unit. Rather, proteins are composed of multiple domains coded by segments of DNA called *exons*, which are assembled epigenetically and frequently evolve independently (Koonin, Aravind et al. 2000). Exons are segments of single-copy DNA separated by nontranscribed segments of DNA called *introns*. Introns are composed of highly repetitive DNA sequences, which are discussed further later.

In Mendelian models of inheritance, evolution depends on the rate of mutation and stochastic drift of the frequencies of alleles in the population. *Stochastic drift* refers to random fluctuations that occur in samples of finite size, such as small isolates like the population of a valley or island. Natural selection is the process whereby some genes increase in their frequency over time because the organisms that carry those genes reproduce more frequently than do others. If only one gene determines the phenotype, then epigenetic inheritance is negligible. When epigenetic inheritance is negligible, characteristics that are acquired by environmental manipulations ("phenocopies") are not inherited. Hence, self-awareness and purposeful adaptation to the environment are irrelevant to evolution of phenotypes determined by a single Mendelian gene or the additive effects of many such genes.

On the other hand, zoologists like Lamarck initially favored models of inheritance by acquisition of adaptations resulting from the "sustained use of any organ" (Lamarck 1809, page 113). The hypothesis of acquired inheritance was supported by many observations that organisms were well adapted to the changing opportunities provided by their environment. In the simplest conditions, plants and animals appeared to adapt in a linear (dose dependent) manner to environmental pressures. For example, if the supply of nutrients in region was poor, plants and animals adapted by becoming more efficient, thereby maintaining functions near to the optimum observed in other regions where the resources were rich. Plants and animals that were reared under conditions of excellent care taking did not do well if relocated to conditions of poor care taking. Some extreme advocates of Lamarckian models, such as Lysenko in Russia, assumed that the characteristics acquired by an organism under extreme conditions could be inherited by subsequent generations. Such assumptions were appealing to political theorists in Russia, who hoped that people would soon adapt to the demands of a communist life style. Such purely environmental approaches to acquired inheritance were practical failures.

## Neo-Darwinian approaches to complex phenotypes

A unified theory of life recognizes the inseparable influence of both genetic and environmental factors—that is, the indissoluble interaction of nature and nurture. Genetic and environmental factors influence all phenotypes, including those with simple Mendelian patterns of inheritance. It is necessary to define what is meant by a complex phenotype for which simple Mendelian models of inheritance are inadequate.

A *complex phenotype* can be defined as one in which the physical or behavioral characteristics of an organism are influenced by combinations of more than one gene and the environment. Empirically, it is found that most common diseases and quantitative traits are complex phenotypes by this definition and that the interactions among multiple genetic and environmental factors are generally nonlinear (Wright 1968, 1977; Falconer and Mackay 1996; Sing, Haviland et al. 1996). Sewall Wright, one of the founders of population genetics, established that inheritance nearly always involved nonlinear interactions among multiple genetic and environmental factors. Wright described the principles of "universal gene–gene interaction" (i.e., epistasis) and "universal gene–environment interaction." These principles have recently been dramatically confirmed in gene-targeting studies in which one particular gene is "knocked-out" in an animal. The phenotype that occurs when a gene is knocked-out can differ greatly depending on the genetic background, the environmental context, and other compensatory mechanisms (Gerlai 2001; Hoffman 2003).

The principles of universal gene–gene and gene–environment interactions mean that development is a nonlinear sequence of transitory causal interactions between changing sets of genes and environmental variables. Consequently, development is a succession of relatively stable states punctuated by periods of rapid change. The pattern of development of organisms as a complex adaptive system is similar in form to the pattern of development of thought as a succession of brain microstates, as discussed in Chapter 6.

The statistical methods for description of complex adaptive systems in general were first developed by Wright to describe what he called the "shifting balance" theory of evolution (1977). Wright viewed evolution as a succession of relatively stable states, separated by periods of instability and change, rather than changing gradually by the addition of small effects of individual genes. Wright described changes in the distribution of adaptive fitness of an organism across time and space as variation in the "fitness landscape." Epigenetic landscapes were visualized with hills and valleys, which corresponded to increases and decreases in reproductive fitness. Reproductive fitness is measured by an organism's success in producing offspring: "any advantage which certain individuals have over others of the same sex and species solely in respect of reproduction"(Darwin 1874). Wright proposed that the fitness of an organism depended on changes in the combinations of many genetic and environmental variables. When the interactions among many genetic and environmental are not linear, there is a "rugged" or bumpy landscape because specific combinations of variables differ greatly in fitness from similar or partial combinations. If the relations are linear, then the fitness landscape is flat or just sloping at a constant angle. In other words, evolution is gradual when the effects of individual genes are additive, as in the classic Mendelian model of evolution described by Ronald Fisher. In contrast, Wright observed in his breeding experiments that fitness landscapes were nearly always rugged because of prominent gene–gene and gene–environment interactions during development. Subsequent research has supported Wright's theory of "punctuated equilibrium."

Conrad Waddington first suggested the idea of fitness landscapes, which he called "epigenetic landscapes," based on his research in both embryological development and genetics (Waddington 1940; Stern 2000). Waddington and Wright had worked extensively on both development of individual organisms and the evolution of populations. Both Waddington and Wright concluded that separate genetic and environmental models could not provide an adequate account of the development of individual organisms or of the evolution of populations of organisms. However, their early work on "epigenetic landscapes" still maintained orthodox neo-Darwinian assumptions, which excluded the possibility of adaptive mutations and other epigenetic phenomena that are recognized as possible today. Nevertheless, it is useful to recognize that some acquired characteristics can be inherited even within a neo-Darwinian paradigm under some conditions.

The inheritance of acquired characteristics

According to Waddington,

> Naturalists cannot fail to be continually and deeply impressed by the adaptation of an organism to its surroundings and of the parts of the organism to each other. These adaptive characters are inherited and some explanation of this must be provided. If we are deprived of the hypothesis of the inheritance of the effects of use and disuse, we seem thrown back on an exclusive reliance on the natural selection of merely chance mutations. It is doubtful, however, whether even the most statistically minded geneticists are entirely satisfied that nothing more is involved than the sorting out of random mutations by the natural selective filter. (1942, page 563)

Waddington cited well-documented examples of acquired inheritance, such as the thickening of the soles of the feet of the human embryo, which even Darwin had attributed "to the inherited effects of pressure." Consequently, Waddington proposed that developmental reactions were coordinated by the interaction of multiple genetic and environmental factors "so as to bring about one definite end-result regardless of minor variations in conditions during the course of the reaction." Waddington called this buffering of development "canalization," thereby likening development to commitment to a particular path, channel, or canal, as described by Chomsky for the development of language (see Chapter 5). The canalization of development is also called "stabilizing selection." Essentially, development can follow any one of several paths, but usually there are inherited constraints that favor an intermediate optimum and select against extreme deviations from it (Waddington 1942; Falconer and Mackay 1996). Waddington proposed that some environmental triggers may activate genes that switch on a particular developmental process or modify the way development is usually buffered by multiple interacting genetic and environmental factors. Excessive or deficient reactivity to such environmental triggers would be disadvantageous, so intermediate phenotypes were usually favored.

Later Waddington demonstrated this process experimentally (1953). He used heat shock to induce an abnormality on the wings of fruit flies. The chosen abnormality did not occur spontaneously in his initial sample of fruit flies without heat shock. After several generations of selection of flies with abnormal wings following heat shock, he produced lines of selected flies that usually produced the abnormality spontaneously. This was interpreted at the time as evidence that heat shock had uncovered genes that were present initially. Heat shock is also one way that is now known to produce adaptive mutations and other epigenetic phenomena, as subsequently described by Barbara McClintock (1978, 1984). In any case, the abnormal wings developed spontaneously and were heritable after selection on treated flies, whereas initially the abnormal wings had not occurred spontaneously at all. Such selection experiments may be difficult to reproduce consistently but do illustrate the possible role of complex gene–environment interaction in development.

Epigenetic development increases in its importance along with the complexity of the adaptive system. As a dynamic system increases in its complexity, that is, in the number of its interactions or connections, it remains stable up to a critical level and then suddenly becomes unstable (Gardner and Ashby 1970; May 1972). For example, the human brain has a large number of connections among its billions of neurons, so epigenetic constraints are important to maintain its stability. Hence, epigenetic interactions play a greater role in humans than in other animals and a greater role in the development of the human brain than in the development of other human organs (Benno 1990; Rakic 1995).

The human genome does not contain sufficient information to specify the structure and connectivity of the mature human brain, which depends on a complex nonlinear succession of epigenetic developments (Stewart 1998). Complex organs like the human brain develop as self-organizing adaptive systems by means of a succession of quasi-stable stages, which Waddington called "competencies." These competencies of development are modified in a discontinuous way by a series that Waddington called "evocations," which induce the next step. Development is generally nonlinear because differentiation can be reversed to an earlier stage, as is now done in cloning by epigenetic reprogramming (Reik and Dean 2002).

In quantitative genetic modeling, epigenetic effects such as Waddington described for the induction of a phenotype by an environmental stress are described as modifications of the threshold for expression of a complex "multifactorial" phenotype (Falconer and Mackay 1996). Such threshold effects are frequent for many common disorders, including personality disorders and other psychopathology (Cloninger, Reich et al. 1975; Reich, Cloninger et al. 1975). The regulation of the developmental mechanisms involved in such multifactorial disorders has been studied in detail for a variety of complex disorders. Examples range from cleft lip and palate in animals using context-dependent selective breeding (Fraser 1980) to human coronary artery disease using context-dependent molecular genetic analysis (Sing, Zerba et al. 1994; Zerba, Ferrell et al. 1996; Turner, Boerwinkle et al. 1999). Quantitative genetic research on the breeding of plants and animals showed that the inheritance of such "regulatory genes" differed in pattern from that of "structural genes," which code for proteins (Fritsch and Fritsch 1998). Specifically, the inheritance of regulatory systems involves nonlinear interactions of multiple genetic and environmental factors, which are characteristic of heritable systems under stabilizing selection (Wright 1977; Sing, Zerba et al. 1994; Falconer and Mackay 1996; Sing, Haviland et al. 1996; Zerba, Ferrell et al. 2000). In other words, epigenetic inheritance is distinguished from inheritance of structural proteins by the prominence of gene–gene interactions ("epistasis") and gene–environment interactions in development. The exact mechanisms underlying the inheritance of epigenetic processes have been identified through molecular biology.

## EPIGENETIC MECHANISMS OF MOLECULAR MEMORY

The human genome is comprised of two copies of twenty-third chromosomes, containing about 3.1 billion base pairs of DNA altogether. About 95% of the genome is comprised of repetitive DNA sequences, and the remainder is single-copy DNA sequences containing about 31,000 protein-encoding genes (Cooper 1999; Baltimore 2001). The repetitive DNA sequences in chromosomes include a variety of types of elements, including mostly satellites of various classes (macrosatellites, minisatellites, and microsatellites) and transposable elements of various classes (transposons, retrotransposons, and retroposons). Each transposable element can contain several regulatory sequences, such as nuclear matrix attachment sites, promoters, enhancers, silencers, RNA splicing sites, recombination sites, origins of chromosomal replication, and sometimes protein-encoding sequences (Von Sternberg 2000). The various sequence classes can differ in the types of regulatory elements that they carry. Hence the genome includes not only the information needed to encode proteins but also the more extensive information needed to regulate expression of that information.

Furthermore, human chromosomes contain DNA in a highly coiled and condensed matrix called *chromatin* (Cooper 1999; Cunliffe 2003). The chromatin must be uncoiled to activate the transcription of DNA to messenger RNA, which in turn is translated into protein. The unfolding of chromatin to reveal active transcription sites is a strongly regulated multistep process. Enzyme activity depends on the three-dimensional configurations of the molecules, which ultimately is what controls the succession of developmental events.

The heritable long-term memory of the cell (the helical DNA molecule) is coiled and uncoiled in three reversible stages. To form chromatin, DNA is first packaged in a highly coiled and condensed fashion in a matrix of proteins contained in structures called *nucleosomes*. The matrix structure is comprised of slightly basic proteins called histones. Chains of nucleosomes make up a 10-nanometer fiber, which is then coiled in the second stage to form a 30-nanometer fiber. Third, there is further coiling to form chromatin (Cooper 1999; Cunliffe 2003).

Likewise, the uncoiling process involves three stages that are each needed to initiate transcription to messenger RNA. The first stage of uncoiling involves the unfolding of large chromosomal compartments or domains involving from 25 to 100 kilobases of DNA. The compartmentalization of DNA is regulated by a complex adaptive system of repetitive elements (Federoff 1999; Wolffe and Matzke 1999), as discussed in the next section. Second, there is a remodeling of the chromatin structure in gene regulatory regions. The higher-order structure, composition, and accessibility of chromatin are remodeled in a strict and dynamic fashion by another epigenetic system directed at the modification of the histone matrix (Wolffe and Matzke 1999; Cunliffe 2003). Third, there are further alterations of nucleosome structure in targeted regions to provide an activated template for transcription (Cooper 1999; Wolffe and Matzke 1999). Unfolding reveals binding sites on the chromosomal DNA for activator proteins. The binding of activator proteins alters the position of nucleosomes for binding of other activator proteins.

Hence, the uncoiled chromatin provides an accessible template for the initiation of transcription. Just as three specific neural networks regulate attention in the brain in synchrony with thoughts in self-aware consciousness, so three specific epigenetic networks regulate the three-dimensional configuration of DNA to control its accessibility for transcription in the cells.

Waddington likened the complex circumstances of DNA to the role played by a telephone directory in a person's social life: "you can't do anything much without it, but having it, you need a lot of other things—telephones, wires, and so on—as well," as cited by Cooper (1999). The chromosomes function within the context of individual cells, which in turn function within the context of the individual organism. The individual organisms function within the context of society. The function and evolution of the genome are strongly dependent on its biopsychosocial context (Sing, Zerba et al. 1994; Roy, Sing et al. 1995; Zerba, Ferrell et al. 1996; Turner, Boerwinkle et al. 1999; Lussier-Cacan, Bolduc et al. 2002).

As an example of the context dependence of gene expression, consider the effects of the apolipoprotein epsilon (ApoE) genotype on risk of common human diseases, such as dementia of the Alzheimer type (DAT) and on cardiovascular disease when other lifestyle variables like drinking, smoking, and obesity are taken into account. ApoE is encoded by a gene on chromosome 19 with different alleles that are associated with different risk for DAT and cardiovascular disease. It is a protein produced by glial cells that has multiple functions in multiple organ systems. According to animal and in vitro studies, the functions of ApoE include brain amyloid deposition and clearance, brain microtubule stability, intracellular signaling, immune modulation, glucose metabolism, oxidative stress, and other cellular processes. These different effects of ApoE result in its complex associations with different diseases and response to cellular insult in ways that remain unclear (Saunders 2000). The gene for ApoE has three common alleles, designated *epsilon2* (*E2*), *epsilon3* (*E3*), and *epsilon4* (*E4*). About half of individuals who get DAT after sixty-five years of age carry the *E4* allele of ApoE because it increases the formation of amyloid plaques in the brain. The *E4* allele increases the risk of late-onset sporadic DAT in a dose-dependent manner, and it is also correlated with earlier age of onset in familial forms of Alzheimer's dementia. In contrast the *ApoE2* allele has a protective effect, decreasing the risk of DAT and increasing its age of onset (Saunders 2000; Wang, Kwon et al. 2000). The ApoE genotype interacts with other unknown genes on chromosomes 9, 10, 12, and 20 to influence the risk of DAT (Warwick, Payami et al. 2000; Myers, Wavrant De-Vrieze et al. 2002; Olson, Goddard et al. 2002). Also, genes for amyloid precursor protein on chromosome 21, presenilin 1 on chromosome 14, and presenilin 2 on chromosome 1 have a major influence the risk of DAT (Olson, Goddard et al. 2002). Furthermore, the *E4* allele impairs functional recovery following a variety of brain insults (Saunders 2000). For example, the risk of DAT in individuals who carry the *E4* allele is much greater in those with a history of severe head injury with loss of consciousness than expected by the sum of the independent effects of *E4* and head injury.

Gene–environmental interactions with ApoE have been even more extensively studied in relation to its effects on cardiovascular disease. Hyperlipidemia, smoking, and obesity are associated with greater risks of cardiovascular disease on average, whereas moderate alcohol intake is associated with lower risk on average. However, these average effects depend on complex interactions among several genetic and environmental factors. For example, moderate alcohol intake is associated with lower total cholesterol levels among men regardless of their ApoE genotype or smoking status. However, among women with the ApoE E4/3 genotype, the beneficial lowering of cholesterol levels by moderate alcohol intake did not occur if the woman was also a smoker (Lussier-Cacan, Bolduc et al. 2002). Furthermore, the influence of differences in ApoE genotypes on expressed plasma apoE levels depend to a large degree on the age of the person, exerting their greatest influence on the differences in plasma ApoE levels between younger and middle-aged individuals (Zerba, Ferrell et al. 1996). The pattern of correlation among expressed plasma levels of cholesterol, triglyceride, ApoE, and apolipoprotein B varied qualitatively with age, gender, and ApoE genotypes (Zerba, Ferrell et al. 2000). Consequently, gene expression must be considered within a developmental context defined by complex interactions with many demographic and lifestyle variables.

Alternative epigenetic states are created by discrete events that generate heritable differences in DNA structure and function (Lewin 1998). Epigenetic processes regulate the expression of genes during development, and may sometimes induce heritable changes that influence evolution by the preservation of information about prior adaptive experience. The cells of the body learn and remember from experience, but these memories are not usually transmitted to the next generation because the germ line (i.e., sperm and eggs) is highly protected from epigenetic changes.

What events do generate differences in gene expression that are heritable during development? The major epigenetic regulatory mechanisms that are heritable are DNA methylation, acetylation of histone in chromatin, and conformational effects on transcription caused by the relocation of transposable elements induced by discrete environmental events (Lewin 1998; Cooper 1999; Von Sternberg 2002; Cunliffe 2003; Darvasi 2003). These three processes are the outstanding features of three complex adaptive systems that regulate each of the three phases of uncoiling of the three-dimensional structure of the DNA–chromatin complex.

### The DNA methylation system

The most direct way to modify access to the DNA code is to modify the constituents of the four-letter code for proteins, which uses configurations of adenine (A), thymine (T), guanine (G), and cytosine (C) nucleotides to store information. In eukaryotic development, the most frequent form of DNA modification is the methylation of cytosine, particularly in the palindromic sequence of cytosine-guanine (CpG). A palindrome reads the same backwards as it does forward, like the word "noon" or the sentence "Live not on evil." The CpG palindrome is usually methylated in mammalian tissues to modify the ease with which it is read (Cooper 1999). In humans, methylation has important roles in gene regulation by silencing target sequences and in imprinting. Unmethylated islands of CpG are often located in gene promoters near the coding sequence.

The effects of DNA methylation during parental imprinting are essential for normal mammalian development, serving to modify the expression of alleles derived from the mother from those derived from the father. Mammalian embryos created from one individual do not develop normally because one and only one allele should be active at certain loci for normal development. A common function of imprinted genes is the control of embryonic growth with paternally expressed genes tending to enhance growth rates and maternally expressed genes reducing them.

Methylation usually inactivates the target sequence, but it also makes it labile to mutation because methylcytosine tends to deaminate to form thymidine, which is not excised by DNA repair mechanisms. Consequently, the increased methylation of DNA in early vertebrates appears to have played a role in the increased number of genes that have evolved in higher vertebrates in comparison to invertebrates. There is extensive methylation of cytosine in vertebrates beginning with jawless fish, but little or no methylation in insects and other invertebrates (Cooper 1999, pages 26–29). The transition from little to extensive methylation appears to have occurred close to the origin of the vertebrates because the vertebrate pattern appears abruptly in jawless fish and not in any invertebrates. The increased number of genes in vertebrates involved the exuberant multiplication of regulatory genes compared with that of structural genes, which are highly conserved (Fritzsch and Fritsch 1998). The increased number of regulatory genes in early vertebrates compared with invertebrates like insects allowed the emergence of increased flexibility in the regulation of gene expression (Fritzsch and Fritsch 1998).

## The chromatin remodeling system

Human chromosomes contain DNA in a highly coiled and condensed form in chains of histone-containing packages coiled into higher-order structures to form chromatin. In essence, 2 meters of DNA are packaged in a dense form within the small space of the cell nucleus. The higher-order structure of chromatin is remodeled during development to control access of transcription factors to target genes. In other words, DNA is stored in dense knots that must be untied to initiate transcription. The remodeling of chromatin depends on a complex series of bio-chemical mechanisms (Cooper 1999; Cunliffe 2003).

The differentiation of cells reflects the gradual process of chromosome remodeling, which is dynamically regulated during development. The inactivation of chromatin causes silencing of transcription, as in the inactivation of the X chromosome in mammals. Once cells differentiate, cellular memory mechanisms involving developmental regulatory proteins maintain cells in a stable epigenetic state. For example, the mammalian *trithorax* gene, *Mll*, is a component of memory for cellular differentiation. It is frequently mutated in leukemias that are characterized by an expanded pool of uncommitted cells with potential to differentiate in many ways (Cunliffe 2003).

Epigenetic modification of chromatin often involves the acetylation or methylation of histones under the control of cellular memory proteins, such as trithorax proteins. The target of these quasi-stable (covalent) modifications are the lysine residues in the amino-terminal, unstructured tails of core histones (Cunliffe 2003). The acetylation of histone leads to activation, whereas methylation leads to inactivation of chromatin. The methylation of different lysine residues generates binding sites for different proteins in mammals, suggesting a code to store the cellular memories needed to guide transcription (Turner 2002). Furthermore, the acetylation of histone is coordinated with the suppression of DNA methylation. Hence, acetylation and methylation of chromatin are an integral part of the epigenetic mechanisms of cellular memory.

The description and interpretation of the histone code for cellular memory is currently growing rapidly, as reviewed in detail elsewhere (Turner 2002). The two meters of DNA are packaged compactly in the cell nucleus by coiling DNA around an octamer of core histones. The information for unravelling the coils is contained primarily in the amino-terminal tails of the four core histones. The tails are exposed on the nucleosome surface, which makes them accessible to a variety of enzyme-catalyzed modifications of selected amino acids that occur after the DNA has been transcribed into an RNA message and the RNA message has been translated into protein (Turner 2002). These "post-translational" modifications influence both the structure and the function of the nucleosomes in a precise spatial and temporal order. The spatiotemporal order specifies a chemical code that defines the epigenetic state of the DNA-histone complex. These modifications influence a complex adaptive cascade of interactions with various structural proteins and RNAs, whose end result is a functionally stable chromatin state that is self-perpetuating and heritable. In this way histone modification is one of the three parts of the heritable epigenetic code (Turner 2002).

## Nucleoprotein compartmentalization

The structure and function of DNA can be modified by the transposition of repetitive elements, thereby modifying the nucleoprotein compartments or domains that are packaged together as well as silencing and activating different segments of the DNA-histone complex (Federoff 1999; Wolffe and Matzke 1999). Changes in compartmentalization modify what genes are expressed and at what rate they are expressed. Mobile or transposable DNA elements contain repetitive DNA sequences along with many regulatory sequences, as noted earlier. A common feature of repetitive sequences is that they have high local concentrations of many protein-binding sites for regulatory factors. The resulting aggregation of many similar nucleoprotein complexes can establish a compartment or domain within the nucleus, thereby altering chromatin configurations in a way that is self-perpetuating and heritable (Wolffe and Matzke 1999; Turner 2002).

There are regional differences in the tolerance of the genome for transpositions because the stability of different DNA regions decreases in proportion to the amount of repetitive DNA or transposable elements (Chiaromonte, Yang et al. 2001). Transposable elements move adaptively in response to cellular conditions, thereby reorganizing patterns of gene expression. Barbara McClintock was among the first to document that transposable elements are mobilized during periods of "genomic shock" or cellular stress, such as irradiation, infection, heat shock, starvation, chemical stress, or *in vitro* culturing (McClintock 1978, 1984). The transposition induces adaptive changes in the epigenetic state of the cell, particularly remodeling the modular organization of the genome. Consequently, transposition events can also facilitate chromosomal rearrangements that further alter the epigenetic state (Federoff 1999).

Such adaptive transpositions can occur in both somatic cells and in the germ line, so the effects are heritable (Federoff 1999; Von Sternberg 2000, 2002; Chiaromonte, Yang et al. 2001). In turn, mobile elements are themselves regulated by the cell by means of DNA methylation and silencing by preferential transposition to inactive chromatin. Hence, mobile elements are one part of an integrated epigenetic system by which cells self-organize their epigenetic state through a succession of discrete quasi-stable adaptations to changes in their environment.

## THE INHERITANCE OF EPIGENETIC EFFECTS

### Mechanisms of inheritance

The three basic mechanisms mediating the inheritance of epigenetic effects at the DNA level during cell duplication are depicted in Figure 7.1. Cell duplication is a life-long process that is essential to provide new cells for growth and for replacement of worn-out cells. One cell duplicates itself, giving rise to two identical daughter cells, each containing the same number and kind of chromosomes as the mother cell. Each chromosome in the cell is made up of two chromatids, one derived from each parent. Early during cell duplication, each chromatid is replicated

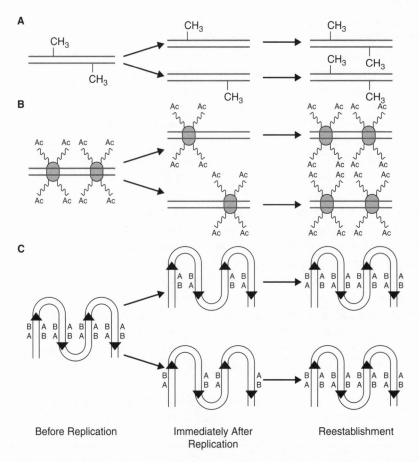

Figure 7.1. Mechanisms of epigenetic inheritance. (Reprinted with permission from Wolffe and Matzke, *Science* 286: 481–486, copyright 1999, American Association for the Advancement of Science.)

to form pairs of identical chromatids. The identical chromatids are pulled to opposite ends of the cell to separate them before cell division. Finally, the cytoplasm of the mother cell divides to form two identical daughter cells, each a reproduction of the original one. The stability of a person's genome throughout their life depends on these basic steps of cell duplication.

Normal mechanisms also allow adaptations that are acquired during epigenesis to be duplicated, so that differentiated cells can maintain their specialized functions. The first mechanism that permits epigenetic inheritance is DNA methylation, as shown in row A of Figure 7.1. When CpG dinucleotides are symmetrically methylated (step 1, before replication), one methyl cytosine will segregate to each daughter chromatid (step 2, immediately after replication). Then each daughter chromatid is rapidly remethylated (step 3, reestablishment) because the enzymes needed to carry out methylation are normally present in mammalian cells to maintain the methylated status of DNA (Wolffe and Matzke 1999).

Another mechanism of epigenetic inheritance is chromatin acetylation, as shown in row B of Figure 7.1. Immature chromatin is normally in an actively acetylated state (step 1), and the associated enzymes needed to carry out acetylation are transferred to the daughter chromatids during replication (step 2). Then the daughter chromatids are rapidly acetylated (step 3), thereby reproducing the parental epigenetic state.

The third mechanism of epigenetic inheritance is compartmentalization of the nucleoplasm by repetitive elements, as shown in row C of Figure 7.1. The presence of repetitive elements is associated with high concentrations of regulatory proteins, as mentioned earlier (step 1). The repetitive elements facilitate the sequestration of free regulatory factors from the nucleoplasm onto both daughter chromatids after replication (step 2). Then the sequestered regulatory factors can reestablish the original epigenetic state (step 3) and maintain it following cell division.

In addition, epigenetic inheritance can sometimes occur from parent to offspring (Federoff 1999; Wolffe and Matzke 1999; Von Sternberg 2002), as in imprinting and paramutation. Paramutation involves an allele at one chromosomal locus altering the activity of an allele at another locus in a way that persists after the two alleles segregate to offspring. This interdependence of segregation is a violation of Mendel's first law. Imprinting and paramutation effects have been demonstrated in susceptibility to human diabetes mellitus (Bennett, Wilson et al. 1997; Moore, Abu-Amero et al. 2001). Such complex epigenetic interactions are exceptions to the patterns of genetic and epigenetic effects that are usually observed. The principles of ordinary Mendelian inheritance are the usual rule, and deviations from them are exceptions. The exceptions are important to understand, particularly when considering complex psychobiological systems.

## The person as a hierarchy of systems

The significance of epigenetic mechanisms for molecular memory is that the whole organism is comprised of a self-organizing hierarchy of systems of learning and memory. At every level of organization (cell, organ, body, society, and cosmos) each system is self-organizing within its context, which in turn defines the next level of organized complexity. Early neo-Darwinian ideas about body function were based on unfounded narratives about cause and effect, which were misleading.

*At every level, the units of life learn and remember, and this intelligence is coordinated as a hierarchy of complex adaptive systems.* Long-term lifestyle choices about diet, exercise, drinking, smoking, and recreation bring about adaptive changes that lead to modification of our epigenetic states, brain microstates, ego states, and overall well-being. For example, starvation and obesity are not just transient modulatory states but involve different quasi-stable changes in the epigenetic state of body tissues, leading to susceptibility to different spectra of diseases and their complications (Turner, Boerwinkle et al. 1999; Lussier-Cacan, Bolduc et al. 2002). Even given the same genome, human monozygotic twins or cloned animals do not have the same succession of experiences. As a result, monozygotic twins do not have the same functional epigenetic states and may differ at every level of the biopsychosocial system (Dennis 2003).

In humans and other vertebrates, the germ line (producing sperm or ova) is distinct from other somatic cells. This differentiation is a mechanism for stabilizing what is inherited so that changes in all parts of the body are not transmitted to the next generation (Koonin, Aravind et al. 2000). Epigenetic states can nevertheless be inherited by offspring and are likely to have a role in adaptive evolution (Federoff 1999; Wolffe and Matzke 1999; Von Sternberg 2002). For example, eukaryotic genomes have expanded in size during evolution through increases in gene number and the accumulation of repetitive sequences, many of which consist of transposable elements (Wolffe and Matzke 1999). The adaptive evolution of epigenetic mechanisms for regulating gene expression may explain the fact that the complexity of life has co-evolved with mechanisms for increasing self-organization and self-awareness.

## COMPARATIVE GENOMICS AND EVOLUTION

Separate genetic or environmental models are inadequate to account for human development or human evolution. Human development involves a transitory succession of quasi-stable configurations of changing genetic and environmental variables. Likewise, evolution involves a succession of quasi-stable configurations punctuated by rapid jumps to a new configuration of genetic and environmental variables. Hence, the well-documented phenomenon of "punctuated equilibria" is the dynamic mechanism by which the development of individuals and the evolution of populations of individuals proceed by a succession of discontinuous jumps on different time scales (Lande 1985; Newman, Cohen et al. 1985; Sneppen, Bak et al. 1995). Furthermore, the punctuated equilibria of complex adaptive systems correspond to the formal dynamics of punctuated equilibria in quantum systems (Hanggi, Talkner et al. 1990).

For example, the dynamic patterns of ontogeny and phylogeny resemble the empirically observed patterns of development of personality and brain microstates. Each of these patterns depends on a complex nonlinear adaptive system (Svrakic, Svrakic et al. 1996; Cloninger, Svrakic et al. 1997). The greater the complexity of the system, the greater is the role of epigenetic development.

A highly complex adaptive system like the human genome clearly has tremendous potential to differentiate in many different ways, as demonstrated in the different organs of the body. What is the nature of the process or processes by which different members of the same species in natural populations resemble one another as much as they do? Why are people so much alike that they can reproduce together, share a more-or-less common culture, and enjoy many of the same activities despite the vicissitudes of development?

The neo-Darwinian view was that genes were active in development and gradually adapted to changes by natural selection on chance mutation and drift. Consequently, the greater the evolutionary distance between two species, the greater the divergence expected at the level of DNA. Neo-Darwinists expected the evolutionary path to be a fairly linear branching tree of life.

Now the epigenetic revolution has forced us to recognize the importance of self-organization in systems that have complex adaptive mechanisms of short- and long-term molecular memory. The rejection of entirely random genetic variation as the substrate of evolution is not a refutation of the theory of natural selection of Darwin but rather a deepening of our understanding (Caporale 1999). The contextual nature of all adaptation at every level in the hierarchy of life implies that the development of each individual organism corresponds generally to the prior evolution of species upon which it builds.

The importance of context-dependent learning in epigenetics has been partially captured in a few memorable phrases. For example, evolution favors the "prepared genome" (Caporale 1999). "Genomes may evolve stereotyped mechanisms to overcome predictable challenges (such as host/pathogen battles), but most challenges are not so predictable. The ability to adapt and evolve can be viewed as a skill, which a genome learns as it moves through time and generations" (Caporale 1999, page 2).

Furthermore, the succession of developmental events in each individual parallels the succession of steps in evolution. In Ernst Haeckel's famous phrase, "ontogeny recapitulates phylogeny." In other words, the contextual nature of epigenetics implies that there is a global path of evolution in which the spiral path of self-aware consciousness is the uniquely human part, and the epigenetic-genetic regulation of cellular memories is the common physical part. That is, a human being on the path of self-aware consciousness is "evolution conscious of itself" (Huxley 1959).

Essentially, the development of life before self-aware consciousness is the early part of development and evolution. In other words, the development and evolution of "instinct" (i.e., prepared skill learning with no self-awareness) represent the early part of the spiral path of consciousness, which involves consciousness below the DFT level of 2.0. The hierarchy of the major evolutionary steps in the development of learning and consciousness in vertebrates is summarized in Table 3.1 (see Chapter 3). Both Sewall Wright (1964) and J. B. S. Haldane (1932), two of the three founders of population genetics, recognized that consciousness at a rudimentary level was an irreducible aspect of all life, although they lacked the scientific tools to demonstrate this aspect of their insight in a testable manner. Now epigenetic research allows us to observe the evolution of specific molecular mechanisms of learning and memory. We can compare the human genome with those of other animals.

Advances in comparative genomics allow us to test the alternative neo-Darwinian and epigenetic views of evolution. Comparative genomics is the comparison of the genomes of different groups of organisms. Comparison of RNA sequences have shown that all life forms can be divided into three primary domains that are very different from one another: eukaryotes (including all animals, plants, fungi, and protists), bacteria, and archaea (i.e., methane-producing microbes that live at extreme temperatures). The genomes of more than thirty species of animals have been sequenced (Koonin, Aravind et al. 2000). Data comparing different animal species are highly incomplete and rapidly accumulating, but initial observations are already highly informative.

Comparisons of the genomes of chimpanzees (*Pan troglodytes*) and modern humans (*Homo sapiens*) are of special interest because chimpanzees are the nearest relatives of human beings but do not have self-aware consciousness (Povinelli 2000). The self-aware consciousness of modern human beings provides a capacity for creativity and integrated intelligence, which has given rise to uniquely human developments in art, science, and spirituality (Mithen 1996). The lineage of modern humans is estimated to have diverged from that leading to Neandertals approximately 0.6 million years ago (Krings, Stone et al. 1997) and from that leading to modern chimpanzees approximately six million years ago (Zhang, Webb et al. 2002). Despite this period of divergence, in early studies of DNA and expressed proteins, King and Wilson found that the average human protein was more than 99% identical to its chimpanzee counterpart (1975). Similarly, the coarse DNA hybridization methods of the time showed that the average nucleotide sequence was almost as similar (98.5%). These findings of genetic similarity raised the question of what made these two species so different in distinguishing modern human features, such as bipedalism, a large brain, language, and self-awareness (Gagneux and Varki 2001; Carroll 2003). King and Wilson suggested the "regulatory hypothesis" that the differences were largely explained by epigenetic differences in the expression of genes, rather than different repertoires of structural genes that code for proteins. Subsequent studies using improved DNA sequencing methods have shown that the average divergence due to base substitution is 1.4% including both repetitive and single-copy DNA, which is only slightly higher than the 1.25% observed in single-copy DNA coding for proteins. There is an additional 3.4% difference due to the presence of insertions and deletions (Britten 2002). However, the sequence divergence in a few DNA regions was in excess of 20%. The regions showing larger divergences involved those known to have higher rates of mutation, such as the palindromic sequence CpG and Alu repetitive elements (Britten 2002). These findings suggest that the biopsychosocial differences between chimpanzees and human beings were caused by a small number of genes or by epigenetic differences in the regulation of gene expression, or both.

Further comparative genomic studies at the Max Planck Institutes in Germany have shown that the differences between chimps and humans depend primarily on the epigenetic state of the brain (Enard, Khaitovich et al. 2002). Wolfgang Enard, Svante Paabo, and their colleagues compared the gene and protein expression profiles of humans, chimpanzees, orangutans (*Pongo pygmaeus*), and rhesus macaques (*Macaca mulatta*). Detailed genomic comparisons with Neandertals and other early humans are limited because fossil DNA is often highly degraded and unlikely to be well preserved beyond 100,000 years (Krings, Stone et al. 1997; Hawks and Wolpoff 2000). Hence the genomes of modern species carry the only available living memories of extinct ancestors. For a further comparison, Paabo and his colleagues studied two mouse species (*Mus musculus* and *Mus spretus*) that have diverged from each other approximately as much as have humans and the great apes. They obtained tissue from the livers and gray matter from the left prefrontal lobes (Brodmann area 9) of three humans, three adult male chimpanzee, and one adult male orangutan that had died of natural causes. In a second experiment, they assayed the extent of expression changes in the brains, blood, and liver of humans, chimpanzees, and macaques.

As expected, the results showed that humans were virtually identical to chimps in gene expression in blood and liver. In contrast, human beings differed quantitatively in the rates of expression in the brain when compared to chimps, and in comparison to the differences between the two species of mouse. The results of the brain protein pattern differences are summarized in Table 7.1. The average divergence in qualitative electrophoretic properties of brain proteins between humans and chimps was the same (7.6%) as that observed between two species of mouse, which shows that the rodent pairs had diverged from each other approximately as much as humans and the chimps. Nevertheless, the rate of gene expression in the left prefrontal cortex of humans is 31.4% greater than that of chimps.

**Table 7.1.** Brain Protein Pattern Differences between Humans and Chimpanzees as Analyzed by Two-Dimensional Gel Electrophoresis

| Comparison | Differences in Row (%) | | |
|---|---|---|---|
| | *Analyzed Spots* | *Qualitative* | *Quantitative* |
| Human–chimp | 538 | 7.6 | 31.4* |
| Mm–Ms | 8767 | 7.6 | 7.5 |

*There is a larger rate of expression of qualitatively similar proteins in the brains of humans than in chimps, or in the differences observed in two mouse species: *Mus musculus* (Mm) or *Mus spretus* (Ms).

Qualitative differences represent changes in electrophoretic mobility of spots, which likely result from amino acid substitutions, whereas quantitative differences reflect changes in the amount of protein.

*Source*: Adapted from Enard et al., 2002.

Similarly, comparison of the relative rates of expression of RNA in the prefrontal cortex of humans was 5.5-fold greater than observed in the chimps, whereas the relative rates of expressed RNA were nearly identical in the blood and liver of chimps. Enard and colleagues (2002) concluded epigenetic changes in protein and gene expression are especially prominent in human brain when compared to chimps and other apes.

The specific epigenetic factor or factors that explain the differences in bio-psychosocial development between primate species still has just begun (Gibbons 1998; Gagneux and Varki 2001; Zhang, Webb et al. 2002; Carroll 2003). A comparative human-chimpanzee clone map is being constructed (Fujiyama, Watanabe et al. 2002). It is necessary to compare the genomes of human beings to the genomes of a broad array of other vertebrates to recognize what makes the human genome unique. Partial comparisons have already been carried out for several vertebrate species by targeting cloned segments of genomes that include a conserved protein-coding sequence. The targeted conserved sequences that correspond to one another in different species are called "orthologs." That is, comparisons can be made across species on specific segments that correspond to one another because they have been conserved during evolution. Such conservation during evolution despite natural selection implies that the sequences are likely to be functionally adaptive (Carroll 2003). When this is done, many of the conserved non-coding sequences have been introns, which suggests that these and other repetitive elements are important in the regulation of gene expression.

Comparative genomic analyses show that the epigenetics of brain systems distinguishes human beings from other vertebrates, including the great apes, who have substantial capacity for cultural inheritance (DeWaal 1999; Whiten, Goodall et al. 1999; Van Schaik, Ancrenaz et al. 2003; Vogel 2003) but not self-aware consciousness (Povinelli 2000). Genetic studies of the inheritance of human personality and related brain processes have also begun to clarify the mechanisms that make modern human consciousness possible (Ding, Chi et al. 2002). Molecular genetic studies of personality and related brain processes provide a direct way of studying the epigenetics of human self-aware consciousness to determine the way differences in gene expression influence information processing in the brain along with the development of personality.

## THE EPIGENETICS OF PERSONALITY

The personality dimensions relevant to the regulation of gene expression in the brain are likely to be interactive with one another because of the nonlinear nature of complex adaptive systems (Cloninger 2000). Accordingly, the Temperament and Character Inventory (TCI) was developed as a set of scales measuring specific psychological constructs. No effort was made to select or combine items in such a way as to give the appearance that the relations between the dimensions were linear or functionally independent, as is often done in tests derived by factor analytic methods. The correlation coefficients observed among the TCI personality dimensions in a sample from the general community are summarized in Table 7.2. Each of the seven dimensions can be described as unique because most of the correlation coefficients among dimensions are negligible (less than .25) and none are strong (greater than .70). Nevertheless, each dimension has a correlation with at least one other dimension, and these vary in magnitude from weak (.25–39) to moderate (.40–59). The observed network of relationships summarized in Table 7.2 allowed accurate prediction of the nonlinear pattern of personality development that we observe in prospective longitudinal studies of 593 individuals in sample representative of general community (Cloninger, Svrakic et al. 1997). The predictability of the spiral form of personality development from the observed correlations indicates that the interrelationships among personality traits reflect the regulatory processes underlying development. In longitudinal studies of 233 boys, we were also able to predict adolescent social maturity and adult psychopathology, such as the risk of alcohol dependence, from independent ratings of temperament at age eleven years (Sigvardsson, Bohman et al. 1987; Cloninger, Sigvardsson et al. 1988). The predictability of adult development is moderate, consistent with the degree of heritability. These observations supported our hypothesis from adoption studies that personality traits are measures of the epigenetic mechanisms underlying vulnerability to mental disorders like substance dependence. At the time, we described epigenetic factors as "neurogenetic adaptive mechanisms" because susceptibility to mental disorders were supposed to involve the genetic regulation of adaptive

**Table 7.2.** Correlations Among the Seven Dimensions of Personality Measured by the Temperament and Character Inventory in a Sample Representative of the General Community of St. Louis

|      | HA     | NS    | RD    | PS    | SD     | CO   |
|------|--------|-------|-------|-------|--------|------|
| HA   | —      | —     | —     | —     | —      | —    |
| NS   | −.08   | —     | —     | —     | —      | —    |
| RD   | −.16   | .08   | —     | —     | —      | —    |
| PS   | **−.25** | −.14  | .03   | —     | —      | —    |
| SD   | **−.47*** | **−.26** | .21   | **.28** | —      | —    |
| CO   | **−.28** | −.10  | **.54*** | .18   | **.57*** | —    |
| ST   | −.08   | .20   | **.28** | .11   | −.10   | .15  |

*Correlations above .25 are indicated in bold, and those above .40, with an asterisk.

HA, Harm Avoidance; NS, Novelty Seeking; RD, Reward Dependence; PS, Persistence; SD, Self-Directedness; CO, Cooperativeness; ST, Self-Transcendence.

*Source*: Adapted from Cloninger et al., 1993.

processes in the brain (Cloninger 1987). Therefore, we carried out further family studies in twins to try to understand more about the genetic and environmental antecedents of personality traits.

Initial twin studies were carried out using only measures of temperament (Heath, Cloninger et al. 1994; Stallings, Hewitt et al. 1996). More recent studies have used the TCI and show that each of the seven TCI dimensions has a unique genetic variance that is not explained by the other dimensions (Gillespie, Cloninger et al. 2003). A sample of 2517 Australian twins aged over fifty between 1993 and 1995 completed the TCI. The correlation between each of the seven dimensions of personality was higher in monozygotic (MZ) twin pairs than in dizygotic (DZ) twin pairs, suggesting significant genetic effects for each dimension. Heritability was derived using a standard multivariate model that is similar to estimating total genetic effects from twice the difference between the correlations of MZ minus DZ twin pairs. For example, for Harm Avoidance the correlations in female MZ twins was .47 and that in female DZ twins was .21, so twice the difference of .26 gives an estimate of 52% heritability. The estimates of heritability for each TCI dimension based on both male and female twins are summarized in Table 7.3. Total genetic effects or heritability varied from 27% to 45%, without correcting for the reliability of the short forms of the TCI used in this study. Each dimension still had significant unique genetic variance when any overlap with other dimensions was taken into account. Both additive genetic and environmental influences that are unique to each individual were significant. Environmental influences shared by twin pairs reared together did not improve the fit of the model to the data, but twin data such as this do not provide sufficient information to evaluate cultural inheritance (Cloninger, Rice et al. 1979), as discussed in Chapter 6.

**Table 7.3.** The Total Genetic Effects (Heritability) of Each of the Seven TCI Personality Dimensions Estimated in 2517 Twins in Australia

|  | Genetic Effects (%) | |
| --- | --- | --- |
| *Personality Dimension* | *Total* | *Unique* |
| Harm Avoidance | 42 | 29 |
| Novelty Seeking | 39 | 32 |
| Reward Dependence | 35 | 20 |
| Persistence | 30 | 23 |
| Self-Directedness | 34 | 25 |
| Cooperativeness | 27 | 16 |
| Self-Transcendence | 45 | 26 |

Unique effects exclude genetic contributions shared with other personality dimensions.

*Source*: Adapted from Gillespie et al. 2003.

These studies of twins did suggest substantial genetic effects on human personality, warranting subsequent molecular genetic studies of linkage and association (Cloninger 1998; Benjamin, Ebstein et al. 2002). Many twin studies suggest heritabilities of about 50% for most complex personality and cognitive traits (Heath, Cloninger et al. 1994). However, these estimates of additive genetic effects are inflated by gene–gene and gene–environmental interactions that have a greater influence on MZ than DZ twins (Cloninger, Rice et al. 1979). In contrast, adoption studies indicate that the heritability of personality is about 20–30% (Loehlin 1992; Cloninger 1998; Plomin, Corley et al. 1998) rather than 50%. The discrepancy between twin and adoption studies suggests that the estimates of heritability in twin studies are inflated by epistasis and gene–environment interactions or that the estimates in adoption studies are reduced by the effects that distinguish the members of two generations, such as age and cohort effects. Either explanation involves nonadditive interactions among multiple genetic and environmental factors. Unfortunately, twin studies have little or no power to test their Mendelian assumptions, such as the assumption that the total genetic effects are additive (Eaves, Eysenck et al. 1989; Plomin, Corley et al. 1998). A practical consequence of these limitations is that the probable nonadditive interactions between genes must be examined directly by measuring specific genetic polymorphisms in molecular genetic studies of linkage and association (Benjamin, Ebstein et al. 2002) and then carrying out studies of gene-environment interaction (Caspi, Sugden et al. 2003; Keltikangas-Jaervinen, Raeikkoenen et al. 2003). There is now substantial direct evidence that personality development depends on the nonlinear effects of gene-gene (Benjamin, Osher et al. 2000; Van Gestel, Forsgren et al. 2002; Strobel, Lesch et al. 2003) and gene-environment (Caspi, Sugden et al. 2003; Keltikangas-Jaervinen, Raeikkoenen et al. 2003) interactions.

The interactions among a few genes that have been extensively studied in relation to personality illustrate the epigenetics of personality and its relationship to psychopathology. Serotonin and dopamine are phylogenetically ancient neurotransmitters that play basic roles in brain function and behavior (Cravchik and Goldman 2000). Extensive diversity in the regulation of serotonin and dopamine function has been studied sufficiently in relation to personality to identify some general epigenetic principles. Some of the genetic polymorphisms that have been studied most extensively are genes that promote, transport, and catabolize these key neurotransmitters. The marked differences in such neurotransmitter functions between individuals is of special interest because they modulate individual differences in personality (Cloninger 1987; Hamer, Greenberg et al. 1999; Ding, Chi et al. 2002; Borg, Andree et al. 2003; Strobel, Lesch et al. 2003).

In the human prefrontal cortex, the enzyme catechol-O-methyltransferase (COMT) is critical in the metabolic degradation of dopamine, and by regulating dopamine availability, it can influence personality and cognitive function. The COMT gene has a common variant (i.e., polymorphism) involving the substitution of valine (Val) by methionine (Met) at position 158. Individuals who are homozygous Met/Met have 4-fold less activity than those with a Val substitution. Individuals with the low activity form of COMT (i.e., Met/Met homozygotes) have been found to have higher scores in TCI Harm Avoidance and to have EEGs with low-voltage alpha activity more frequently than others (Enoch, Xu et al. 2003). The relationship between Harm Avoidance and the COMT polymorphism is shown in Figure 7.2. The association of the low-activity (Met/Met) form of COMT with high Harm Avoidance is also consistent with its association with behavioral disorders. The disorders associated with high Harm Avoidance and low activity of COMT include late onset (type 1) alcoholism (Tiihonen, Hallikainen et al. 1999) and heavy social drinking (Kauhanen, Hallikainen et al. 2000) but not early onset (type 2) alcoholism (Hallikainen, Lachman et al. 2000). Low activity of COMT is also associated with greater sensitivity to chronic pain and anxiety as a result of decreased activation of mu-opioid receptors (Zubieta, Heitzeg et al. 2003). At the other extreme, low childhood Harm Avoidance is predictive of type 2 alcoholism with early onset of antisocial behavior and polysubstance dependence (Cloninger 1987; Cloninger, Sigvardsson et al. 1988).

Individuals with early-onset (type 2) alcoholism with impulsive-aggressive behavior are more likely to be homozygous for the less active short allele of the promoter of the human serotonin transporter (5-HTTLPR) than either type 1 alcoholics or healthy controls (Hallikainen, Saito et al. 1999). The short allele also interacts nonlinearly with stressful life events to increase susceptibility to depression, illustrating the importance of gene–environment interaction (Caspi,

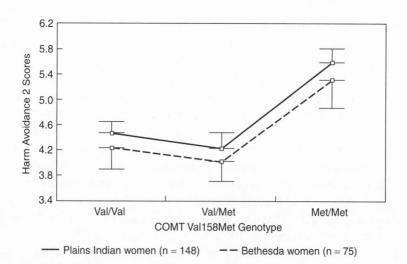

Figure 7.2. The relationship between worry and fearfulness subscales of Harm Avoidance with the COMT Val158Met polymorphism. (Reprinted with permission from Enoch et al., *Psychiatric Genetics* 13: 33–41, copyright 2003, Lippincott Williams & Wilkins.)

Sugden et al. 2003). The short allele has been associated with anxiety-related traits such as neuroticism, which confound high Harm Avoidance with the low Self-Directedness and low Cooperativeness seen in personality disorders. The less active form of the serotonin transporter promoter may be more strongly associated with low TCI Self-Directedness and low TCI Cooperativeness than with the temperament trait of Harm Avoidance (Hamer, Greenberg et al. 1999).

Furthermore, the high activity forms of COMT (Val/Val or Val/Met) have increased dopamine catabolism in the prefrontal cortex, which impairs prefrontal brain physiology, and have been found to slightly increase the risk of schizophrenia (Egan, Goldberg et al. 2001). The relationship of COMT genotype to perseverative errors in the Wisconsin Card Sorting Test, which measures function of the dorsolateral prefrontal cortex, is shown in Figure 7.3. The subjects included 175 patients with schizophrenia, 219 unaffected siblings, and 55 healthy controls. The genotype explained 4% of the variance in perseverative errors, that is, having difficulty switching strategies when an error is made. The relationship was further supported by studies of prefrontal physiology on fMRI during a working memory task and by a family study showing the increased transmission of the Val allele to schizophrenic offspring (Egan, Goldberg et al. 2001).

These results are impressive, but the small proportion of explained variance and the nonadditive effects of the alleles in both Figures 7.2 and 7.3 indicate that interactions with other regulatory factors are important. Such findings about a single gene have often proven to be inconsistently replicable when they are studied by

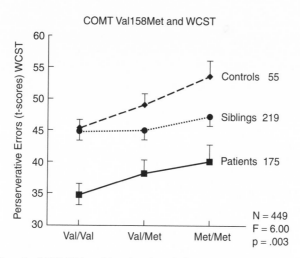

Figure 7.3. Level of COMT in schizophrenics, their sibs, and controls. (Reprinted with permission from Egan et al., *PNAS* 98: 6917–6922, copyright 2001, National Academy of Sciences.)

many independent groups, as has been the case with the association of the DRD4 dopamine receptor and Novelty Seeking (Kluger, Siegfried et al. 2002; Schinka, Letsch et al. 2002).

Such inconsistent results need to be evaluated within the general context of the role of personality dimensions as moderator variables in nonlinear adaptive systems. As a result of their nonlinear function as moderators, the inheritance of personality is expected to involve gene–gene and gene–environment interactions (Kluger, Siegfried et al. 2002; Keltikangas-Jaervinen, Raeikkoenen et al. 2003). For most quantitative traits, individuals with intermediate values are usually adapted better than individuals with extremely high or low values. In contrast, individuals at the each extreme of a quantitative trait are more prone to disorders and are less well adapted than intermediate individuals. For example, type 1 and type 2 alcoholism may be at opposite extremes of the epigenetic regulation of alcohol consumption, with type 1 alcoholics being mature but excessively Harm Avoidant and type 2 alcoholics being immature and excessively Novelty Seeking. Other intermediate personality profiles provide sufficient checks and balances to maintain normative drinking, but both extremes increase susceptibility to problems. Unless the relevant interacting biopsychosocial variables are simultaneously measured, results with individual variables in different samples are expected to be inconsistent despite their validity in some contexts.

For example, Harm Avoidance has been shown clearly to be a nonlinear adaptive process in studies of the modulation of the eyeblink startle reflex. The strength of the human startle reflex varies according to whether the subject is thinking about pleasant or unpleasant stimuli when startled by a sudden, loud noise. The modulation of the eye-blink startle response by Harm Avoidance has been studied by having subjects view a series of slides that are classified as pleasant, unpleasant or neutral, and presenting the loud noise unpredictably during and between slides. Electromyographic measures of the eye-blink response show that pleasant slides reduce and unpleasant slides increase the amplitude of the startle (see Figure 7.4). In addition, TCI Harm Avoidance is a nonlinear moderator of these effects: only subjects high in Harm Avoidance had significantly enhanced startle responses when viewing unpleasant slides, whereas only subjects low in Harm Avoidance showed significantly attenuated startle responses when viewing pleasant slides (Corr, Wilson et al. 1995). This interaction between startle and Harm Avoidance has been replicated in an independent sample (Corr, Kumari et al. 1997).

Furthermore, the prediction of differential susceptibility to affect induction by high and low TCI Harm Avoidance, as well as related measures from other inventories, has also been demonstrated independently (Zelenski and Larsen 1999). When pictures of happy faces are shown to individuals who are low in Harm Avoidance (as indicated by being stable extraverts), there is activation of the region around the left amygdala, uncus, and hippocampus (Canli, Zhao et al. 2001; Canli, Sivers et al. 2002). Happy faces do not activate the amygdala in individu-

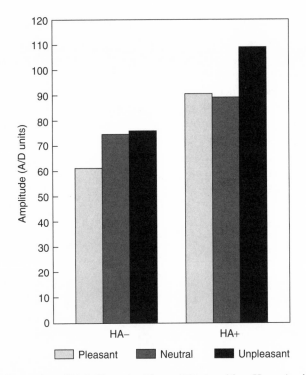

Figure 7.4. Interaction of high Harm Avoidance (HA+) and low Harm Avoidance (HA–) and magnitude of eye-blink startle (Reprinted from Corr et al., Personality and Individual Differences, 19: 543–553, "Personality and affective modulation of the startle reflex," copyright 1995, with permission from Elsevier.)

als who are high in Harm Avoidance. On the other hand, when fearful faces are shown to individuals who are high in Harm Avoidance (as indicated by being neurotic introverts), there is activation of the region around the right amygdala. However, fearful faces do not activate the amygdala in individuals who are low in Harm Avoidance (Canli, Sivers et al. 2002; Hariri, Mattay et al. 2002). In related work, high Harm Avoidance predicted greater magnitude of activation of the right insula following punishment during a task to make decisions about risks (Paulus, Rogalsky et al. 2003).

Similarly, Novelty Seeking is associated with individual differences in exploratory and consummatory behaviors, such as eating disorders and substance dependence. High Novelty Seeking has been associated in many studies with bulimea, early-onset alcoholism, and polysubstance abuse (Cloninger, Przybeck et al. 1994; Howard, Kivlahan et al. 1997). Furthermore, recent findings reveal that Novelty Seeking is associated with susceptibility to initiation of drinking, as shown in recent work by my colleague Rick Grucza. Four stages of ethanol use and problems were distinguished. First, the "uninitiated" individuals were those who had never been drunk and never had any problems from alcohol abuse or dependence. Second, "social" drinkers had a history of heavy drinking or having been drunk, but no problems. Third, "problem" drinkers had at least one indicator for alcohol abuse or dependence according to *DSM-3R* criteria. In the fourth stage of drinking, individuals with alcohol "dependence" satisfied the diagnostic criteria for alcohol dependence according to *DSM-3R*. In Figure 7.5, Novelty Seeking related to the number of alcoholic parents (zero, one, or two) while controlling for personal drinking history. Novelty Seeking increases with the number of alcoholic parents among individuals with alcohol dependence or problem drinking. In contrast, Novelty Seeking decreases with the number of alcoholic parents among individuals who are "uninitiated." Novelty Seeking is unrelated to the number of alcoholic parents among social drinkers.

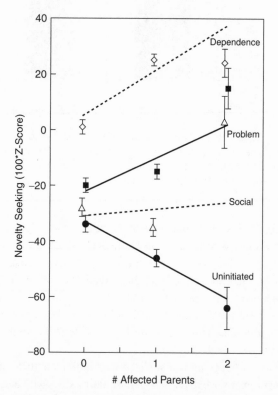

Figure 7.5. Linear regression plots of Novelty Seeking versus number of affected parents for individuals at four stages of alcohol use and dependence. Uninitiated (filled circles), social or recreational drinkers (open triangles), problem drinkers (filled squares), and dependent drinkers (open diamonds). Error bars are ±0.5 standard error and determine the relative weights of each point in estimating the regression line (i.e., the error bar is inversely proportional to the weight). Novelty Seeking is adjusted for age, gender, and education before regression analysis

In addition, the odds ratio (OR) for alcohol problems or dependence to the level of Novelty Seeking does increase along with the number of alcoholic parents, as shown in Figure 7.6. In other words, susceptibility to alcohol abuse and dependence increases in proportion to the level of Novelty Seeking, controlling for the number of alcoholic parents. On the other hand, the likelihood of never getting drunk decreases in proportion to the level of Novelty Seeking, controlling for the number of alcoholic parents. Therefore, being uninitiated in drinking is not simply the absence of alcohol problems. Low Novelty Seeking is associated with a greater likelihood that a person will not be exposed to drinking at all. Social drinking is an intermediate normative pattern of drinking characterized by Novelty Seeking that is neither too high nor too low.

Molecular genetic studies on Novelty Seeking confirm the importance of nonlinear gene–gene and gene–environment interactions in Novelty Seeking. A polymorphism of the dopamine transporter is associated with individual differences in initiating and continuing to smoke cigarettes, an effect which is mediated by the joint association of cigarette smoking and the dopamine transporter with Novelty Seeking (Sabol, Nelson et al. 1999). In addition, the dopamine receptor DRD4 exon 3 seven-repeat allele has been associated with high Novelty Seeking and increased risk of opiate dependence (Kotler, Cohen et al. 1997). Other work has shown that Novelty Seeking is associated with the ten-repeat allele of the dopamine transporter DAT1 when the DRD4 seven-repeat allele is absent (Van Gestel, Forsgren et al. 2002).

Novelty Seeking also depends on the three-way interaction of DRD4 with COMT and the serotonin transporter locus promoter's regulatory region (5-HTTLPR). In

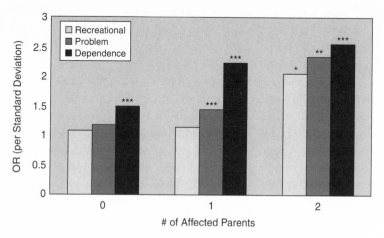

Figure 7.6. Results of multinomial logistic regression analysis illustrating the association between novelty seeking and alcohol use/dependence for each of three levels of familial risk. For each odds ratio plotted, the baseline is the uninitiated group.

the absence of the short 5-HTTLPR allele (5HTTLPR L/L genotype) and in the presence of the high activity COMT Val/Val genotype, Novelty Seeking scores are higher in the presence of the DRD4 seven-repeat allele than its absence (Benjamin, Osher et al. 2000). Furthermore, within families, siblings who shared identical genotype groups for all three polymorphisms (COMT, DRD4 and 5-HTTLPR) had significantly correlated Novelty Seeking scores (intraclass correlation = .39 in 49 subjects, $p < .008$). In contrast, sibs with dissimilar genotypes in at least one polymorphism showed no significant correlation for Novelty Seeking (intraclass coefficient = .18 in 110 subjects, $p = .09$). Similar interactions were also observed between these three polymorphisms and Novelty Seeking in an independent sample of unrelated subjects (Benjamin, Osher et al. 2000) and has been replicated by independent investigators (Strobel, Lesch et al. 2003). A similar three-way interaction has been described for the temperament dimension Persistence with dopamine receptor genes type 4 (D4DR) and type 3 (D3DR), and the serotonin receptor gene type 2c (5-HT2c) (Ebstein, Segman et al. 1997).

Gene–environment interaction has also been demonstrated for TCI Novelty Seeking in prospective population-based studies (Ekelund, Lichtermann et al. 1999; Keltikangas-Jaervinen, Elovainio et al. 2003; Keltikangas-Jaervinen, Raeikkoenen et al. 2003). The Temperament and Character Inventory was administered to two large birth cohorts of Finnish men and women, and the individuals who scored in the top 10% and bottom 10% of TCI Novelty Seeking were genotyped for the exon 3 repeat polymorphism of the type 4 dopamine receptor gene (DRD4). The four-repeat and seven-repeat alleles were most common in the Finnish sample (Ekelund, Lichtermann et al. 1999; Keltikangas-Jaervinen, Elovainio et al. 2003), as is usual throughout the world (Ding, Chi et al. 2002). The two-repeat and five-repeat alleles, which are rare in the Americas and Africa, were more than three times as frequent (16% versus 5%) in Finns who were very high in Novelty Seeking than in those who were very low in Novelty Seeking (Ekelund, Lichtermann et al. 1999), and this difference was confirmed in an independent sample (Keltikangas-Jaervinen, Elovainio et al. 2003). The association with the two-repeat and five-repeat alleles was strongest for the two most adaptive aspects of Novelty Seeking (see Table 3.3), exploratory excitability and impulsive decision making (Keltikangas-Jaervinen, Elovainio et al. 2003). Finnish men and women with the two-repeat and five-repeat alleles of the exon three DRD4 polymorphism were higher in Novelty Seeking as adults if they experience a hostile childhood environment, as measured by maternal reports of emotional distance and a strict authoritarian disciplinary style with physical punishment (Keltikangas-Jaervinen, Raeikkoenen et al. 2003). The effect of a hostile childhood environment on Novelty Seeking was significant for the total Novelty Seeking score and for the spiritual aspect of Novelty Seeking (exploratory excitability) but not for the intellectual aspect of Novelty Seeking (impulsive decision making). The mother's reports of childhood environment were obtained when the children were aged 18 to 21 years, and genotyping and personality assessment of Novelty Seeking was done independently 15 years later. If children had the two-repeat or five-repeat alleles of the DRD4 polymorphism, their TCI Novelty Seeking scores were high if they were reared in a hostile childhood environment and their Novelty Seeking was low if they were reared in a kind and cooperative environment. Children with certain genotypes are likely to evoke a characteristic pattern of responses from their parents and others, and to select for themselves certain aspects from the available environments (Scarr and McCartney 1983). However, therapeutic environments, such as kind and cooperative parenting, can evoke positive adaptation by modifying gene expression, which depends on the orchestrated interaction of many genes and environmental influences (Keltikangas-Jaervinen, Raeikkoenen et al. 2003).

Such complex gene–gene and gene–environmental interactions are well documented for other common diseases, such as coronary artery disease and hypertension (Sing, Haviland et al. 1996; Zerba, Ferrell et al. 2000). For example, a hostile childhood environment is correlated with many variables that are associated with coronary artery disease, such as marital dissatisfaction, type A personality, emotional distance, and a high level of job involvement among fathers (Keltikangas-Jaervinen, Raeikkoenen et al. 2003). The importance of gene–gene and gene–environmental interactions in common diseases and quantitative traits has stimulated work to develop more realistic methods of analysis that go beyond the assumptions of the Cartesian-Mendelian paradigm (Sing, Haviland et al. 1996; Templeton, Weiss et al. 2000; Nelson, Kardia et al. 2001).

What are the consequences of such complex epigenetic effects for brain activity? Fortunately, the relationship between individual differences in Persistence and the activity of related brain networks has been worked out in detail recently (Gusnard, Ollinger et al. 2003). In fMRI studies, blood oxygenation level differences (BOLD) indicate changes in metabolic activity of the region, as described in Chapter 6. Persistence was found to be strongly correlated ($r = .79$) with activation of a well-known circuit for regulation of reward-seeking behavior in a recent fMRI study (Gusnard, Ollinger et al. 2003). The circuit includes the ventral striatum, anterior cingulate Brodmann area 24), and orbitofrontal cortex (Brodmann area 47) bilaterally. Subjects were asked to rate pictures as pleasant, unpleasant, or neutral. As the percentage of neutral pictures in the picture set increased, subjects who were more persistent rated more pictures as pleasant at the expense of neutral picture ($r = .34$, $p < .05$). This selection bias was independent of the percentage of neutral pictures in the sets. There was also a nonlinear interaction between the percentage BOLD change and the percent of neutral pictures. The same distributed neural circuit was up-regulated (i.e., became more metabolically active) when persistent individuals viewed a high percentage of neutral pictures, but it was down-regulated in impersistent individuals when they viewed a high percentage of neutral pictures (see Figure 7.7).

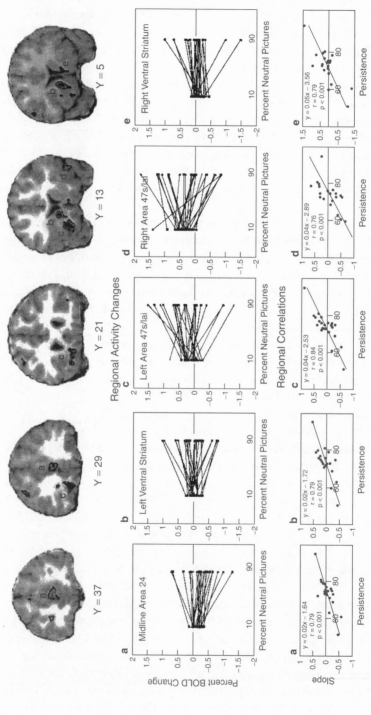

Figure 7.7. Persistence and regional brain activity. (Reprinted with permission from Gusnard et al., *PNAS* 100: 3479–3474, copyright 2003, National Academy of Sciences.)

These findings show that the regulation of gene expression by personality is mediated by nonlinear adaptive systems made up of multiple genetic and environmental factors. Personality is comprised of multiple heritable dimensions comprised of unique but partially overlapping sets of epistatic genes. These epigenetic systems modulate brain states by modifying the transitory connections between changing distributed networks of neurons. The prominence of gene–gene and gene–environmental interactions is characteristic of most common diseases and quantitative phenotypes, which involve intermediate adaptive optima maintained by stabilizing selection.

## EVOLUTION OF CREATIVITY IN MODERN HUMAN BEINGS

Natural selection does not favor intermediate values for all phenotypes, or there would be no vertical evolution. Recent work on the psychobiology and evolution of the DRD4 locus in human beings illustrates how advantageous traits like creativity may have evolved in modern human beings. The DRD4 dopamine receptor gene on chromosome 11p is very rich in GC dinucleotides and is one of the most variable human genes known (Ding, Chi et al. 2002). Most of its diversity is the result of variation in a forty-eight–base pair tandem repeat in exon 3 that encodes the third intracellular loop of the DRD4 dopamine receptor. The number of tandem repeats in this genetic segment has been observed to vary from two to eleven in humans, and the resulting proteins vary from 32 to 176 amino acids at the corresponding position. The frequency of different alleles has been examined in thirty-six different populations around the world (Chang, Kidd et al. 1996). The frequency of the four-repeat allele is 64%, occurring in every population with a range from 16% to 96%. The seven-repeat allele is the second most common, occurring in 20% globally, followed by the two-repeat allele with 8%. Other variants are rare. This polymorphic segment is functionally important because this part of the receptor couples to G proteins and mediates postsynaptic effects of dopamine that modulate attention, emotion, and self-aware behavior (Swanson, Oosterlaan et al. 2000; Ding, Chi et al. 2002; Fossella, Sommer et al. 2002). The presence of the seven-repeat allele has been associated with individual differences in personality measured by TCI Novelty Seeking (Benjamin, Ebstein et al. 2002), TCI Self-Transcendence (Comings, Gade-Andavolu et al. 2000; Comings, Gonzales et al. 2000), and with attention deficit/hyperactivity disorder (ADHD) (Swanson, Oosterlaan et al. 2000). Adults with the seven-repeat allele were more likely to be high in TCI measures of contemplative and spiritual thinking than other adults in one study (Comings, Gonzales et al. 2000). Efficiency of conflict resolution in reaction time experiments has also been associated with DRD4 variants that enhance the activation of the executive attention network, particularly the anterior cingulate (Fan, Fossella et al. 2003). In another study the reactions of hyperactive children with the seven-repeat allele were normal in speed and variability of response, whereas the reactions of hyperactive children without the seven-repeat allele were slow and variable(Swanson, Oosterlaan et al. 2000). Hence the presence of the seven-repeat variant of the DRD4 gene may be useful in distinguishing hyperactive children who are divergent in their thinking because they are gifted or creative from others who have deficits in attention (Hallowell and Ratey 1994; Cramond 1995), but further investigation is needed, particularly in view of the small effect sizes observed and the complexity of traits like self-transcendence that are influenced by multiple other gene products such as the serotonin 5-HT$_{1a}$ receptor (Borg, Andree et al. 2003). Also in different parts of the world, Novelty Seeking is associated with different DRD4 alleles. For example, among Finns the two-repeat and five-repeat alleles, not the seven-repeat allele, are associated with the most adaptive aspect of Novelty Seeking, which is measured by the exploratory subscale (Ekelund, Lichtermann et al. 1999; Keltikangas-Jaervinen, Elovainio et al. 2003).

The frequency of the DRD4 alleles varies widely in different parts of the world. In particular, the seven-repeat allele has an extremely low incidence in Asian populations (2%) and a high frequency in the Americas (48%). The two-repeat allele is most frequent in Asia (18%) and uncommon in Africa (2%) and the Americas (3%). The seven-repeat allele differs greatly in its DNA sequence organization from the common shorter repeats, suggesting it arose as a rare mutation or was imported to modern human beings from a closely related lineage of early humans (Ding, Chi et al. 2002). The relatively high worldwide population frequencies of the four-repeat and seven-repeat alleles suggest that they are over 300,000 years old and arose before the global dispersion of modern humans. Variability within the seven-repeat allele, however, suggests that it arose much more recently, only about 30,000 to 50,000 years ago. The seven-repeat allele of the DRD4 gene appears to have increased to high frequency in many, but not all, modern human populations as a result of positive selection as people migrated outward from Africa (Ding, Chi et al. 2002).

The migration of modern human beings out of Africa has been suggested to account for the spread of art, science, and spirituality throughout the world (Mithen 1996). The DRD4 locus may have an essential role in self-aware consciousness, but it is not yet certain how its associations with creativity and spirituality depend on interactions with other genes. The seven-repeat allele is certainly not needed for self-awareness because Asians and Americans are self-aware and differ greatly in its relative frequency. Rather the variant alleles of the DRD4 locus appear to modulate individual differences in aspects of self-aware consciousness, like creative and contemplative personality traits, which differ in their context-dependent biopsychosocial advantages. The path of evolution is indicated by the positive selection for extreme values of particular traits like contemplative thinking and creative exploration, which will be considered further in the next and final chapter.

## REFERENCES

Baltimore, D. (2001). "Our genome unveiled." *Nature* 409: 814–815.

Benjamin, J., R. P. Ebstein, et al., eds. (2002). *Molecular genetics and the human personality*. Washington, D.C., American Psychiatric Association.

Benjamin, J., Y. Osher, et al. (2000). "Association of tridimensional personality questionnaire (TPQ) traits and three functional polymorphsms: Dopamine receptor D4 (DRD4), serotonn transporter promoter region (5–HTTLPR) and catechol O-methyltransferase (COMT)." *Molecular Psychiatry* 5: 96–100.

Bennett, S. T., A. J. Wilson, et al. (1997). "Insulin VNTR allele-specific effect in type 1 diabetes depends on identity of untransmitted paternal allele." *Nature Genetics* 17: 350–352.

Benno, R. H. (1990). Development of the nervous system: Genetics, epigenetics, and phylogenetics. *Developmental behavior genetics: Neural, biometrical, and evolutionary approaches*. M. E. Hahn, J. K. Hewitt, N. D. Henderson and R. H. Benno, eds. New York, Oxford University Press: 113–143.

Bernardi, G. (1995). "The human genome: Organization and evolutionary history." *Annual Review of Genetics* 29: 445–476.

Borg, J., B. Andree, et al. (2003). "The serotonin system and spiritual experiences." *American Journal of Psychiatry*: 160: 1965–1969.

Britten, R. J. (2002). "Divergence between samples of chimpanzee and human DNA sequence is 5%, counting indels." *Proceedings of the National Academy of Sciences USA* 99: 13633–13635.

Canli, T., H. Sivers, et al. (2002). "Amygdala response to happy faces as a function of extraversion." *Science* 296: 2191.

Canli, T., Z. Zhao, et al. (2001). "An fMRI study of personality influences on brain reactivity to emotional stimuli." *Behavioral Neuroscience* 115: 33–42.

Caporale, L. H. (1999). "Chance favors the prepared genome." *Annals of New York Academy of Science* 870: 1–21.

Carroll, S. B. (2003). "Genetics and the making of Homo sapiens." *Nature* 422: 849–857.

Caspi, A., K. Sugden, et al. (2003). "Influence of life stress on depression: Moderation by a polymorphism in the 5-HTT gene." *Science* 301: 386–389.

Chang, F. M., J. R. Kidd, et al. (1996). "The world-wide distribution of allele frequencies at the human dopamine D4 receptor locus." *Human Genetics* 98: 91–101.

Chiaromonte, F., S. Yang, et al. (2001). "Association between divergence and interspersed repeats in mammalian noncoding genomic DNA." *Proceedings of the National Academy of Sciences USA* 98: 14503–14508.

Cloninger, C. R. (1987). "Neurogenetic adaptive mechanisms in alcoholism." *Science* 236: 410–416.

Cloninger, C. R. (1987). "A systematic method for clinical description and classification of personality variants: A proposal." *Archives of General Psychiatry* 44: 573–587.

Cloninger, C. R. (1998). The genetics and psychobiology of the seven factor model of personality. *The biology of personality disorders*. K. R. Silk, ed. Washington, D.C., American Psychiatric Association: 63–84.

Cloninger, C. R. (2000). "Biology of personality dimensions." *Current Opinions in Psychiatry* 13: 611–616.

Cloninger, C. R., T. R. Przybeck, et al. (1994). *The temperament and character Inventory: A guide to its development and use.* St. Louis, Missouri, Washington University Center for Psychobiology of Personality.

Cloninger, C. R., T. Reich, et al. (1975). "The multifactorial model of disease transmission: II. Sex differences in the familial transmission of sociopathy (antisocial personality)." *British Journal of Psychiatry* 127: 11–22.

Cloninger, C. R., J. Rice, et al. (1979). "Multifactorial inheritance with cultural transmission and assortative mating. II. A general model of combined polygenic and cultural inheritance." *American Journal of Human Genetics* 31: 176–198.

Cloninger, C. R., S. Sigvardsson, et al. (1988). "Childhood personality predicts alcohol abuse in young adults." *Alcoholism: Clinical and Experimental Research* 12: 494–505.

Cloninger, C. R., N. M. Svrakic, et al. (1997). "Role of personality self-organization in development of mental disorder and disorder." *Development and Psychopathology* 9: 881–906.

Comings, D. E., R. Gade-Andavolu, et al. (2000). "A multivariate analysis of 59 candidate genes in personality traits: The Temperament and Character Inventory." *Clinical Genetics* 58: 375–385.

Comings, D. E., N. Gonzales, et al. (2000). "The DRD4 gene and the spiritual transcendence scale of the character temperament index." *Psychiatric Genetics* 10: 185–189.

Cooper, D. N. (1999). *Human gene evolution.* San Diego, California, Academic Press.

Corr, P. J., V. Kumari, et al. (1997). "Harm avoidance and affective modulation of the startle reflex: A replication." *Personality and Individual Differences* 22: 591–593.

Corr, P. J., G. D. Wilson, et al. (1995). "Personality and affective modulation of the startle reflex." *Personality and Individual Differences* 19: 543–553.

Cramond, B. (1995). *The coincidence of attention deficit hyperactivity disorder and creativity.* Storrs, Connecticut, University of Connecticut, The National Research Center on the Gifted and Talented.

Cravchik, A. and D. Goldman (2000). "Neurochemical individuality: Genetic diversity among human dopamine and serotonin receptors and transporters." *Archives of General Psychiatry* 57: 1105–1114.

Crow, J. F. (2001). "The beanbag lives on." *Nature* 409: 771.

Cunliffe, V. T. (2003). "Memory by modification: the influence of chromatin structure on gene expression during vertebrate development." *Gene* 305: 141–150.

Darvasi, A. (2003). "Genomics: Gene expression meets genetics." *Nature* 422: 269–270.

Darwin, C. (1874). *The descent of man and selection in relation to sex.* New York, Merrill and Baker.

Dennis, C. (2003). "Altered states." *Nature* 421: 686–688.

DeWaal, F. B. M. (1999). "Cultural primatology comes of age." *Nature* 399: 635–636.

Ding, Y. C., H. C. Chi, et al. (2002). "Evidence for positive selection acting at the human dopamine receptor D4 gene locus." *Proceedings of the National Academy of Sciences USA* 99: 309–314.

Draghici, S., P. Khatri, et al. (2003). "Global functional profiling of gene expression." *Genomics* 81: 98–104.

Eaves, L. J., H. J. Eysenck, et al. (1989). *Genes, culture, and personality: An empirical approach.* London, Academic Press.

Ebstein, R. P., R. Segman, et al. (1997). "5-HT2c serotonin receptor gene polymorphism assocaited with the human personality trait of reward dependence: Interaction with dopamine D4 receptor (D4DR) and dopamine D3 receptor (D3DR) polymorphisms." *American Journal of Medical Genetics* 74: 65–72.

Egan, M. F., T. E. Goldberg, et al. (2001). "Effect of COMT Val108/158Met genotype on frontal lobe function and risk for schizophrenia." *Proceedings of the National Academy of Sciences USA* 98: 6917–6922.

Ekelund, J., D. Lichtermann, et al. (1999). "Association between novelty seeking and the type 4 dopamine receptor gene in a large Finnish cohort sample." *American Journal of Psychiatry* 156(9): 1453–1455.

Enard, W., P. Khaitovich, et al. (2002). "Intra- and interspecific variation in primate gene expression patterns." *Science* 296: 340–343.

Enoch, M. A., K. Xu, et al. (2003). "Genetic origins of anxiety in women: A role for a functional catechol-O-methyltransferase polymorphism." *Psychiatric Genetics* 13: 33–41.

Falconer, D. S. and T. F. C. Mackay (1996). *Introduction to quantitative genetics.* New York, Prentice Hall.

Fan, J., J. Fossella, et al. (2003). "Mapping the genetic variation of executive attention onto brain activity." *Proceedings of the National Academy of Sciences USA* 100: 4706–7411.

Federoff, N. V. (1999). "Transposable elements as a molecular evolutionary force." *Annals of New York Academy of Science* 870: 251–264.

Fisher, R. A. (1918). "The correlation between relatives on the supposition of Mendelian inheritance." *Transactions of the Royal Society of Edinburgh* 52: 399–433.

Fossella, J., T. Sommer, et al. (2002). "Assessing the molecular genetics of attention networks." *BMC Neuroscience* 3: 14.

Fraser, F. C. (1980). "The William Allan Memorial Award Address: Evolution of a palatable multifactorial threshold model." *American Journal of Human Genetics* 31: 796–813.

Fritzsch, B. and B. Fritsch (1998). "Of mice and genes: Evolution of vertebrate brain development." *Brain, Behavior, and Evolution* 52: 207–217.

Fujiyama, A., H. Watanabe, et al. (2002). "Construction and analysis of a human-chimpanzee comparative clone map." *Science* 295: 131–134.

Gagneux, P. and A. Varki (2001). "Genetic differences between humans and great apes." *Molecular Phylogenetics and Evolution* 18: 2–13.

Gamow, G. (1966). *Thirty years that shook physics: The story of quantum theory.* New York, Dover Publications.

Gardner, M. R. and W. R. Ashby (1970). "Connectance of large dynamic (cybernetic) systems: Critical values for stability." *Nature* 228: 784.

Gerlai, R. (2001). "Gene targeting: technical confounds and potential solutions in behavioral brain research." *Behavior and Brain Research* 125: 13–21.

Gibbons, A. (1998). "Which of our genes makes us human?" *Science* 281: 1432–1436.

Gillespie, N. A., C. R. Cloninger, et al. (2003). "The genetic and environmental relationship between Cloninger's dimensions of temperament and character." *Personality and Individual Differences* 35: 1931–1946.

Gusnard, D. A., J. M. Ollinger, et al. (2003). "Persistence and brain circuitry." *Proceedings of the National Academy of Sciences USA* 100: 3479–3484.

Haldane, J. B. S. (1932). *The inequality of man: Essay on science and ethics.* London, Chatto.

Hallikainen, T., H. Lachman, et al. (2000). "Lack of association between the functional variant of the catechol-O-methyltransferase (COMT) gene and early-onset alcoholism associated with severe antisocial behavior." *American Journal of Medical Genetics* 96: 348–352.

Hallikainen, T., T. Saito, et al. (1999). "Association of low activity serotonin transporter genotype and early onset alcoholism with habitual impulsive violent behavior." *Molecular Psychiatry* 4: 385–388.

Hallowell, E. M. and J. J. Ratey (1994). *Answers to distraction.* New York, Pantheon Books.

Hamer, D. H., B. D. Greenberg, et al. (1999). "Role of the serotonin transporter gene in temperament and character." *Journal of Personality Disorders* 13: 312–327.

Hanggi, P., P. Talkner, et al. (1990). "Reaction-rate theory: Fifty years after Kramers." *Reviews of Modern Physics* 62: 251–332.

Hariri, A. R., V. S. Mattay, et al. (2002). "Serotonin transporter genetic variation and the response of the human amygdala." *Science* 297: 400–403.

Hawks, J. and M. H. Wolpoff (2000). "Paleoanthropology and the population genetics of ancient genes." *American Journal of Physical Anthropology* 114: 269–272.

Heath, A. C., C. R. Cloninger, et al. (1994). "Testing a model for the genetic structure of personality: A comparison of the personality systems of Cloninger and Eysenck." *Journal of Personal and Social Psychology* 66: 762–775.

Hoffman, H. A. (2003). "Functional genomics of neural and behavioral plasticity." *Journal of Neurobiology* 54: 272–282.

Howard, M. O., D. Kivlahan, et al. (1997). "Cloninger's tridimensional theory of personality and psychopathology: Applications to substance use disorders." *Journal of Studies of Alcohol* 58: 48–66.

Huxley, J. (1959). Foreword. *The phenomenon of man.* P. Teilhard de Chardin, ed. New York, Harper & Row: 11–28.

Jablonka, E. and M. J. Lamb (2002). "The changing concept of epigenetics." *Annals of New York Academy of Science* 981: 82–96.

Kauhanen, J., T. Hallikainen, et al. (2000). "Association between functional polymorphism of catechol-O-methyltransferase gene and alcohol consumption among social drinkers." *Alcoholism: Clinical and Experimental Research* 24: 135–139.

Keltikangas-Jaervinen, L., M. Elovainio, et al. (2003). "Association between the type 4 dopamine receptor gene polymorphism and Novelty Seeking." *Psychosomatic Medicine* 65: 471–476.

Keltikangas-Jaervinen, L., K. Raeikkoenen, et al. (2003). "Nature and nurture in novelty seeking." *Molecular Psychiatry* (advance online publication, October 21, 2003): 1–4.

King, M. C. and A. C. Wilson (1975). "Evolution at two levels in humans and chimpanzees." *Science* 188: 107–116.

Kluger, A. N., Z. Siegfried, et al. (2002). "A meta-analysis of the association between DRD4 polymorphism and novelty seeking." *Molecular Psychiatry* 7: 712–717.

Koonin, E. V., L. Aravind, et al. (2000). "The impact of comparative genomics on our understanding of evolution." *Cell* 101: 573–576.

Kotler, M., H. Cohen, et al. (1997). "Excess dopamine D4 receptor (D4DR) exon III seven repeat allele in opioid-dependent subjects." *Molecular Psychiatry* 2: 251–254.

Krings, M., A. Stone, et al. (1997). "Neanderthal DNA sequences and the origin of modern humans." *Cell* 90: 19–30.

Lamarck, J. B. (1809). *The zoological philosophy.* London, MacMillan.

Lande, R. (1985). "Expected time for random genetic drift of a population between stable phenotypic states." *Proceedings of the National Academy of Sciences USA* 82: 7641–7645.

Lederberg, J. (2001). "The meaning of epigenetics." *The Scientist* 15: 6.

Lenski, R. E. and J. E. Mittler (1993). "The directed mutation controversy and Neo-Darwinism." *Science* 259: 188–194.

Lewin, B. (1998). "The mystique of epigenetics." *Cell* 93: 301–303.

Lewin, R. (1998). *Principles of human evolution: A core textbook.* London, Blackwell Science.

Loehlin, J. C. (1992). *Genes and environment in personality development.* Newbury Park, Sage Publications.

Lussier-Cacan, S., A. Bolduc, et al. (2002). "Impact of alcohol intake on measures of lipid metabolism depends on context defined by gender, body mass index, cigarette smoking, and apolipoprotein E genotype." *Arteriosclerosis, Thrombosis and Vascular Biology* 22: 824–831.

Makalowski, W. (2001). "The human genome structure and organization." *Acta Biochimica Polonica* 48: 587–598.

May, R. M. (1972). "Will a large complex system be stable?" *Nature* 238: 413–414.

McClintock, B. (1978). Mechanisms that rapidly reorganize the genome. *The discovery and characterization of transposable elements.* J. A. Moore, ed. New York, Garland: 593–616.

McClintock, B. (1984). "The significance of responses of the genome to challenge." *Science* 226: 792–801.

Mithen, S. (1996). *The prehistory of the mind: The cognitive origins of art, religion, and science.* London, Thames and Hudson, Ltd.

Moore, G. E., S. N. Abu-Amero, et al. (2001). "Evidence that insulin is imprinted in the human yolk sac." *Diabetes* 50: 199–203.

Morton, N. E. (1982). *Outline of genetic epidemiology.* Basel, Karger.

Myers, A., F. Wavrant De-Vrieze, et al. (2002). "Full genome screen for Alzheimer disease: Stage II analysis." *American Journal of Human Genetics* 114: 235–244.

Nelson, M. R., S. L. Kardia, et al. (2001). "A combinatorial partitioning method to identify multilocus genotypic partitions that predict quantitative trait variation." *Genome Research* 11: 458–470.

Newman, C. M., J. E. Cohen, et al. (1985). "Neo-Darwinian evolution implies punctuated equilibria." *Nature* 315: 400–401.

Olson, J. M., K. A. Goddard, et al. (2002). "A second locus for very-late-onset Alzheimer disease: A genome scan reveals linkage to 20p and epistasis with the amyloid precursor protein region." *American Journal of Human Genetics* 71: 154–161.

Paulus, M. P., C. Rogalsky, et al. (2003). "Increased activation in the right insula during risk-taking decision making is related to harm avoidance and neuroticism." *NeuroImage* 19: 1439–1448.

Plomin, R., R. Corley, et al. (1998). "Adoption results for self-reported personality: Evidence for nonadditive genetic effects?" *Journal of Personal and Social Psychology* 75: 211–218.

Povinelli, D. J. (2000). *Folk physics for apes: The chimpanzee's theory of how the world works.* New York, Oxford University Press.

Rakic, P. (1995). "A small step for the cell, a giant leap for mankind: A hypothesis of neocortical expansion during evolution." *Trends in Neuroscience* 18: 383–388.

Rakyan, V. K., J. Preis, et al. (2001). "The marks, mechanisms and memory of epigenetic states in mammals." *Biochemical Journal* 356: 1–10.

Rao, D. C., N. E. Morton, et al. (1979). "Path analysis under generalized assortative mating." *Genetical Research, Cambridge* 33: 175–188.

Reich, T., C. R. Cloninger, et al. (1975). "The multifactorial model of disease transmission: I. Description of the model and its use in psychiatry." *British Journal of Psychiatry* 127: 1–10.

Reik, W. and W. Dean (2002). "Epigenetic reprogramming: Back to the beginning." *Nature* 420: 127–128.

Roy, M., C. F. Sing, et al. (1995). "Impact of a common mutation of the LDL receptor gene, in French-Canadian patients with familial hypercholesterolemia, on means, variances and correlations among traits of lipid metabolism." *Clinical Genetics* 47: 59–67.

Sabol, S. Z., M. L. Nelson, et al. (1999). "A genetic association for cigarette smoking behavior." *Health Psychology* 18: 7–13.

Saunders, A. M. (2000). "Apolipoprotein E and Alzheimer disease: An update on genetic and functional analyses." *Journal of Neuropathology and Experimental Neurology* 59: 751–758.

Schinka, J. A., E. A. Letsch, et al. (2002). "DRD4 and novelty seeking: results of meta-analyses." *American Journal of Medical Genetics* 114: 643–648.

Shapiro, J. A. (1999). "Genome system architecture and natural genetic engineering in evolution." *Annals of New York Academy of Science* 901: 224–236.

Sigvardsson, S., M. Bohman, et al. (1987). "Structure and stability of childhood personality: Prediction of later social adjustment." *Journal of Child Psychology and Psychiatry* 28: 929–946.

Sing, C. F., M. B. Haviland, et al. (1996). "Genetic architecture of common multifactorial diseases." *Ciba Foundation Symposium* 197: 211–229.

Sing, C. F., K. E. Zerba, et al. (1994). "Traversing the biological complexity in the hierarchy between genome and CAD endpoints in the population at large." *Clinical Genetics* 46: 6–14.

Sneppen, K., P. Bak, et al. (1995). "Evolution as a self-organized critical phenomenon." *Proceedings of the National Academy of Sciences USA* 92: 5209–5213.

Stallings, M. C., J. K. Hewitt, et al. (1996). "Genetic and environmental structure of the Tridimensional Personality Questionnaire: Three or four temperament dimensions?" *Journal of Personal and Social Psychology* 70: 127–140.

Stern, C. D. (2000). "Conrad H. Waddington's contributions to avian and mammalian development, 1930–1940." *International Journal of Developmental Biology* 44: 15–23.

Stewart, I. (1998). *Life's other secret: The new mathematics of the living world.* Harmondsworth, England, Penguin Books.

Strobel, A., K. P. Lesch, et al. (2003). "Further evidence for a modulation of novelty seeking by DRD4 exon III, 5-HTTLPR, and COMT Val/Met variants." *Molecular Psychiatry*: 8:371–372.

Svrakic, N. M., D. M. Svrakic, et al. (1996). "A general quantitative theory of personality development: Fundamentals of a self-organizing psychobiological complex." *Development and Psychopathology* 8: 247–272.

Swanson, J. M., J. Oosterlaan, et al. (2000). "Attention deficit/hyperactivity disorder children with a 7–repeat allele of the dopamine receptor D4 gene have extreme behavior but normal performance on critical neuropsychological tests of attention." *Proceedings of the National Academy of Sciences USA* 97: 4754–4759.

Templeton, A. R., K. M. Weiss, et al. (2000). "Cladistic structure within the human lipoprotein lipase gene and its implications for phenotypic association studies." *Genetics* 156: 1259–1275.

Thieffry, D. and L. Sanchez (2002). "Alternative epigenetic states understood in terms of specific regulatory structures." *Annals of New York Academy of Science* 981: 135–153.

Tiihonen, J., T. Hallikainen, et al. (1999). "Association between the functional variant of the catechol-O-methyltransferase (COMT) gene and type 1 alcoholism." *Molecular Psychiatry* 4: 286–289.

Turner, B. M. (2002). "Cellular memory and the histone code." *Cell* 111: 285–291.

Turner, S. T., E. Boerwinkle, et al. (1999). "Context-dependent associations of the ACE I/D polymorphism with blood pressure." *Hypertension* 34: 773–778.

Van Gestel, S., T. Forsgren, et al. (2002). "Epistatic effects of genes from the dopamine and serotonin systems on the temperament traits of novelty seeking and harm avoidance." *Molecular Psychiatry* 7: 448–450.

Van Schaik, C. P., M. Ancrenaz, et al. (2003). "Orangutan cultures and the evolution of material culture." *Science* 299: 102–105.

Van Spreybroeck, L. (2002). "From epigenesis to epigenetics: The case of C. H. Waddington." *Annals of New York Academy of Science* 981: 61–81.

Vogel, G. (2003). "Animal behavior: Orangutans, like chimps, heed the cultural call of the collective." *Science* 299: 27–28.

Von Sternberg, R. (2000). "Genomes and form: the case for teleomorphic recursivity." *Annals of New York Academy of Science* 901: 224–236.

Von Sternberg, R. (2002). "On the roles of repetitive DNA elements in the context of a unified genomic-epigenomic system." *Annals of New York Academy of Science* 981: 154–188.

Waddington, C. H. (1940). *Organizers and genes*. Cambridge, England, Cambridge University Press.

Waddington, C. H. (1942). "Canalization of development and the inheritance of acquired characteristics." *Nature* 150: 563–565.

Waddington, C. H. (1953). "Genetic assimilation of an acquired character." *Evolution* 7: 118–126.

Wang, J. C., J. M. Kwon, et al. (2000). "Effect of APOE genotype and promoter polymorphism on risk of Alzheimer's disease." *Neurology* 55: 1644–1649.

Warwick, D. E., H. Payami, et al. (2000). "The number of trait loci in late-onset Alzheimer disease." *American Journal of Human Genetics* 66: 196–204.

Whiten, A., J. Goodall, et al. (1999). "Culture in chimpanzees." *Nature* 399: 682–685.

Wolffe, A. P. and M. A. Matzke (1999). "Epigenetics: Regulation through repression." *Science* 286: 481–486.

Wright, S. (1964). Biology and the philosophy of science. *Process and divinity: The Hartshorne festschrift*. W. L. Reese and E. Freeman, eds. LaSalle, Illinois, Open Court Publishing Co.: 101–126.

Wright, S. (1968). *Evolution and the genetics of populations: Genetic and biometric foundations*. Chicago, Illinois, University of Chicago Press.

Wright, S. (1977). *Evolution and the genetics of populations: Experimental results and evolutionary deductions*. Chicago, Illinois, University of Chicago Press.

Zelenski, J. M. and R. J. Larsen (1999). "Susceptibility to affect: A comparison of three personality taxonomies." *Journal of Personality* 67: 761–791.

Zerba, K. E., R. E. Ferrell, et al. (1996). "Genotype-environment interaction: Apolipoprotein E (apoE) gene effects and age as an index of time and spatial context in the human." *Genetics* 143: 463–478.

Zerba, K. E., R. E. Ferrell, et al. (2000). "Complex adaptive systems and human health: the influence of common genotypes of the apolipoprotein E (ApoE) gene polymorphism and age on the relational order within a field of lipid metabolism traits." *Human Genetics* 107: 466–476.

Zhang, J., D. M. Webb, et al. (2002). "Accelerated protein evolution and origins of human-specific features: FOXP2 as an example." *Genetics* 162: 1825–1835.

Zubieta, J. K., M. M. Heitzeg, et al. (2003). "COMT val158met genotype affects mu-opioid neurotransmitter responses to a pain stressor." *Science* 299: 1240–1243.

# 8

# THE IRREDUCIBLE TRIAD OF WELL-BEING

## THE HIERARCHY OF LIFE SYSTEMS

### The unity of life

The DNA code was hailed as the key to the secrets of life when its self-replicating structure was recognized (Watson and Crick 1953). DNA is the pervasive mechanism of heritable long-term memory for the cells of all the domains of life discovered on earth, even though pathogenic prion proteins are also self-replicating without nucleic acids. Hence, DNA indicates a pervasive unity and order for all known forms of normal life.

The DNA sequence of the human genome has often been described as the book of life because of the pervasive role of DNA as a genetic code for the structural proteins of the body. Nevertheless, the fact that over 90% of human DNA is not protein encoding means that the DNA protein code is only one part of the description of life (Consortium 2001; Venter, Adams et al. 2001). The histone code for regulation of gene expression is incomplete, and the adaptive regulation of repetitive elements is largely unknown. Moreover, the genome operates within the context of the cell, the cell within the context of the body, the body within the context of the self, the self within the context of society, and society within the context of the cosmos. Hence, the cosmos is encompassed within a universal field, which is nondual, nonlocal, and noncausal in its characteristics. *In other words, all life develops and evolves within a universal unity of being encompassing a nested hierarchy of complex adaptive systems.*

The hierarchical organization of life that we have discovered or uncovered in a step-by-step process in prior chapters is summarized in Table 8.1. The increasing levels of complexity are indicated by the five major transitions from the physics of matter to the biology of cells, from biology to the psychophysiology of organisms, from psychophysiology to social science, from social science to philosophy, and from philosophy to spirituality. The hierarchy is recursive because each level is nested within the succeeding level, which is its context. Matter is most simply described in terms of its physics and chemistry. The physics and chemistry of matter operate within the context of the biology of abundant cellular life, with which matter is in constant flux. Cells develop within the context of the differentiated body with biomorphogenesis of various specialized organs including the brain. In human beings, the brain–body complex develops within the context of the self, which is a mind–body complex. Each individual self develops within the context of society, which in turn develops in a spiritual context. *Hence, the hierarchical organization of life is an ever-expanding upward spiral of complexity within the coherence of the universal unity of being.*

The spiral pattern of growth and development observed in human consciousness is pervasive throughout all of ontogeny and phylogeny, including even plants and ancient sea animals. The spiral is most ubiquitous mathematical form in development of all life forms. The logarithmic spiral is also called the Fibonacci spiral in honor of the mathematician Fibonacci of Pisa. In 1202, Fibonacci described the numerical sequence that is most ubiquitous in growth and development (Stewart 1998). The patterns of development of repetitive elements like leaves, flowers, or seed heads in plants have been extensively studied. The "phyllotaxic" patterns are so regular that a physicist can compare their order with that of crystals (Douady and Couder 1996). All botanical forms can be explained by developmental processes in which there is a succession of discontinuous events producing bifurcations in which new primordial cells are produced where and when there is enough space for their formation (Douady and Couder 1996). The great diversity of whorls and spiral patterns occurring in nature is the result of this succession of discontinuous events. About 90% of all plants exhibit a spiral pattern of leaf arrangement that involves a numerical sequence called the Fibonacci series (1, 2, 3, 5, 8, 13, 21, 34, 55, 89, 144 . . .) in which each successive number beginning with 3 is the sum of the prior two numbers (Cook 1979).

Other rare sequences follow the same iterative principles but begin with different starting numbers. For example, the Lucas series begins with 2 and 1 to give the sequence 2, 1, 3, 4, 7, 11 . . . , so that beginning with 3, both Fibonacci and Lucas numbers are the sum of the prior two numbers in the sequence. These numbers occur in the pattern of arrangement of leaves when we count the number of

**Table 8.1.** Hierarchical Organization and Spiral Development of Being

| Levels of Self-Aware Organization | Levels of the Irreducible Triad* | | | Levels of Context (Phase Space) |
|---|---|---|---|---|
| | Information (1) Light (Nonduality) | Biomorphogenesis (2) Life (Nonlocality) | Coherence (3) Love (Noncausality) | |
| Spirituality | Nondual (universal) order (well-being) | Nonlocal (third stage of) self-awareness (understanding) | Creative states (noncausal freedom) (coherence seeking) | Nonduality (truth/good) (unity of being) |
| Philosophy | Social order | Truth seeking (second stage of self-awareness) | Moral states | Spirit of truth |
| Sociology, psychology | Self (order seeking) | Self-development (first stage of self-awareness) | Ego states | Society |
| Psychophysiology | Brain–body (physical order) | Mental development | Brain states | Self (mind–body complex) |
| Biology, genetics | Cell milieu (cell life) | Epigenesis (biomorphogenesis) | Epigenetic states | Brain–body complex |
| Chemistry, physics | Matter | Movement | Quantum states | Cellular life |

*What is nondual (nonlocal and noncausal) is a whole that cannot be reduced because there is nothing else and no part is adequate to define the whole. There can only be stepwise growth in awareness by exploration of one's context, leading ultimately to awareness of one's fundamental nature.

times we go around the stem, going from leaf to leaf, as well as counting the leaves we meet until we encounter a leaf directly above the starting one. For example, if we make three clockwise rotations around the stem before we meet a leaf directly above the first leaf, meeting five leaves along the way, then there are 3/5 clockwise rotations per leaf. For example, common examples of Fibonacci numbers are 1/2 for elm and linden, 1/3 for beech and hazel, 2/5 for oak and apple, 3/8 for poplar and pear, and 5/13 for pussy willow and almond, where $t/n$ means that there are $t$ turns for $n$ leaves.

Whenever development or speciation is the result of a sequence of discontinuous events causing bifurcations, a Fibonacci series will result (Douady and Couder 1996). The regularities of form indicate that development and evolution are frequently based on discontinuous jumps in which there are bifurcations producing a new form while retaining all the old forms as part of the context or phase space of life. Cellular differentiation is a self-organizing dynamic system, as described in Chapter 7.

Fibonacci spirals and related whorls are also pervasive in the development of all plants (e.g., spirals in seed heads) and animals (e.g., proportions of limbs), as well as in the forms of galaxies throughout the universe. The ratio of successive Fibonacci or Lucas numbers to the one preceding it is called the Golden Ratio, which is approximately 1.618034. Alternatively, the ratio of the smaller to the larger number (that is, 0.6180399 . . .) was called the *golden section* or *divine proportion*. The only way to divide a line so that its parts are in proportion to the whole is by the golden section; then the ratio of the larger part to the whole (i.e., 0.618) is the same as the ratio of the smaller part to the larger part. The golden section is symbolized by the Greek letter Phi in honor of the Greek sculptor Phidias (493–430 BC) who based the entire design of the Parthenon on this proportion. Phidias also used Phi in creating his statue of Athena, which became the symbol of Athens because it beautifully combined the creative wisdom of the psyche and the indomitable strength of the body in just balance. The golden ratio has played a prominent role in figure drawing and aesthetics throughout history because of its frequency of occurrence in normal morphogenesis throughout phylogeny and cosmogenesis. It is prominent in the normal proportions of the human figure, as noted in the works of Phidias, Leonardo da Vinci, and Botticelli (Cook 1979). Even earlier, the Egyptians used the golden ratio in the design of the pyramids.

There is even more fundamental evidence of the unity of being from modern physics. Physics assumes that physical laws are universal, applying uniformly throughout all space and time. For example, the standard model of particle physics depends on the assumption of a universal field from which all things continually arise and to which they return, as described in Chapters 1 and 5. The assumption of the universal unity of being is accepted as an empirical fact because all available information supports its validity. Hence, the assumption of the positive philosophy that there is universal unity to all being (i.e., all that is or can be) is not only plausible but also strongly preferred to all alternative assumptions.

Recognition of the dynamic properties of complex adaptive systems provides an empirically testable alternative to dualistic models. Essentially, the transitions between quasi-stable states involve abrupt transitions between two points of equilibrium in a rugged adaptive landscape. The same formal dynamics occurs in the discrete transitions of quantum states (Hanggi, Talkner et al. 1990), epigenetic states (Lande 1985), personality or ego states (Svrakic, Svrakic et al. 1996), or speciation events during evolution (Newman, Cohen et al. 1985; Sneppen, Bak et al. 1995).

*The science of well-being is founded on the understanding that there is an indissoluble unity to all that is or can be. The universal unity of being is recognized widely as an empirical fact, as well as an essential organizing principle for any adequate science.* The universal unity of being is not an arbitrary philosophical assumption, and it is not an optimistic assumption. Rather the universal unity of being is the only viewpoint consistent with any coherent and testable science. Any coherent science must recognize its interdependent position within the nested hierarchy of adaptive systems within which everything operates. *Psychology, like particle physics, must postulate a universal field in which all aspects of each person are bound together at the same nodal point in space and time.*

## The irreducible triad

The spiral of biomorphogenesis is a three-dimensional form moving flexibly and adaptively within time, as previously described in detail for human self-aware consciousness in Chapter 3. It is not surprising that we observed the effects of three epigenetic systems of cellular development in Chapter 7, three complex adaptive systems of human attention in Chapter 3, and three dynamic systems of psychosocial development of character in Chapters 2 and 6. Likewise philosophy is divided into three basic branches for being, knowledge, and conduct, as described in Chapter 1. More generally, the coordinated effects of three fundamental forces on the level of self-aware organization of life are described in Table 8.1.

First, any complex system must have *order* if it is an aspect of the universal unity of being. Order is defined as the global adaptive optimum, which is the norm-favoring tendency inherent in all complex adaptive systems, as described by Waddington and Wright (see Chapter 7). *Order* can also be defined in terms of the level of information content of a system. The greater the level of information content, the greater is the order of the system. The level of self-aware organization of life increases in proportion to its level of information content in a stepwise manner in the succession of inorganic matter to cellular life, the differentiated brain–body complex, the personal order of the self, the social order, and ultimately the universal order. This progressive increase in level of information content reaches its limit at the level of nonduality, which is designated as the spiritual level in Table 8.1. The level of order is sometimes described in terms of the degree of lightness, goodness, or recollection of truth in philosophical or spiritual terms because all of these terms indicate the presence of order rather than chaos. However, order and perfection are static and unchanging, but life is adaptive and flexible. Additional energies influence biomorphogenesis, which can be defined in terms of the development and evolution of life in space and time.

Second, any living system must be adaptive, that is, capable of *biomorphogenesis*. The progressive increase in adaptive self-organization increases in proportion to the level of understanding in self-aware consciousness in Table 8.1. Life increases from the movement of inanimate matter to the biomorphogenesis of cellular life, and then mental development among vertebrate animals, culminating in the three stages of human self-aware consciousness. Biomorphogenesis leads to the third stage of human self-understanding, which involves nonlocal awareness. Nonlocal awareness is the basis for understanding of truth, which leads to wisdom. However, variation in the levels of information content and biomorphogenesis are inadequate to account for the flexibility inherent in the three-dimensional spiral of living systems.

Third, any living being must be flexible and creative in its adaptive self-organization. Otherwise life would be mechanistic and predictable from prior conditions, rather than free and creative. Hence, the level of flexibility of self-aware organization increases in proportion to the level of coherence of the system, as indicated in Table 8.1. *Coherence* is defined in terms of nonresistance to the biomorphogenic movement toward order, which ultimately leads to a state of noncausality in which movement is free, impartial, and creative without influence from prior conditions. A person at the third stage of self-aware consciousness who is fully coherent may also be described as being free, creative, and loving. In Table 8.1, there is a progressive increase in noncausality from the quantum states of inanimate matter to epigenetic states of cellular life, brain states of the body, ego states of the self, moral states of members of society, and ultimately the creative states of the spiritual level of human self-aware consciousness. Each of these states is a step in a recursive hierarchy because each end-state of one level is what develops in the succeeding level in the hierarchy until the spiritual level is reached. At the nondual level, our fundamental spontaneity is recognized as love, which is impartial and free of all past conditioning, fear, struggle, and conflict. Nonduality is complete and beyond all fear because there is no other. What is nondual is also nonlocal and noncausal, as in all quantum systems. In other words, what is nondual is a whole that cannot be reduced because there is nothing else and no part is adequate to define the whole. There can be only stepwise growth in awareness of one's context, leading ultimately to awareness of one's fundamental nature. Consequently, information, biomorphogenesis, and coherence are an irreducible triad of forces at the foundation of the universal unity of being.

Essentially, the development within each level is an exploration of the possibilities inherent in the context of that level. In the terms used in Chapter 7, the exploration of one's context is the exploration of the epigenetic or fitness landscape, which is a search for what possible configurations lead to the global optimum of adaptive fitness. The exploration of one's context to discover the global adaptive optimum is also called the exploration of one's phase space, which is all the possible configurations of a fitness landscape (Stewart 1998, page 111). Hence, the purpose of life can be described as learning what is most adaptive by the thorough exploration of all possibilities. The level of self-aware consciousness refers to one's understanding of the consequences of alternative behaviors. We are free to do this in an efficient manner by following the path of order to full coherence as well as we can recognize it. Alternatively, we can follow a less direct route, but all routes eventually lead to increases in spiritual awareness.

## THE DYNAMICS OF BIOPSYCHOSOCIAL SYSTEMS

Despite the overall unity and interdependence evident in evolved forms of life, most people think of themselves as functioning separately from one another. Likewise, in ordinary cognition, people regard most material objects in the world as discrete and separate except under rare conditions that are not relevant to daily life. Such dualistic assumptions often influence people's expectations about the dynamics of connected sets of adaptive systems like those that make up cells within body, organs within a person, individual people within society, and so on.

Statisticians have studied the dynamics of complex adaptive systems in detail in recent years. Until very recently, people had assumed that the connections in networks are either "regular" or "random" (Watts and Strogatz 1998). In a regular network, the connections are strongly clustered among nearby elements so that the average number of steps in the path between elements is large. The local clustering of regular networks is often described as "cliquishness," just as an exclusive cluster of friends is called a clique. In contrast, in a "random" network, there are random connections among a large proportion of elements so that the average number of steps in the path between connected elements is small. Regular networks with many local connections or cliques are stable, whereas random networks with many long-range connections are unstable, as described in Chapter 7 (May 1972; Watts and Strogatz 1998).

Increased complexity is achieved in living organisms by the development of connections that are intermediate in pattern to those of regular or random networks (Wagner 2000; Wagner and Fell 2001; Wuchty 2001). These networks with intermediate patterns of connectivity are called "small-world" (Watts and Strogatz 1998) or "scale-free" networks (Albert, Jeong et al. 1999; Wuchty 2001). In a small-world or scale-free network, a few shortcuts or "superhighways" connect different cliques, with the result that the average number of steps between elements throughout the network is small even though there is still much local cliquishness. Examples of such small-world connections are the superhighways of the American road system, the core transit backbone of the Internet, and the long conducting tracts of the human central nervous system. In the human central nervous system, the long conducting tracts are monoaminergic tracts that begin in the brain stem and extend forward throughout the limbic and neocortical system, and the long conducting tracks from the cortex and brain stem that extend through the length of the spinal cord. The small-world effects of such efficient long-range connection patterns were first described in social studies of networks of friends, giving rise to the observation that no two people have more than "six degrees of separation" (Milgram 1967; Guare 1990). Similar sociological results have been obtained for networks of film actors or scientists working together (Watts and Strogatz 1998). In addition, the connection patterns of most biological systems are characterized by the dynamics of small world networks. For example, small-world dynamics is typical of the evolution of connections among genetic and metabolic pathways (Wagner and Fell 2001) and among different protein domains in all domains of life (Wuchty 2001). All the neuronal connections of the worm *Caenorhabditis elegans* are known and have a small-world pattern (Watts and Strogatz 1998). In addition, small-world dynamics is characteristic of the interactions of whole organisms in food chains or what are more precisely called *food networks* (Albert, Jeong et al. 1999; Albert and Barabasi 2002). In general, small-world dynamics is characteristic of most psychosocial behaviors, such as patterns of visiting Internet sites or the spread of fads (Watts and Strogatz 1998; Albert, Jeong et al. 1999).

One of the remarkable characteristics of small world networks is that the close connection among all components of the network is not prominent from a local perspective. What stands out to local inspection is the cliquishness or local clusters. Only a few shortcuts or long superhighways connecting these cliques is sufficient to allow the whole network to function as a "scale-free" network in which what appears to be a distant site actually functions as an inseparable part of each and every cluster regardless of location.

A thorough review of the statistical properties of small-world and scale-free networks is presented elsewhere (Albert and Barabasi 2002). In a "scale-free" network, there is a small-world pattern at each level in a hierarchy of coupled complex adaptive systems, like that described in Table 8.1. Therefore, there is rapid communication both within each level of the hierarchy and between levels of the hierarchy. The overall result is that the whole system approaches (but does not reach) the formal dynamics of a "nonlocal" field as a limit. Only "entangled" quantum systems have truly nonlocal dynamics in which events at a distance are simultaneous with no time lag at all, as discussed in Chapter 5. Nevertheless, small-world (or nearly nonlocal) dynamics allows synchronous rapid shifts in fads of social opinion, the thoughts of individuals, brain microstates, and cellular epige-netic states, as described in Chapters 6 and 7, giving rise in a stepwise manner to increasing order and coherence as the adaptive systems learn and develop.

Living systems are a nested hierarchy of complex dynamic systems that have small-world and scale-free properties. In particular, the development of human thought is scale invariant, which is crucial to recognize in clinical work. The scale invariance of thought means that each step in personal growth along the path of the psyche has the same phases as the overall stages of self-aware consciousness described in Chapter 3: (1) acceptance, (2) growing in awareness, (3A) enlarging of consciousness, and (3B) commitment. The small-world properties of psycho-biological systems explain the "nearly nonlocal" dynamics of complex living systems. The small world properties also explain the ease with which most people are misled by Cartesian-Mendelian thinking: most connections involve cliques that are local, even though the dynamics of the whole hierarchy is nearly nonlocal for most psychosocial and biological systems. The scale-invariant dynamics of living systems suggest that there are some basic parameters that pervade each level of the hierarchy. Identification of such scale-invariant parameters can allow a truly unified description of biological, psychological, and social phenomena, as de-scribed in the next section.

## THE TOPOLOGY AND FUNCTIONS OF THE HUMAN PSYCHE

Dualistic thinking has been so commonplace in psychology that it is essential to remind oneself frequently that we all live and develop within a universal unity of being, which has properties of nonlocality and noncausality. To acknowledge the fundamental properties of nonlocality and noncausality in psychobiological systems, we need a model of the nature of human beings that acknowledges our material, mental, and spiritual characteristics within a integrated and *scale-invariant* struc-ture. Here I describe the functions of the human psyche only in sufficient detail to make predictions that can be tested empirically in studies of creativity. Further de-tails that are needed for the clinical assessment and treatment of psychopathology will be described elsewhere. A person cannot properly understand or treat psycho-pathology until he or she has an adequate model of normal psychology.

I suggest that an adequate model of human nature must recognize that each person is a unified whole comprised of body, mind, and spirit, and that each per-son is an inseparable part of an all-encompassing cosmic order. Each person is a finite but inseparable part of an infinite and encompassing whole within which he or she is growing in awareness. From this perspective, life can be recognized as an exploration of infinite possibilities. The development of increasingly complex life forms is the way by which finite aspects of the whole become increasingly aware of the fundamental nature of the infinite whole. In the stepwise process of evolution, we will see that there has been a stepwise increase from local causal systems to small-world systems that are nearly nonlocal and, in human beings, a further progression from small-world systems to quantum systems that are truly nonlocal and noncausal in their dynamics.

A person is a psychobiological unity composed of many interdependent systems, and this integrated whole is more than the sum of its parts because the parts do not function separately (Lief 1948; Meyer 1957). Like a hologram, at whatever scale of space and time we look, the same picture of life emerges, even though the clarity and depth of details may vary slightly (Bohm and Hiley 1993). This scale-free hierarchical model is founded on the observations that there is a unity to all life, which has the three irreducible properties of order, consciousness, and coherence. The levels of order, consciousness, and coherence that we can observe vary according to the location of a particular living organism along the spiral path of development that I have called the path of the psyche. *The functions and path of the psyche are the proper foci of study for the fields of psychology and psychological medicine.*

The functions and development of the human body, mind, and psyche can be understood in concrete terms by analogy to the topological features of the worldwide Internet. The internet behaves like a scale-free hierarchy of coupled small-world dynamic systems (Albert, Jeong et al. 1999; Claffy, Monk et al. 1999; Huberman and Adamic 1999). The global infrastructure of the Internet consists of a complex array of telecommunications carriers and providers. Individual sites in homes and businesses are supported by thousands of small and medium-sized Internet service providers (ISPs), which are in turn interconnected by "arteries" maintained by the core transit (backbone) providers. At its heart is a mesh of interconnected backbone networks that are rapidly evolving to provide the basis for future growth in national and international communication. The interconnections between ISPs are illustrated in Figure 8.1, which is based on actual data about part of the Internet from monitoring on December 3, 1998. The connectivity pattern observed has the properties of a scale-free network in which there are a moderate number of shortcuts ("superhighways") connecting more densely interconnected cliques.

As a result of the topology of its connections, the Internet exhibits lawful logarithmic growth and communication patterns, as illustrated in Figure 8.2. To construct a topographical model of the Internet, Albert and her colleagues constructed a robot that added to its database all links (URLs) to other sites found on a document and recursively followed these to retrieve the related documents and URLs (Albert, Jeong et al. 1999). They used the data to measure the probability $P(k)$ that a document has a certain number $k$ of outgoing links $P_{out}(k)$ and incoming links $P_{in}(k)$. The logarithm of the probabilities of occurrence are plotted against the logarithm of the number of links in Figure 8.2 for outgoing links (8.3a) and for incoming links (8.3b). The linear slope of the relationships in Figure 8.2 is

Netname:

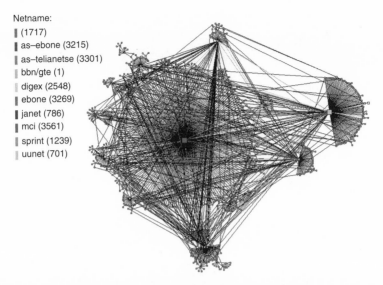

- ▌ (1717)
- ▌ as–ebone (3215)
- ▌ as–telianetse (3301)
- ▌ bbn/gte (1)
- ▌ digex (2548)
- ▌ ebone (3269)
- ▌ janet (786)
- ▌ mci (3561)
- ▌ sprint (1239)
- ▌ uunet (701)

Figure 8.1. Connections between Internet service providers in December 1998, illustrating a scale-free dynamic network. (Reproduced by permission of Claffy et al. 1999.)

characteristic of the dynamics of "small-world" networks, but not regular or random networks (Watts and Strogatz 1998; Albert, Jeong et al. 1999; Strogatz 2001).

The Internet is a "scale-free" hierarchy of coupled "small-world" dynamic systems. In other words, the connectivity of the Internet is dominated by a small number of highly connected Web pages with a few shortcuts connecting these cliques. Furthermore, the probability of finding very popular addresses among incoming suggested links is substantial, thereby creating a tendency for communications to flock to popular sites. Similarly, although the operator of each web site has complete freedom in choosing the number of links on a documents and the addresses to which they point, these choices obey scaling laws that are characteristic of coupled complex self-organizing systems with small-world and scale-free properties.

The topology of the Internet provides a useful analogy for a topological model of the development of a human being. As previously described in Chapter 2, the psyche is the most spiritual aspect of a human being, whereas the soma is the most material aspect of a human being. As a scale-free aspect of being, the psyche of an individual person is like a specific site in the Internet, which is functionally defined by its connectivity pattern. Different sites vary in the number of their connections and the frequency with which they are visited. Furthermore, the soma or body of an individual person is like the material content at a particular site, which varies in form, function, and outgoing links. Thoughts, which are at the

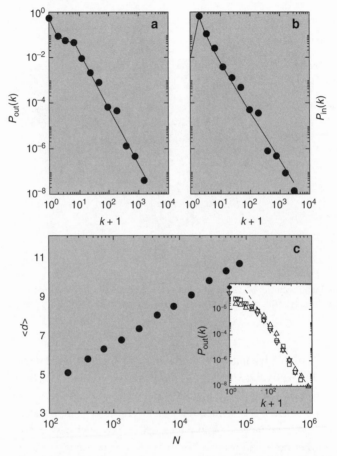

Figure 8.2. Lawful logarithmic growth patterns of the Internet. (Reproduced by permission of Albert and Barabasi, 1999.)

interface of the soma and the psyche, are like the computer screen reflecting the information available to consciousness. The operator of a particular Web site corresponds to a person (i.e., the self or ego state), who maintains the binding of the psyche and the soma together in space and time, thereby allowing the development of thought in the various stages of self-aware consciousness.

The development of each individual is a complex dynamic process that is characterized by a transitory sequence of changing combinations of psychosomatic systems that have small-world and scale-free dynamics. The nearly nonlocal dynamics and topological structure of the Internet provides an analogy for a topological model of human biopsychosocial development in terms of its fundamental mechanisms (Cloninger 2002).

First, let us consider the functions of the psyche. The functions of the psyche are recollection, understanding, and will, as previously discussed in Chapter 2. These three functions can be shown to correspond to the effects of fields of information, biomorphogenesis, and coherence in Table 8.1. Specifically, from the perspective of Table 8.1 and our analogy to small-world networks, the level of information content corresponds to the memory function of the psyche. Individuals vary in their ability to recollect information contained in the cosmic order. The level of order of a person's memories of reality greatly influences the ability to recognize the way to well-being. In the terminology of small-world networks, the level of elevation of the psyche is its "coordination number" or "connectivity level." The greater the level of elevation of the psyche, the more extensively and more closely it is connected with the whole unity of being. In Erikson's psychodynamic terms, the higher the level of elevation of the psyche, the greater will be the "social radius" or "sphere of influence" of that individual. In other words, the higher the level of awareness and influence, the greater is the "magnitude" of the psyche (Augustine 388). In practice, the level of the psyche can be estimated from a mental status examination from a person's worldview, as described in Chapter 5. The higher the level of elevation of the psyche, the more elevated is a person's world view, average level of thought, and capacity for well-being. However, greater connectivity is necessary, but not sufficient, for understanding and coherence. The level of elevation of the psyche is not the same as the level of thought because we must take into account processes other than memory that influence the functions of the psyche.

Second, the level of resonance of a person with the biomorphogenic field depends on his or her degree of understanding. Listening to the psyche allows a person to grow in awareness by purifying their rational intuition. The ability to know what is truly satisfying has a strong impact on a person's level of well being. In my experience, the range of a person's affect on mental status examination provides an estimate of their overall level of listening to their psyche. As the level of listening to the psyche increases, the range of affect changes from anhedonia, in which only negative emotions are experienced, to well-being, in which only positive emotions are experienced. TCI scores on Self-Transcendence also indicate a person's level of listening to the psyche.

Pure rational intuition involves direct self-aware perception of what is real and true without misunderstanding as a result of preconceptions, prejudices, fears, desires, and conflicts. Similarly, an important quantity describing the process of searching for information on the Internet is the shortest possible path between two documents based on incoming links listed on retrieved documents. The average size of the shortest path between any two documents is called the diameter of the Internet, which is designated as <d> in Figure 8.2c. The diameter is defined as the smallest number of URL links that must be followed to navigate from one document to the other. Despite the huge size of the Internet, the average diameter was only nineteen links in 1999. Even a 1000% increase in the size of the web is expected to change <d> very little (from nineteen to twenty-one) because <d> increases only with the logarithm of number of sites on the web, as shown in Figure 8.2c (Albert, Jeong et al. 1999). In other words, the Internet is a small-world network, which is typical of social and biological systems (Albert, Jeong et al. 1999; Albert and Barabasi 2002).

The relatively small value of the shortest route between two points on the Internet indicates that an intelligent ("smart") agent, who can interpret the links and follow only the relevant one, can find desired information quickly and efficiently by navigating the Internet using his or her intuitive understanding. However, a robot that locates information based on matching strings of information or keywords does not have the intuitive understanding needed to select the shortest path. Albert and colleagues found that a robot that searches by matching strings of information or keywords needs to search about 10% of the whole Internet on average to find a particular document. Robots cannot benefit from the highly interconnected nature of the Web because their only successful strategy is to index as much of the Web as possible. Experimental studies have shown that intelligent people have only limited awareness of the connections within their own social networks (Dodds, Muhamad et al. 2003; Granovetter 2003). Hence, intuitive understanding is an essential and irreducible feature of the development of consciousness in living systems in addition to the level of order or connectivity of living adaptive systems. Individuals who are low in listening to their psyche will be ineffective in using available small-world networks, as in the case of depressed individuals. However, as listening to the psyche increases in contemplation, then communication approaches nonlocality in a progressive stepwise manner. Nonlocality requires quantum-like coherence, which depends on a third dynamic property of complex living systems.

The third irreducible feature of the unity of being is coherence. The level of coherence of social and biological systems depends on the degree of freedom of will. Freedom of will permits coherence, which involves flexibly coordinated adaptive responses that are independent of prior conditions. TCI scores of Cooperativeness measure individual differences in the influence of freedom of will on human thought. Like the elevation of the psyche and the diameter of awareness, the dynamics of free will can also be understood by analogy to the Internet. Although the overall dynamics of communication on the Internet obeys scaling laws, as shown in Figure 8.1a,b, the operators of individual Web sites have freedom to chose the number of links on the documents they produce and the addresses to which they point. Likewise, Internet users have freedom to choose which links to pursue.

Nevertheless, individuals vary in their exercise of their potential freedom of will (Table 8.2). Viewers may develop conditioned habits so that they only connect with identified links with which they have had prior experiences that are rela-

**Table 8.2.** Basic Parameters Underlying Mental Health and Its Disorders

| Parameter Name | Parameter Description |
|---|---|
| Psyche level | Level of information content (i.e., order) of a person's memories of the coherence of the cosmic order, indicated by effects on long-term average level of thoughts or world view on mental status examination. |
| Listening to psyche | Level of understanding of the path of the psyche (i.e., life's developmental processes) from intuitive awareness, indicated by effects on thought measured by TCI Self-Transcendence and on mental status exam by the range of affect from well-being (full positive emotionality) to anhedonia (narrow negative emotions), reflecting the degree of letting go of struggles and conflict about being controlled or controlling. |
| Freedom of will | Degree of coherence with understanding of the path of the psyche, allowing freedom from prior conditioning and fear, as indicated by effects on thought measured by TCI Cooperativeness and on mental status exam by flexibility in legislative functions, such as fluidity of speech and spontaneity of volitional choices in behavior. |
| Following the path | Level of following the path of the psyche, allowing awareness of reality or truth without distortion and deception, which depends on the configuration of order, listening, and free will, as indicated by effects on thought measured by TCI Self-Directedness and on mental status exam by a person's level of reality testing and sense of spontaneous agency and responsibility rather than being controlled by external influences. |
| Ego level | Strength of binding of psyche and soma, allowing continuity of self-aware consciousness when normal, dissociation if low, and defensive struggling, grandiosity and pride if inflated. |
| Serenity level | Degree of calmness and impartiality, allowing psyche to enlighten thoughts so that there is overall well-being from coherence of all aspects of being, as indicated by the calmness and appropriateness of affect on mental status exam. |
| Thought level | Level of coherence of self-awareness in conscious thought, as measured by Diagnosis of Frequency of Thought. |
| Relationship level | Level of awareness in human relationships, as measured by Diagnosis of Human Relationships, indicated by the level of thoughts and feelings that a relationship elicits in a particular person. |

tively satisfying. Navigation on the Web is dominated by very popular addresses, which are often, but not always, part of the optimal path. Hence optimal solutions often depend on openness to novel routes. As self-aware consciousness increases, individuals are increasingly able to recognize and understand their problems. As intuitive understanding increases, people are able to let go of old habits that reduce their freedom and adaptability.

Creativity and freedom of will indicate underdetermination of activity by prior conditions (Walker 2000). That is, flexibility in adaptation depends on the coordination of spontaneity in coupled small-world networks. The activities of different brain networks, for example, often show large-scale or global patterns of coherence (Freeman 1995). The spatial and temporal properties of such global coherence cannot be explained except by small-world dynamics or quantum coherence. Small-world dynamics is clearly present in neuronal systems, even in worms, and appears adequate to explain most biological and social phenomena, including friendship networks involving the second stage of self-aware consciousness.

However, small-world dynamics appears inadequate to explain the phenomena of nonlocality and noncausality associated with contemplative thinking, such as creativity. Transfer of information between fields that do not usually communicate can be explained by small-world dynamics of a few enterprising individuals, but true invention or creativity involves more than rapid transfer between cliques on the Internet. Freedom of will and creativity ultimately imply noncausality, which means that no prior conditions predict what is produced. According to standard dictionaries, creativity is defined as "bringing into being out of nothing," which is impossible according to the assumptions of causal realism (Boden 1994, page 75). Noncausality is the characteristic that distinguishes the nonalgorithmic nature of human creativity from all forms of algorithmic information processing that can be achieved by computer simulation (Penrose 2001). Art, science, and spirituality are the unique features of human self-aware consciousness and underlie the development of our civilization. The emergence of these indicators of human creativity abruptly in modern human beings suggests a qualitatively new process at work that is not present in other primates, as described in Chapter 7.

I think we must seriously consider the possibility that the third stage of human self-aware consciousness depends on actual quantum coherence. The observation of quantum coherence in the brain is unlikely under ordinary conditions, which are accurately described as "warm, wet, and noisy." However, the context of self-aware consciousness is ultimately the biomorphogenic field itself, which is intrinsically creative. Therefore, creativity implies quantum coherence within a universal field, just as particle physics must postulate to explain the constant flux of particles to and from a universal field.

Psychology would have to postulate that the human brain is capable of quantum-like coherence to explain the quantum phenomena of nonlocality and noncausality observed in the third stage of self-aware consciousness. Is there any supporting empirical evidence to support this postulate? In fact, quantum coherence has been induced in the living human brain, even providing a novel method for magnetic resonance imagining (MRI) (Warren, Ahn et al. 1998; Rizi, Ahn et al. 2000). Quantum dipole couplings of protein spins in molecules separated by distances ranging from ten microns to one millimeter (which are huge distances at the quantum level) yield detectable MRI signals under certain conditions. In human MRI, the sites of maximal quantum coherence appear in the frontal, parietal, and occipital cortex, as well as periaqueductal gray matter (Rizi, Ahn et al. 2000).

Such induced quantum coherence supports the possibility that the brain may be capable of intrinsic quantum coherence, as has been proposed (Hameroff and Penrose 1995). However, the spontaneous occurrence of quantum coherence in contemplation or creative states has not been directly studied. We must be cautious about attributing quantum properties of nonlocality and noncausality to even the most elevated stage of human self-aware consciousness. Let us examine what empirical evidence there is for such phenomena in the history of science.

## THE NONCAUSAL NATURE OF HUMAN CREATIVITY

### Empirical Findings

Fortunately, we are in a better position to test specific hypotheses about the relationship of quantum phenomena to human consciousness than past investigators. We can now make specific hypotheses about the topology of creative cognition in relation to the level of self-aware consciousness. As mentioned earlier, I hypothesize that intuition is an underlying aspect of all human self-aware consciousness, and that rational intuition becomes purified in contemplation (i.e., the third stage of self awareness). Creative thinking involves intuitive leaps that are facilitated in the higher stages of self-aware consciousness. The vast majority of creative work in science and art has involved thought in the intellectual plane. Because fewer people attain the higher levels of self-awareness, we can expect that most people will make discoveries at moderately elevated levels of thought. The most creative individuals are those with a high level of elevation of their psyche, that is, a "high coordination" number. The most creative individuals are expected to make unique discoveries of outstanding quality and originality of insight, which is the evidence for their creativity. In addition, the most creative individuals are also expected to participate in more multiple independent discoveries, which may be made at nearly the same time by less creative individuals (this is the evidence of variability in level of connectivity).

Fortunately, there has been extensive biopsychosocial research on creativity, as led by individuals with diverse interests such as Arthur Koestler (Koestler 1964), Howard Gardner (Gardner 1993), Robert Sternberg (Sternberg 1988), and Dean

Simonton (Simonton 1978, 1979, 1994, 1999). Psychological research on creativity includes studies of cognition, personality, and development, as well as how these domains are influenced by biological and social variables.

The well-known phenomenon of multiple independent discoveries in science provides quantitative data that allows tests of alternative models of the process of creative invention and discovery. A representative list of multiple independent discoveries in science is given in Table 8.3. Table 8.3 gives examples involving two, four, or six to nine independent discoveries to illustrate the variation in degree of creativity as a function of the number of independent discoverers. Multiple discoverers are not at all uncommon, even for major discoveries in science, as shown in Table 8.3. In addition, the majority of applications for new patents are rejected because of prior discoveries, which are presumably unknown to the applicant (Garfield 1980a, 1980b).

The characteristics of "multiple" independent discoveries have been compared with unique ("singleton") discoveries from psychological and sociological perspectives (Merton 1961; Simonton 1994). The psychological processes leading to such discoveries have also been studied in depth from the perspective of cognition, personality, and development (Koestler 1964; Gruber 1974; Sternberg 1988, 1990; Simonton 1994). The biogenetic (Simonton 1994; Eysenck 1995), sociological (Merton 1961; Merton 1973), and psychodynamic (Jung 1957; Von Franz 1992) aspects have also been described.

Key facts that have been established about creative discoveries are summarized in Table 8.4. First, great unique discoveries are frequently inspired by visual imagery leading to sudden flashes of insight that occur in contemplative states of thought (Hadamard 1945; Koestler 1964). Often there are serendipitous accidents in which a person has a sudden flash of insight, as in the discovery of buoyancy by Archimedes or the discovery of a way to hold the charge of static electricity in a so-called Leyden jar by the Dutch physicist Pieter van Musschenbroeck of the University of Leiden (see Table 8.3). Systematic studies of the relationship of creativity to contemplative thinking have already been described in detail in Chapter 6. Nevertheless, some additional examples of contemplation and serendipity in relation to scientific discoveries may help to clarify the functional significance of these findings.

For example, Kekule's dream of snakes grasping their tails to form a circle inspired his intuitive discovery of the chemical model of the carbon ring of benzene:

> I turned my chair to the fire and dozed. Again the atoms were gamboling before my eyes. . . . all twining and twisting in snake-like motion. But look! What was that? One of the snakes had seized hold of its own tail, and the form whirled mockingly before my eyes. As if by a flash of lightning I awoke. (Simonton 1994, page 97)

Similarly, the French mathematician Henri Poincare was unable to find the formula for certain arithmetic transformations until he intuitively glimpsed the solution in a contemplative state.

**Table 8.3.** Representative Examples of Multiple Independent Discoveries and
Inventions in Science, Selecting Examples Involving Two, Four, or Six to Nine
Independent Discoverers to Illustrate the Range of Creativity, All Drawn from a Prior
Systematic Review of Eight Fields of Science

| Discovery or Invention | Independent Discoverers (Date) |
|---|---|
| TWO DISCOVERERS | |
| Nebular hypothesis (origin of solar system) | Kant (1755), Laplace (1796) |
| Calculus | Newton (1671), Leibniz (1676) |
| Principle of buoyancy | Archimedes (250 BC), Stevinus (1608) |
| Molecular theory of gases | Avogadro (1811), Ampere (1814) |
| Leyden jar (holds static charge) (1746) | von Kleist (1745), van Musschenbroek |
| Theory of gene mutations | Korschinsky (1899), DeVries (1900) |
| FOUR DISCOVERERS | |
| Discovery of sunspots | Galileo, Fabricus, Scheiner, Harriott (all in 1611) |
| Introduction of decimal | Burgi (1592), Piticus (1608), Kepler (1616), Napier (1616) |
| Method of liquefying gases | Cailletet, Pictet, Wroblowski, Olzewski (all 1877–1884) |
| Equivalence of heat and energy | Carnot (1830), Sequin (1839), Joule (1840), Mayer (1842) |
| Invention of telegraph | Henry (1831), Morse (1837), Cooke-Wheatstone (1837), Steinheil (1837) |
| Laws of genetic inheritance | Mendel (1865), DeVries (1900), Correns (1900), Tschermarck (1900) |
| SIX OR MORE DISCOVERERS | |
| Telescope | Lippershey, Della Porta, Digges, Johannides, Metius, Drebbel, Fontana, Janssen, Galileo (1558–1609) |
| Thermometer | Galileo, Drebbel, Sanctorious, Paul, Fludd, von Guericke, Porta, DeCaus (1592–1617) |
| Logarithmic criteria for convergence of a series | Abel, DeMorgan, Bertrand, Raabe, Duhamel, Bonnet, Paucker (1832–1851) |
| Cellular basis of both animal and vegetable tissue | Schwann, Henle, Turpin, Dumortier, Purkinje, Muller, Valentin (1839) |
| Electric railroad | Davidson, Jacobi, Lilly-Colton, Davenport, Page, Hall (1835–1850) |
| Self-exciting electric dynamo | Hjorth, Varley, Siemens, Wheatstone, Ladd, Wilde (1866–67) |

*Source*: From review by Ogburn 1922.

**Table 8.4.** Consensus Findings about Multiple Independent Discoveries in Science by Both Sociologists and Neo-Darwinian Psychologists

1. Creative discoveries are frequently inspired by sudden intuitions or visual imagery during contemplation.
   The quantity and quality of creative discoveries are positively correlated in two ways (2 and 3 below).
2. Unique discoveries that are not duplicated by others are often made by scientists who are highly prolific and high ranking in professional stature.
3. Highly prolific scientists are more often involved in multiple independent discoveries than expected according to the overall quantity of discoveries.
4. There is often delayed recognition of highly creative discoveries, with multiple independent rediscoveries at a later time.

> Then I turned my attention to the study of some arithmetical questions apparently without much success and without a suspicion of any connection with my preceding researches. Disgusted with my failure, I went to spend a few days at the seaside, and thought of something else. One morning, walking on the bluff, the idea came to me, with just the same characteristics of brevity, suddenness and immediate certainty, that the arithmetic transformations of indeterminate ternary quadratic forms were identical with those of nonEuclidian geometry. (Simonton 1994, page 94)

Poincare then realized that his unconscious was not only creatively imaginative but also capable of valid mathematical insight (Von Franz 1992, page 1). Moreover, his description of illuminative thought allowing the connection to previously disconnected areas of research illustrates an important aspect of the functional dynamics of contemplation. Contemplative thinking facilitates divergent thinking, that is, the ability to connect what are conventionally regarded as disparate phenomena (Sternberg 1988, 1990, Simonton 1994), as discussed by Godel in Chapter 1. Divergent thinking differs from eccentric thinking in that it is actually integrative, increasing the coherence of the expanded whole. In other words, the nonlocal characteristics of awareness in contemplation create insightful intuitive leaps that establish "small-world" networks in thought. These bridges between previously disconnected areas of thought provide the long-range connections that are often needed for scientific or artistic progress at a lower level of self-aware consciousness.

Second, individuals can be ranked according to their level of creativity. Discoverers of high rank are both highly prolific and generate uniquely outstanding discoveries (Simonton 1994, pages 115–122). Third, highly prolific discoverers are more likely to be involved in multiple independent discoveries, even taking into account the number of their discoveries (Merton 1961, 1973; Simonton 1978, 1979, 1994). Hence, the rank or level of the discovery is positively correlated with the frequency of connection with multiple discoveries. For example, Kelvin and Freud were each involved in over thirty multiple discoveries with others during the course of their prolific careers (Merton 1961). The principle that creative rank is correlated with involvement in multiple discoveries was first clearly demonstrated by Robert Merton in work with Elinor Barber on 264 multiple independent discoveries (Merton 1961) and has been confirmed consistently in other series (Simonton 1978, 1979, 1994). However, the highly creative scientist is distinguished by discoveries that are not duplicated by others, as stated in the second finding summarized in Table 8.4 (Simonton 1994). It is not really accurate to say that the highly creative scientist is "the functional equivalent of a considerable array of other scientists of varying degrees of talent," as was concluded by Robert Merton in arguing for the social inevitability of scientific discoveries. Rather, the intuitive awareness that leads to divergent insight allows some individuals to serve as trailblazers and pathfinders. Trailblazers provide a foundation from which others can build with more conventional thinking, as is often observed in discoveries that are made independently by more than four individuals (see Table 8.3).

Fourth, many highly original discoveries are made "ahead of their time," that is, before there is an extensive intellectual basis for the intuitive leap required to integrate the novel finding with what is scientifically acceptable at the time. This is illustrated by the delay before independent duplication following original discoveries by Archimedes, Avogadro, and Mendel in Table 8.3. For example, around 250 BC Archimedes described his recognition that a person feels lighter when floating in water in proportion to the weight of the volume he displaces. However, the hydrostatic principle of buoyancy was not rigorously understood in terms of statistical physics until 1608 when the Dutch mathematician Stevinus independently developed rigorous proofs based on recent advances in the physics of fluids.

Likewise, in 1811 the Italian physicist Avogadro observed that gases chemically combine in simple proportions by volume, which led him to the intuition that equal volumes of gases contain the same number of molecules when they are at the same temperature and pressure. This intuition was formulated as Avogadro's law, which is a fundamental principle of chemistry to this day. However, Avogadro's intuition was not generally accepted until after 1858 when the Italian chemist Cannizzaro constructed a logical system of chemistry based on Avogadro's law.

Delayed recognition of novel ideas that are inconsistent with contemporary assumptions and methods of proof lead to long gaps in time before many highly creative findings are independently rediscovered (Merton 1961; Garfield 1980a, 1980b). In Merton's study of 264 multiple discoveries, only 20% were found to have taken place within a one-year interval. In fact, a decade or more elapsed between discoveries in nearly one-third of multiples. Furthermore, when there is an initial prolonged delay, there are often multiple synchronous rediscoveries at a later date after the foundation of tools needed for discovery and their connections are more fully developed. For example, as shown in Table 8.3, the original principles of Mendelian inheritance were first published in 1865. On the basis of rigorous breeding experiments and careful statistical analysis, Mendel concluded that paired genes that are present in the parent separate (i.e., segregate) during the formation of the gametes. He also showed that different traits could be inherited independently as a result of independent assortment of genes. However, his results were ignored for the next 35 years for two reasons. Neither Charles Darwin nor the leading Swiss botanist of the time, Karl von Nageli, endorsed the findings as important when Mendel sent copies of his publication to them for consideration (Henig 2000). In Mendel's time, most hybridists accepted von Nageli's theory of blending inheritance and doubted the possibility of the constancy of particulate inheritance of genes. Furthermore, when the work was originally published, little was known about the cell, and the processes of mitosis and meiosis were completely unknown. Flemming did not describe the mechanism of mitosis until 1878, and cell theory did not become a major force in physiology until the publication of Max Verworn's *General Physiology* in English in 1899. Following these scientific developments, Mendel's work was rediscovered in 1900 when three botanists independently recognized the importance of Mendel's work on the basis of their own research and cited his earlier publication. Advances in the theory of the cell and its differentiation allowed the Dutch botanist Hugo De Vries to develop the theory of gene mutation in 1900 (see Table 8.3), and from this he was able to deduce the laws of Mendelian inheritance. The delay between Mendel and De Vries is only one of many examples of rediscovery at a later time when additional tools and concepts have been established to help understand original concepts that challenge traditional thinking.

Hence, multiple independent discoveries in science are not always evidence of "synchronicity" because they are really not simultaneous. Information about the timing of discoveries is useful to help understand the complex interactions among the personal characteristics of scientists (i.e., the role of "genius"), the social *zeitgeist* ("spirit of the times"), and the role of rare events that occur by chance (Simonton 1979).

## Interpretive models and analyses

Extreme sociocultural and neo-Darwinian models have had strong advocates who describe plausible but untested narratives to explain creativity. However, these dualistic models do not allow for objective tests of their basic assumptions, as was described in Chapter 6. For example, some early sociologists regarded the frequent occurrence of multiple independent discoveries as evidence of sociocultural determinism (Ogburn and Thomas 1922). They suggested that when the sociocultural milieu was right, the emergence of particular discoveries was inevitable. They acknowledged the role of the individual inherited genius but regarded such individuals as "a medium of social change" and "the product of their times" because a culture always had individuals to fill whatever social roles were required (Duncan 1964, pages 33–43). In other words, the social milieu, not individual inherited genius, made particular discoveries inevitable when the time was right.

Later, neo-Darwinian advocates pointed out that the consensus findings summarized in Table 8.4, showing a correlation between the quantity and quality of discoveries, were compatible with a neo-Darwinian interpretation (Simonton 1994; Eysenck 1995). The creative genius evolved through "blind-variation and selective-retention" according to neo-Darwinists, giving rise to prolific production of creative discoveries, both unique and multiple. Furthermore, the argument that the social milieu was determinative was undermined by the fact that multiple independent discoveries were usually separated in time by many years (consensus finding 4).

However, consensus about the observations summarized in Table 8.4 means that most investigators of creativity recognize that multiple genetic and environmental influences were interacting in a complex nonlinear manner (Merton 1961; Simonton 1994, 1999). The simple early models of social determinism and hereditary genius have been abandoned in favor of multifactorial models that recognize the interaction of genetic and environmental factors. Despite this consensus, the ideological conflicts inherent in dualistic multifactorial models have resulted in persistent controversy and different interpretations of the available data.

For example, Merton acknowledged that the achievements of a great discoverer may influence their times, but concluded that the frequency of multiple co-discoverers provided convincing evidence for the inevitability of scientific discoveries (Merton 1961). Once the necessary cultural base has accumulated certain discoveries were largely predetermined. For example, if neither Newton nor Leibniz had developed calculus, someone else would have done so eventually. Hence, Merton did not recognize any difference between the trail-blazing role of socially divergent originality associated with unique discoveries or low-grade multiples, and the more ordinary thinking associated with high-grade multiples.

Hence, both social determinists and neo-Darwinists acknowledged some role for genetic and environmental factors, but their interpretation of the role of chance rare events was different. Many social scientists came to regard discoveries as "ripe apples picked by blind men" (Price 1963). In contrast, some social scientists have recognized chance events as unpredictable variables in a self-organizing developmental process in which people are at least partially self-aware and self-directed (Bandura 1982). The suggestion that blind men can pick ripe fruits clearly contradicts the claim of transcendentalists like Thoreau, who said that only a "genius" can pick the "ripe fruits" of artistic creations.

On the other hand, neo-Darwinists regarded discoveries as the fruit of prepared genotypes produced by differential retention of "blind variations" (Simonton 1978, 1994). Both camps agree that frequency of occurrence of discoveries decreases monotonically as the number of independent co-discoverers increases in all series of multiple discoveries (Price 1963; Simonton 1994). Therefore, alternative theories must explain why larger numbers of co-discoverers are increasingly rare.

It is instructive to observe how this controversy was generated. Derek Price, a historian of science, suggested the "ripe apple" model using a Poisson statistical distribution to predict the frequency of multiple discoveries. Price asked (1963), "If there are 1000 apples in a tree, and 1000 blindfolded men reach up at random to pick an apple, what is the chance of a man's getting one to himself, or finding himself grasping as well the hand of another picker, or even more than one?" The expected distribution of multiple discoveries was then compared to the actual distribution observed by Merton and Barber in a series of 264 multiple discoveries. A Poisson distribution is often used as a model of "regular" complex systems in which a particular event is rare. Price suggested that the observed frequencies agreed fairly well with those expected frequencies from a Poisson distribution for the frequencies of two to four discoverers, but under-predicted the frequency of larger numbers of discoverers. Actually, the observed data differed significantly from the expectations of the Poisson distribution, but the suggestion was still made that making discoveries was like blind men picking ripe apples.

Simonton reexamined the same data of Merton (1961) and the Ogburn series of 148 multiples (Ogburn and Thomas 1922). Using the Poisson distribution, Simonton found that the mean value of 1.4 gave the best fit for the Merton data and 1.2 for the Ogburn data. Simonton noted that the observed data differed significantly from the expectations of the Poisson distribution. Nevertheless, Simonton argued eloquently that an important role for rare chance events had been demonstrated and was best interpreted as evidence of neo-Darwinian evolution because of the findings in Table 8.5 (Simonton 1978, 1979, 1994). He even suggested that the underprediction of larger numbers of discoverers might be explained by low-grade multiples being less often reported than high-grade multiples. However, this *post hoc* explanatory narrative is based on the unproven assumption that the Poisson distribution is the appropriate description of the process of creative discovery (Simonton 1978). Of course, the dynamics of small-world and scale-free networks were only described in 1999. Therefore, the true significance of the underprediction of high-grade multiple discoveries could not have been properly interpreted until very recently.

My colleague Nenad Svrakic and I have further analyzed the same two data sets considered by Simonton because we noted that the Poisson distribution actually did not provide a good fit to the observed frequency of multiple discoveries, particularly the number of discoveries made by large numbers of people independently. It is the tails of distributions that are most informative for distinguishing alternative interpretations because most distributions are similar near their mode.

To try to understand the dynamics of multiple discoveries, I examined the detailed listing of 148 multiple discoveries provided by Ogburn and Thomas (1922). Although not exhaustive in scope, this list was based on a systematic review of discoveries and inventions in the history of eight fields of science, including astronomy, mathematics, chemistry, physics, electricity, biology, medicine, and

**Table 8.5.** Observed Distribution of Multiple Discoverers in
the Merton-Barber Series Compared with the Best-Fitting
Levy and Poisson Distributions

| No. of Co-discoverers | Observed | Poisson (mu = 1.4) | Levy (power = 3.15) |
|---|---|---|---|
| 2 | 179 | 156 | 179 |
| 3 | 51 | 73 | 50 |
| 4 | 17 | 26 | 20 |
| 5 | 6 | 7 | 10 |
| 6 | 8 | 2 | 6 |
| 7 | 1 | 0 | 3 |
| 8 | 0 | 0 | 2 |
| 9 | 2 | 0 | 2 |
| $\chi^2$ | | 20 $df = 2$ | 7.25 $df = 7$; (2.1, $df = 4$) |

technology. From the findings summarized in Table 8.4, I thought that three hypotheses about the relations between level of creativity, level of thought, and degree of multiplicity in discovery had not been adequately considered in prior analyses of multiple discoveries. First, creative discoveries and invention vary markedly in their degree of originality. Second, the degree of creativity is directly related to the degree of elevation of the thought that inspires the invention or discovery. Third, the number of co-discoverers is likely to be inversely related to the degree of creativity or originality of the invention and its underlying level of thought. Therefore, it is useful to consider discoveries according to the number of co-discoverers to be able to consider the nature of the discovery and available psychosocial information about the discoverers (see Table 8.3).

The discoveries appeared to vary in their psychological and social characteristics depending on the number of independent discoverers. The degree of creativity appeared to decrease as the number of others who made the same discovery increased, which is not surprising because originality and uniqueness are fundamental signs of creativity. The average scientific eminence of the discoverers also appeared to decrease along with increasing number of other discoverers, although eminent scientists like Galileo may also be involved in discoveries along with less eminent scientists. The positive philosophers, such as Archimedes and Leonardo, and other eminent scientists, like Newton, Leibniz, and Avogadro, usually made unique inventions or occurred in multiples of two. When information was available, the average Diagnosis of Frequency of Thought (DFT) level of thought at the time of inspiration was inversely related to number of eventual discoverers, as shown in Figure 8.3. For example, the discovery of the principle of buoyancy by Archimedes led him to run down the streets of Syracuse in Sicily naked and shouting the now famous phrase "Eureka!" ("I've found it"). Archimedes' sudden

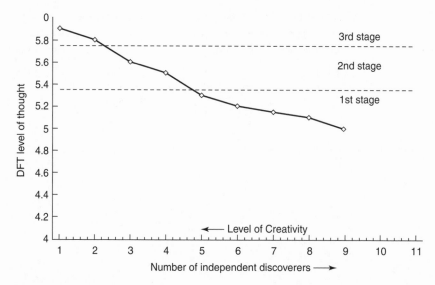

Figure 8.3. The relationship between the level of creativity and the average DFT level of the thought that inspired a discovery. I postulate that the level of creativity decreases as the number of independent discoverers increases.

insight was characteristic of contemplative thinking. In contrast, the process of effortful deductive reasoning from earlier discoveries in a synthetic manner is typical of discoveries involving more than two discoverers.

Each of the postulated relationships between creative rank, thought level, and degree of multiplicity suggest the power–law pattern observed in scale-free dynamic systems, as discussed earlier. However, psychological details were not consistently available, so I looked for an objective way to test the postulated pattern of scale-free dynamics. I hypothesized that the pattern of creative discoveries was what is expected from intelligent foraging for knowledge, as described previously for human behavior in searching the Internet. The dynamics of foraging behavior is expected to be a scale-free dynamic behavior based on previous studies of the foraging activity of many animals, including ants, flies, turtles, and birds (Viswanathan, Afanasyev et al. 1996) or price fluctuations from trade on the stock market (Casti 1997). If this hypothesis is true, the statistical distribution of multiple creative discoveries should follow a power–law distribution (Albert and Barabasi 2002), which has a greater probability of many co-discoveries than is found in a Poisson distribution (Viswanathan, Afanasyev et al. 1996; Casti 1997).

Power–law distributions have a long skewed tail, as observed in scale-free dynamic networks. For example, the length of the flight of an albatross foraging for food has a Levy distribution, which is a power–law distribution in which the power is 2 (Casti 1997). Systematic observations have been made on the distance an albatross flies when it searches for food at different times (Viswanathan,

Afanasyev et al. 1996; Casti 1997). Most of the time an albatross flies about randomly for short periods of time within areas with plenty of food, but they also make frequent long excursions to new areas to adapt intelligently when food becomes scarce locally. Such long excursions connect different small-world areas in which foraging is easy and random. However, a dumb or blind albatross is unlikely to survive long in nature if they stay in a depleted small habitat. Hence, the prevalence of these longer flights is what distinguishes a scale-free (power–law) process from processes that are either Gaussian (symmetrical bell shaped) or Poisson (asymmetrical curves that fall to zero rapidly in the skewed tail).

A power–law distribution is also characteristic of patterns of discovery in games of hide-and-seek in which people try to avoid spending too much time searching in unproductive areas. In terms of our original analogy to search behavior on the Internet, the co-occurrence of many independent discoverers of the same invention corresponds to a very popular Internet site. When a person with a high coordination number develops a site on the Internet, the site is likely to be popular because many other individuals will later tend to flock to the same site. The establishment of a new site on the Internet is analogous to a new "insight" from contemplative thinking, which establishes a new path leading to fuller understanding. Later explorers of the Internet may arrive at the popular site without knowing the original developer of the site because the original developer is connected to many others who provide the necessary individual linkages by which a person may reach the site independent of the developer. In this way a person with a highly connected psyche (i.e., a popular albatross) may serve as a "trail blazer," marking a new path. Subsequently, other people may independently flock to the same site without even being directly aware of each other or of the originator of the site. Such flocking behavior corresponds to the occurrence of a high-grade multiple. Therefore, we expected that high-grade multiples (i.e., five or more independent discoveries), which correspond to flocking behavior on the Internet, would differ from unique discoverers in their psychosocial features. We expected that very low-grade multiples (i.e., multiples of two only) would be similar to the divergent creative thinking of unique discoverers.

The observations of Merton about 264 multiple independent discoveries are compared with the frequencies of multiples expected from the best-fitting power–law and Poisson distributions in Table 8.4. The fit to the observed data is also depicted in Figure 8.4. The power–law distribution agrees well with the data throughout the whole range of number of co-discoverers ($\chi^2 = 7$, $df = 7$, showing no appreciable difference between observed and expected). In contrast, the best-fitting Poisson distribution is a poor fit ($\chi^2 = 20$, $df = 2$, $p < .001$) because it predicts too few multiples of 2 and too few multiples of more than 4. Therefore, the observed distribution of multiple discoveries is what is expected in a scale-free dynamic system in which there is intelligent foraging for knowledge. In other words, many discoveries are dominated by rare chance events. m··-¹

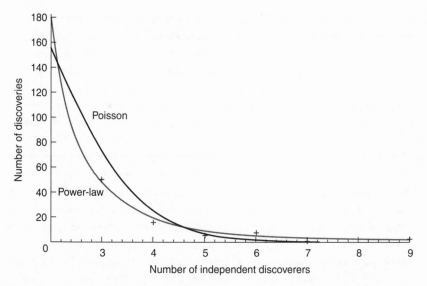

Figure 8.4. The distribution of 264 multiple independent scientific discoveries observed by Merton and Barber compared with the best fitting Levy and Poisson distributions (Levy power = 3.15, Poisson mean = 1.4).

man picking ripe fruit in places of abundance. There are also frequent long-range searches for knowledge carried out by persistent intelligent investigators over long periods of time.

To check on the replicability of the scale-free dynamics of creativity, we analyzed the Ogburn series of 148 multiples in the same way and obtained nearly identical results. In the power–law distribution, the probability of the number of independent co-discoverers is the inverse of the number of co-discoverers raised to a power $w$. For the Merton-Barber series the power $w$ is 3.15 and for the Ogburn-Thomas series the power is 3.0. By comparison, the value of $w$ was about 2.0 for the flight time of foraging albatrosses (Viswanathan, Afanasyev et al. 1996) and about 2.1– 2.45 for searches on the Internet (Albert, Jeong et al. 1999). From these statistics, the dynamics of scale-free systems in nature appear to vary within approximately two to three dimensions corresponding roughly to the order of the power function. Specifically, the flight of the albatross is essentially a search in two dimensions (specifically, distance and time), whereas human creativity is a search in three psychological dimensions, just as I postulated earlier in this chapter.

Hence, the observed dynamics is consistent with our earlier observations of the prevalence of three-dimensional spiral forms in the development and evolution of scale-free networks, which are characteristic of biopsychosocial systems. Human creativity is an integral aspect of the spiral hierarchy of complex adaptive systems that comprise life. Creativity has developed as an expression of the drives

go allows us to grow in understanding of hope, which leads to increasing
ss, serenity, and well-being.

ce, increasing lightness corresponds to the elevation of thought along the
path of the psyche. The greater degree of following the path of the psyche
ces thought so that there is increased TCI Self-Directedness. The eleva-
the psyche is also analogous to empirical measures of coordination num-
degree of connectivity in the Internet, as described earlier in this chapter.
e psychological terms, to increase in order or connectivity means to increase
er, trust, and hope, which are the distinguishing properties of lightness.
ond, to grow in awareness, we must listen to our psyche, which means to
understand our own nature rather than blaming, criticizing, and judging.
n the absence of dualistic judging can we face the truth inherent in reality
pproach it little by little without conflict or distortion. Hence, growing in
ness corresponds to the process of transcendence, as described by Carl Jung
1960). The greater degree of listening to the psyche influences thought so
ere is increased TCI Self-Transcendence. Such nonjudgmental measurement
at truth we can recognize allows us to grow in understanding of faith, which
to increasing integration of intelligence and eventually to wisdom. Increas-
eath of awareness corresponds to the widening diameter of the spiral path
psyche. This is also analogous to empirical measures of the diameter of the
et described in this chapter. In more psychological terms, to grow in self-
consciousness means to be more calm, serene, faithful, and open.
rd, to grow in love, we must be free of prior conditioning and work in the
e of others unconditionally. Such increasingly unconditional service allows
grow in understanding of charity, compassion, and eventually to uncondi-
love. Love is the absence of fear, egoism, and elitism. Such altruism is based
ontaneous kindness and is *not a defense* against selfishness and cruelty, as is
suggested in psychoanalysis. Increasing depth of the spiral path leads to
ed effort to dominate or inhibit conflicts, the reduced striving to be better
others (and oneself!), and increased spontaneity of love. The greater free-
of will influences thought so that there is increased TCI Cooperativeness. In
of the analogy to search behavior on the Internet, increasing depth of aware-
corresponds to freedom of choice of viewing sites, as discussed earlier in
hapter. In more psychological terms, to grow in freedom means to be more
y loving, charitable, humble, and creative, which are naturally expressed by
ing at the service of others.
ese steps are the basic principles of coherence therapy, which I will describe
tail in a companion book on clinical applications of the science of well-being.
ever, in addition, for clinical practice we need to understand why everyone does
ecome wise and lead a happy life. The downward spiral is the result of igno-
, misunderstanding, and fears that lead to struggles, problems, and conflicts,
scussed in Chapter 3. How do these obstacles to well-being arise if the natural

for order, truth, and coherence that motivate the development and evolution of
increasing self-aware consciousness of the universal unity of being.

Conclusions

We are finally in a position to draw major conclusions about the dynamics of
human creativity and the nature of its source. For example, we can now make
objective statements about the dualistic question of the direction of effects in
complex dynamic systems. A recurrent debate throughout the twentieth century
was whether cultural progress and creativity were attributable to the inherited
characteristics of great persons or to sociocultural determinism. The unpredictability of creative progress was interpreted in conflicting ways: as the blind variation of random mutations (by neo-Darwinists) or the picking of ripe apples by
blind men (by social determinists). This debate about the source of cultural progress
is a special form of the dualistic controversy of nature versus nurture.

So who wins the debate? Human creative discovery has the dynamics of a scale-
free dynamic system, which means that the question under debate was mistaken
because of an artificial dualism. The answer is that neither side wins. Also, neither side loses! Rather, cultural progress depends on the elevation of thought in
self-aware consciousness. The nondualistic awareness of contemplative thinking
inspires creative insights, which establish *conceptual bridges* between what previously seemed like disparate clusters of knowledge. In turn, these conceptual
bridges create a scale-free hierarchy of small-world networks that facilitate further self-organization by means of ordinary levels of thought (i.e., at lower levels
of consciousness). In other words, both the revolutionary intuitions of individuals with elevated levels of self-aware consciousness and the more conventional
thinking of ordinary cognition contribute in important ways to psychosocial development of individuals and to the biological and cultural evolution of society
as a whole.

However, contemplative thought is the medium through which the psyche enlarges the scope of information in self-aware consciousness. Contemplation brings
order, truth, and coherence, which are the irreducible three driving forces of the
motor of the psyche. Contemplation is not an emergent property of social order;
it is the means by which order, truth, and coherence are communicated among
individuals in society. In other words, order is not an property whose emergence
is driven by lower-level forces; rather, living systems are self-organizing along a
path leading to the ever-increasing realization of coherence with the information
that has always been inherent in all things. In turn, increasingly enlightened individuals shape, and are shaped by, their culture in a complex dynamic process of
reciprocal interactions. To paraphrase Julian Huxley, a human being is truly evolution growing in consciousness of itself by movement along the path of the psyche.

In summary, we can draw four new and fundamental conclusions from the consistent empirical evidence of the scale-invariant dynamics of human creative inventions. First, it has long been recognized that creative inventions are the fuel for the progressive expansion of human culture (Ogburn and Thomas 1922; Merton 1961). Now we can conclude that contemplation (i.e., listening to the psyche) is the source of human creativity. Second, the introduction of such creations into the culture provides bridges that make the world increasingly coherent. In other words, creative inventions make the world into a scale-invariant hierarchy of small-world networks because the inventions provide bridges that allow individuals who are less creative to participate with greater awareness of the expanding world. Creative inventions allow the discoverer to share his or her expanded self-awareness with everyone. Consequently, everyone can contribute to cultural progress to varying degrees, which depend on their level of self-aware consciousness.

Third, the small-world networks of brain microstates, ego states, and moral states are increasingly quantum-like but can only approach the quantum properties of nonlocality and noncausality as a limit. Nonlocality and noncausality are characteristics of universal fields at the quantum level. Listening to the psyche allows communication with the source of creativity, which is necessarily noncausal because it is not determined by antecedent conditions. Therefore, the conclusion follows logically that what has been called the psyche is a specific node in the universal field of superconscious life, which is the source of human self-aware consciousness. From this perspective, the psyche necessarily has the property of superconsciousness, in the sense that it is the nondualistic source of all information that emerges into human self-aware consciousness. The potential of the psyche for nondual awareness in contemplation is not a hypothesis *a priori*—rather it is a conclusion based on confirmed predictions about the frequency of human creative inventions.

The spiral path of self-aware consciousness provides a practical bridge between material particles and immaterial waves in the field of superconsciousness. The bridge between the soma and the psyche provides the means for living systems to grow in self-aware consciousness. Of course, the dual aspects of the unity of human beings, who are composed of both soma and psyche, has profound implications. Little is known about the organization and function of the psyche, but the limited information that is available is essential to guide future research and clinical practice concerned with the development of well-being.

Fourth, the universal field of superconsciousness is characterized by three interdependent forces, which underlie the self-organizing effects of information, biomorphogenesis, and coherence. In psychological terms, the three forces motivating development are the human needs for order, awareness, and well-being. In more inspiring terms, light, life, and love guide the growing awareness of the universal unity of being. These three energies appear to be irreducible aspects of all living systems. Efforts to understand life or consciousness in reduced terms are necessarily inadequate oversimplifications, which can l ful, particularly in psychology. Reductive approaches are cause they undermine the insights needed for the devel well-being.

These four major conclusions have vast implications fo ing, and clinical practice in psychological medicine, as well fields of science and education. I think these conclusion empirically and theoretically. Nevertheless, as always ha conclusions actually expose many other questions, which ture investigation so that we can clarify, test, and refine ou ever, the implications of these fundamental findings for th of well-being are so immediate and strong that I will desc because this will also help to clarify the significance of the

## IMPLICATIONS FOR THE FUTURE

### Clinical practice

Coherence of personality is the natural development of foll psyche, which was described in detail in Chapter 3. Follc psyche brings increasing order (i.e., well-being or nondual of truth (i.e., wisdom or nonlocal awareness), and freedor sharing of gifts, or noncausal service). Therefore, the step self-aware consciousness is a path that leads spontaneously to and creativity, under certain conditions that we must know a foundation for the clinical practice of the science of well-be

The conditions for the development of well-being, wisdo the natural spontaneity characteristic of the upward spiral of s ness described in Chapters 3 and 6. Essentially, the upward spi occurs spontaneously when three conditions are simultaneou

First, to reduce resistance to the order and information in we must let go of all our struggles so that we become calm. ( corresponds to the process of sublimation, as described by Si that it is a spontaneous tendency of life, *not a defense* agains antness, and heaviness. Sublimation cannot be a defense be essential precondition for the psyche to enlighten our subcon we let go of our struggles in a stepwise manner, the valenc becomes more pleasant and enjoyable. As we become more s receptive to enlightenment, which maintains growth through Recognition of this positive feedback relationship between s enment allows us to understand the paradoxical benefit of letting

spontaneity of living systems is toward increasing order, awareness, and coherence? The brief answer is that systems evolving toward coherence are not yet fully coherent, so even human rational intuition can only approach wisdom gradually. The significance of this obvious fact can be appreciated by considering the process of cultural development stimulated by the introduction of creative discoveries and inventions. Contemplative thinking begins at DFT level of 5.8, but at this level rational intuition is still impure or partially incoherent. Intuition is not described as purified or wise until the DFT level is over 7.8, as described in detail in Chapter 5. Consequently, many human discoveries and inventions that are introduced into society represent partial truths mixed with misinformation and misunderstanding. The quality of human creations can be rated according to their degree of lightness, that is, conformity to the principles of the positive philosophy described in Chapter 1. Furthermore, they can be rated according to their degree of shadow, that is, conformity to the principles of the negative philosophy. Human creations involve varying degrees of shadow, that is, untruth and misinformation. The level of shadow of human creations refers to the degree of disorder, distrust, and despair from which all our narcissism and defensive struggles arise. In our analogy of searching for information on the Internet, the degree of shadow corresponds to encountering misinformation that misdirect a person from following the path toward higher order. For example, unwanted e-mail, commonly called "spam," is increasing exponentially on the Internet despite efforts to filter and block its distribution. More than 40% of e-mail messages in 2003 were spam, which is frequently filled with unrealistic claims and advertisements (Hansell 2003).

Even if information encountered is correct, infidelity in listening to the psyche can lead to misapprehension of reality, which leads to apprehensiveness, fears, lack of serenity along with distortion and delusion in thought. Even if people are aware of reality, they may fail to adapt flexibly to changing conditions because of selfishness or prior conditioning, which leads to varying degrees of conflict, selfishness, and even hate.

Both the facilitators and the obstacles to the development of well-being are directly understandable in terms of the three irreducible energies that modulate the spiral path of self-aware consciousness. Consequently, treatments that ignore any aspect of the body, mind, or psyche are inadequate to facilitate the development of biopsychosocial health and well-being.

Much is already known about the biomedical and psychosocial treatment of mental disorders. However, many patients with mental disorders are unresponsive to available treatments or, at best, respond partially (Brodaty, Luscombe et al. 2001). When treatments are partially effective, they usually require lifelong or recurrent treatment because the underlying vulnerability is not corrected. The limitations of available therapies are further exacerbated by the stigma attached to having a "mental disease or defect" and by the costs and constraints on access to treatment under "managed care."

In studies of antidepressants, about 50% of depressed subjects improve with anti-depressants within 6 weeks, whereas about 30% improve with placebos (Walsh, Seidman et al. 2002). The proportion of adult outpatients with major depressive disorder who improved with placebos in published trials has also been increasing substantially between 1981 and 2000 (Walsh, Seidman et al. 2002), suggesting the possibility of a systematic change in people's degree of hopeful self-awareness. Measurement of the level of hopeful self-awareness, as measured by high TCI Self-Directedness and low TCI Harm Avoidance, may explain why many improve with placebos, as well as why many do not improve with antidepressants (Tome, Cloninger et al. 1997). Relief of depression depends on increased hopefulness, which is mea-sured by TCI personality traits that are moderately heritable, particularly high Self-Directedness and low Harm Avoidance (Farmer, Mahmood et al. 2003). Both the brain and the psyche have substantial influences on human thought, but the effects of the psyche on thought have nearly always been neglected because ways of mea-suring self-awareness quantitatively were not available until now.

Fortunately, recognition of the path of the psyche and the principles of coher-ence therapy provide a means to define the fundamental parameters for differen-tial diagnosis, as well as integrating and extending the scope and depth of available treatments. Rather than describing mental disorders in terms of thousands of de-scriptive items, as in *ICD-10* and *DSM-IV*, my goal has been to identify a small number of basic parameters that can be efficiently evaluated in every person. In addition, these basic parameters provide a solid foundation for understanding the mechanisms of biopsychosocial development and for treatment planning (Cloninger 2002). The goal of coherence therapy is more rapid, more complete, and less expensive treatment that actually results in stepwise growth in self-awareness, culminating in stable well-being. Medication and other biological therapies may be helpful, but in many cases, it is possible to improve self-awareness sufficiently that the need to continue medications is eliminated. The application of the prin-ciples of the science of well-being to assessment and treatment in clinical prac-tice will be explored in detail in a companion book.

## Implications for understanding consciousness

Unfortunately, even to the present day, there is much confusion in discussions of consciousness because the level of self-awareness is not specified. For example, the otherwise insightful descriptions of human emotion by Antonio Damasio per-petuate dualistic thinking about consciousness by pitting Spinoza against Descartes as if they were opponents on different sides of a dualistic controversy (Damasio 1994, 1999, 2003). Essentially Damasio, like Freud, is writing from the perspec-tive typical of the second stage of self-aware consciousness, as I discussed in Chapter 5. Damasio's theory of emotion retains the dualistic conflicts of all the lower stages, including an emphasis on the sensory origins of emotions, as originally described by William James and discussed in Chapter 1. According to Damasio, "intuition occurs only after we acquire knowledge and use reason to analyze it" (Damasio 2003, page 174); that is, intuition is an algorithmic product of reasoning, rather than the basis of self-aware consciousness. Damasio's statement is inconsistent with the standard meaning of intuition as what occurs without reasoning or prior training. Biological reductionism cannot explain individual differences in the creative gifts shown by prodigies and savants. It simply cannot explain the nonalgorithmic nature of intuition. In other words, dualistic science can explain many things but not the creative scientist!

Furthermore, according to Damasio (2003, page 184), "spiritual experiences . . . are biological processes of the highest level of complexity." Hence, Damasio reduces spirituality to biology. Like Freud, Damasio admits that he does not know the way to the happy life, and like Freud, he nevertheless recommends a "combative stance" in which reason must overpower the "machinery of emotion and feeling"(Damasio, 2003, page 275). We have seen repeatedly that such a combative stance can only perpetuate endless conflict and self-struggle, as discussed in detail in Chapters 1–4. We cannot achieve coherence by combat; rather, we can only grow in awareness of its presence by letting go of all of our struggles with our self and others.

Like all of the positive philosophers since Plato, Spinoza recognized the path of the psyche with its distinct ways of knowing. Spinoza clearly distinguished each of the levels of human self-aware consciousness in his *Ethics* (Part II, proposition XL, Note II), although not all of his interpreters have appreciated this fact. For example, Spinoza described the absence of self-aware consciousness as forming ideas "from particular things represented to our intellect fragmentarily, confusedly, and without order through our senses." He then distinguished the three stages of self-aware consciousness, which he calls "knowledge of the first kind, opinion, or imagination" (i.e., first stage), "reason and knowledge of the second kind" (i.e., second stage), and "a third kind of knowledge, which we will call intuition" (i.e., third stage). Hence, Spinoza described mental processes that involve each of these distinct levels of knowledge as developmental stages in the progressive self-awareness of the universal unity of being. Spinoza's understanding of the stages of self-aware consciousness is similar to the description of Hegel that I have described and illustrated. The occurrence of a somatic sensory basis for emotion, as described by William James, is the most fragmentary way of knowing in Spinoza's philosophy of mind. Consequently, there is an especially revealing irony in Damasio's error of confusing the dualistic theory of emotion of the negative philosopher William James with the nondualistic theory of mind of the positive philosopher Spinoza. In Spinoza's nondualistic theory of mind, somatic feelings of particular things occur only as a fragmentary and inadequate basis for knowledge. In other words, for Spinoza, feelings based on sensations are manifestations of immature thinking that occur in the absence of self-aware consciousness.

Like Descartes's error of splitting body and mind, Damasio's error of reducing thought to the algorithmic processing of physical sensations can be easily corrected. Both errors can be corrected by recognition of the primary role of intuition in self-aware consciousness and a more consistent recognition of the unique properties of each level in the hierarchy of self-aware consciousness. Human thought is influenced both by sensations of the body and by intuitions of the psyche. Consequently, human consciousness is not a homogeneous phenomenon. Rather, each level of self-aware consciousness involves distinct psychosomatic processes. In the absence of self-aware consciousness, human thought is dominated by the algorithmic processing of physical sensations. However, in the third stage of self-aware consciousness thought is dominated by pure rational intuition of the universal unity of being.

I am not saying that recognition of the path of the psyche by some people will put an end to all controversy. Differences between people in their level of self-aware consciousness ensure that controversy will continue in the minds of some people until the consciousness of everyone has developed fully. A person simply cannot (and should not) accept what he or she cannot recognize intuitively. Intuitive recognition depends on the level of self-aware consciousness, which differs markedly between individuals as they move along the path of the psyche at variable rates.

Diversity in the level of self-aware consciousness exists between individuals as well as between ages within the same individual. The variation in self-awareness serves to educate all of us about the nature of life as a path of development in which we can do what we can to serve others with love and respect for our mutual need for freedom. This need to combine tolerance and service brings up a particularly urgent need for the application of what we have learned about the science of well-being in service to young or immature individuals.

## Implications for research

Reductive models, whether biomedical or psychosocial, are inadequate approaches to a science of well-being. Such simplifying approaches present a misleading dualistic concept of reality (Heisenberg 1971; von Weizsacker 1980; Schmahl and von Weizsacker 1998), which can be truly harmful because dualism is the foundation of the world views that lead to all struggles, fears, and conflicts. Only an integrated biopsychosocial approach can be adequate to account for available epigenetic and psychophysiological data about human development. Only an integrated biopsychosocial approach appears to be considered adequate by a majority of people in the world today, as shown by the increasing quest for well-being through complementary therapies. Likewise, only an integrated approach based on the nested hierarchies of life systems is adequate to account for available clinical and psychosocial information.

However, it is difficult for many people to let go of their familiar dualistic assumptions about such clinical and psychosocial data. Fortunately, advances in psychobiology now present us with better tools and concepts to bridge the gap between practical scientific research and the wisdom of the positive philosophy.

The methods for studying the biopsychosocial levels of the first two stages of self-aware consciousness are already strong. However, human creativity depends on the third stage of self-aware consciousness, which is distinguished by the quantum or quantum-like properties of nonlocality and noncausality. Although this conclusion has often been resisted in the past, the supporting evidence for human creativity in the path of the psyche has now become at least moderately strong in my opinion. My conclusion is based in part on psychophysiological studies and in part on studies of the dynamics of multiple independent discoveries in science. Hence, the evidence for quantum characteristics of human creativity goes well beyond subjective reports and dogmatic assertions. The most undeniable evidence for the quantum phenomena of free will and creativity as characteristics of modern human beings is the impressive advance in art, science, and spirituality that distinguish modern human beings from all other animals including early hominids (Mithen 1996).

Fortunately, we now have a solid scientific foundation for a science of well-being that is adequate to begin characterizing biopsychosocial development in terms of its fundamental mechanisms. *The Science of Well-Being* is intended to provide a nondualistic perspective that describes a realistic path to full mental health and happiness. You may not agree with my conclusions, but I do hope that the questions I have raised and the data I have presented have deepened your understanding of questions about which we must all keep an open mind.

## REFERENCES

Albert, R. and A. L. Barabasi (2002). "Statistical mechanics of complex networks." *Reviews of Modern Physics* 74: 47–97.

Albert, R., H. Jeong, et al. (1999). "Diameter of the World-wide Web." *Nature* 401: 130.

Augustine (388). The magnitude of the soul. *Writings of Saint Augustine*. New York, Cima Publishing Co.: 51–59.

Bandura, A. (1982). "The psychology of chance encounters and life paths." *American Psychologist* 37: 747–755.

Boden, M. A. (1994). *Dimensions of creativity.* Cambridge, Massachusetts, MIT Press.

Bohm, D. and B. J. Hiley (1993). *The undivided universe: An ontological interpretation of quantum theory.* London, Routledge.

Brodaty, H., G. Luscombe, et al. (2001). "A 25–year longitudinal, comparison study of the outcome of depression." *Psychological Medicine* 31: 1347–1359.

Casti, J. (1997). "Flight over Wall Street." *New Scientist* 154(19 April): 38–42.

Claffy, K., T. E. Monk, et al. (1999). Internet tomography. *Nature*, Web Matters, 7 January 1999, http://www.nature.com/nature/webmatters/tomog.html.

Cloninger, C. R. (2002). Implications of comorbidity for the classification of mental disorders: The need for a psychobiology of coherence. *Psychiatric Diagnosis and Classification.* M. Maj, W. Gaebel, J. J. Lopez-Ibor, and N. Sartorius, eds. Chichester, England, John Wiley & Sons, Ltd.: 79–106.

Consortium, I. H. G. S. (2001). "Initial sequencing and analysis of the human genome." *Nature* 409: 860–921.

Cook, T. A. (1979). *The curves of life: being an account of spiral formations and their application to growth in nature, to science, and to art, with special reference to the manuscripts of Leonardo da Vinci.* New York, Dover Publications.

Damasio, A. R. (1994). *Descartes' error: Emotion, reason, and the human brain.* New York, GP Putnam.

Damasio, A. R. (1999). *The feeling of what happens: Body and emotion in the making of consciousness.* New York, Harcourt Brace.

Damasio, A. R. (2003). *Looking for Spinoza: Joy, sorrow, and the feeling brain.* London, Harcourt.

Dodds, P. S., R. Muhamad, et al. (2003). "An experimental study of search in global social networks." *Science* 301: 827–829.

Douady, S. and Y. Couder (1996). "Phyllotaxis as a dynamical self organizing process." *Journal of Theoretical Biology* 178: 255–312.

Duncan, O. D., Ed. (1964). *William F. Ogburn on culture and social change: Selected papers.* Chicago, Illinois, The University of Chicago Press.

Eysenck, H. J. (1995). Genius: The natural history of creativity. Cambridge, England, Cambridge University Press.

Farmer, A., A. Mahmood, et al. (2003). "A sib-pair study of the Temperament and Character Inventory in major depression." *Archives of General Psychiatry* 60(5): 490–496.

Freeman, W. J. (1995). *Societies of brains: A study of the neuroscience of love and hate.* Hove, Lawrence Erlbaum Associates.

Gardner, H. (1993). *Creating minds: An anatomy of creativity seen through the lives of Freud, Einstein, Picasso, Stravinsky, Eliot, Graham, and Gandhi.* New York, Basic Books.

Garfield, E. (1980a). "Multiple independent discovery and creativity in science." *Current Contents* 44: 5–10.

Garfield, E. (1980b). "Delayed recognition or premature discovery—Why?" *Current Contents* 21: 5–10.

Granovetter, M. (2003). "Ignorance, knowledge, and outcomes in a small world." *Science* 301: 773–774.

Gruber, H. E. (1974). *Darwin on man: A psychological study of scientific creativity.* New York, E. P. Dutton & Company.

Guare, J. (1990). *Six degrees of separation.* New York, Vintage Books.

Hadamard, J. (1945). *The psychology of invention in the mathematical field.* Princeton, New Jersey, Princeton University Press.

Hameroff, S. and R. Penrose (1995). "Orchestrated reduction of quantum coherence in brain microtubules, a model of consciousness." *Neural Network World* 5: 793–812.

Hanggi, P., P. Talkner, et al. (1990). "Reaction-rate theory: Fifty years after Kramers." *Reviews of Modern Physics* 62: 251–332.

Hansell, S. (2003). Internet is losing ground in battle against spam. *New York Times.* New York: A1 and C6, April 22.

Heisenberg, W. (1971). *Physics and beyond.* New York, Harper and Row.

Henig, R. M. (2000). *The monk in the garden: The lost and found genius of Gregor Mendel, the father of genetics.* New York, Houghton Mifflin.

Huberman, B. A. and L. A. Adamic (1999). "Growth dynamics of the World-wide Web." *Nature* 401: 131.

Jung, C. G. (1957). *Psychology of the unconscious: A study of the transformations and symbolisms of the libido, a contribution to the history of the evolution of thought.* New York, Dodd Mead.

Jung, C. G. (1960). The transcendent function. *The collected works of C. G. Jung, Volume 8.* H. Read, M. Fordham, G. Adler, and W. McGuire, eds. Princeton, New Jersey, Princeton University Press: 67–91.

Koestler, A. (1964). *The act of creation.* New York, Macmillan.

Lande, R. (1985). "Expected time for random genetic drift of a population between stable phenotypic states." *Proceedings of the National Academy of Sciences USA* 82: 7641–7645.

Lief, A., Ed. (1948). *The commonsense psychiatry of Dr. Adolf Meyer: Fifty-two selected papers edited, with biographical narrative.* New York, McGraw-Hill Book Company.

May, R. M. (1972). "Will a large complex system be stable?" *Nature* 238: 413–414.

Merton, R. K. (1961). "Singletons and multiples in science." *Proceedings of the American Philosophical Society* 105: 470–486.

Merton, R. K. (1973). The sociology of science. Chicago, Illinois, University of Chicago Press.

Meyer, A. (1957). Psychobiology: A science of man. Springfield, Illinois, C C Thomas.

Milgram, S. (1967). "The small world problem." *Psychology Today* 2: 60–67.

Mithen, S. (1996). *The prehistory of the mind: The cognitive origins of art, religion, and science.* London, Thames and Hudson, Ltd.

Newman, C. M., J. E. Cohen, et al. (1985). "Neo-Darwinian evolution implies punctuated equilibria." *Nature* 315: 400–401.

Ogburn, W. F. and D. Thomas (1922). "Are inventions inevitable? A note on social evolution." *Political Science Quarterly* 37: 83–98.

Penrose, R. (2001). "Consciousness, the brain, and spacetime geometry: An addendum. Some new developments on the Orc OR model for consciousness." *Annals of New York Academy of Science* 929: 105–110.

Price, D. J. D. (1963). *Little science, big science.* New York, Columbia University Press.

Rizi, R. R., S. Ahn, et al. (2000). "Intermolecular zero-quantum coherence imaging of the human brain." *Magnetic Resonance in Medicine* 43: 627–632.

Schmahl, F. W. and C. F. von Weizsacker (1998). "Medicine and modern physics." *Lancet* 351: 1291–1292.

Simonton, D. K. (1978). "Independent discovery in science and technology." *Social Studies of Science* 8: 521–532.

Simonton, D. K. (1979). "Multiple discovery and invention: Zeitgeist, genius, or chance?" *Journal of Personal and Social Psychology* 37: 1603–1616.

Simonton, D. K. (1994). *Greatness: Who makes history and why.* New York, Guilford Press.

Simonton, D. K. (1999). *Origins of genius: Darwinian perspectives on creativity.* New York, Oxford University Press.

Sneppen, K., P. Bak, et al. (1995). "Evolution as a self-organized critical phenomenon." *Proceedings of the National Academy of Sciences USA* 92: 5209–5213.

Sternberg, R. J., ed. (1988). *The nature of creativity: Contemporary psychological perspectives.* New York, Cambridge University Press.

Sternberg, R. J., ed. (1990). *Wisdom: Its nature, origins, and development.* Cambridge, England, Cambridge University Press.

Stewart, I. (1998). *Life's other secret: The new mathematics of the living world.* Harmonds-worth, England, Penguin Books.

Strogatz, S. H. (2001). "Exploring complex networks." *Nature* 410: 268–276.

Svrakic, N. M., D. M. Svrakic, et al. (1996). "A general quantitative theory of personality development: Fundamentals of a self-organizing psychobiological complex." *Development and Psychopathology* 8: 247–272.

Tome, M. B., C. R. Cloninger, et al. (1997). "Serotonergic autoreceptor blockade in the reduction of antidepressant latency: personality and response to paroxetine and pindolol." *Journal of Affective Disorders* 44: 101–109.

Venter, J., M. Adams, et al. (2001). "The sequence of the human genome." *Science* 291: 1304–1351.

Viswanathan, G. M., V. Afanasyev, et al. (1996). "Levy flight search patterns of wandering albatrosses." *Nature* 381: 413–415.

Von Franz, M. L. (1992). *Psyche and Matter.* Boston, Massachusetts, Shambhala.

von Weizsacker, C. F. (1980). *The unity of nature.* New York, Farrar Straus Giroux.

Wagner, A. (2000). "Robustness against mutations in genetic networks of yeast." *Nature Genetics* 24: 355–361.

Wagner, A. and D. A. Fell (2001). "The small world inside large metabolic networks." *Proceedings of the Royal Society London B Biological Science* 268: 1803–1810.

Walker, E. H. (2000). *The physics of consciousness: Quantum minds and the meaning of life.* Cambridge, MA, Perseus Books.

Walsh, B. T., S. N. Seidman, et al. (2002). "Placebo responses in studies of major depression: variable, substantial, and growing." *Journal of the American Medical Association* 287(14): 1840–1847.

Warren, W. S., S. Ahn, et al. (1998). "Imaging contrast enhancement based on intermolecular zero quantum coherences." *Science* 281: 247–251.

Watson, J. D. and F. H. C. Crick (1953). "Molecular structure of nucleic acids." *Nature* 171: 737–738.

Watts, D. J. and S. H. Strogatz (1998). "Collective dynamics of 'small-world' networks." *Nature* 393: 440–442.

Wuchty, S. (2001). "Scale-free behavior in protein domain networks." *Molecular Biology and Evolution* 18: 1694–1702.

# APPENDIX

The Quantitative Measurement of Thought

PLANE 2

2-7 (Lack of Hope)
- 2.9 Basic confidence and responsibility (mocking/flattering or exhibiting)
- 2.8 Primary narcissism (passive-avoidance or shyness/risk-taking or grandiosity)

2–5 (Lack of Self-Respect)
- 2.7 Negative fantasy (superstition)/positive, fantasy (romanticism)
- 2.7 Focusing on negative only (devaluation)/focusing on positive only (idealization)
- 2.6 Cautiousness (anticipatory worry and pessimism)/careless ignoring of risk
- 2.6 Basic trust (helpless/exploitative, taking advantage)

2–4 (Lack of Self-Acceptance)
- 2.5 Criticism or dislike of self and others/validation
- 2.5 Harm Avoidance (feel sick and/or anxious/denial of sickness and/or anxiety)
- 2.4 Mistrust (ignore information/ honor and validation seeking)
- 2.4 Worry/compensation

2–3 (Lack of Tolerance)
- 2.3 Condemnation or opposition (reaction formation)/seductive or extreme flattery
- 2.3 Do not like to experience emotionally (isolation of affect)/negativism
- 2.2 Feeling vulnerable to harm (fear of uncertainty)/feeling invulnerable
- 2.2 Hate or unacceptability (mind goes blank or repression)/eroticism

2–2 (Lack of Trust)
- 2.1 Worthlessness/exploitation
- 2.1 Hopelessness (fatigability)/ostentation (anxious show-off)
- 2.0 Total distrust/dishonesty
- 2.0 Emptiness (controlled, passivity, lack of agency) or fear of annihilation/hate-filled lust (wish to rape and victimize)

PLANE 3

3–7    (Lack of Charity)
  3.9 Feeling powerful and purposeful(giving direction/sarcasm)
  3.8 Industrious and exploratory power-seeking/skeptical rigidity

3–5    (Lack of Discretion or Forethought)
  3.7 Bored or seeking thrills and fun/liking stability, indifferent to thrills or boredom
  3.7 Impulsive, innovative, liberal, accepting transience/traditional, conservative
     permanence
  3.6 Argumentative, liking to debate/compliant or deferential
  3.6 Secondary narcissism (feelings of superiority and pride/feelings of inferiority)

3–4    (Lack of Forbearance or Nonviolence)
  3.5 Curiosity or courage/conforming or stoical (slowness to complaint or interest)
  3.5 Novelty seeking (quick to explore/slow to explore)
  3.4 Anger or quick loss of temper/slowness to lose temper
  3.4 Initiative (self-efficacy) with envy, jealousy, or aggravation/slowness to envy

3–3    (Lack of Flexibility)
  3.3 Excessive wants/excessive frugality
  3.3 Extravagance/reserve (minimal wants)
  3.2 Autonomy with competition and seeking control/regulation (feeling trapped)
  3.2 Greed, self-aggrandizement/guilt and blaming others when unsuccessful or
     incredulity (derealization) when successful

3–2    (Lack of Self-Control)
  3.1 Opposition or acting out/feeling offended or wrongly opposed
  3.1 Obsession/compulsion
  3.0 Disorderliness, leading to acts of aggression (fight) when frustrated/regimenta-
     tion, leading to retreat (flight, escape) when frustrated with fear for self and
     feelings of powerlessness, humiliation, or shame
  3.0 Selfish desire for gratification with craving, gluttony, addiction/aimlessness
     (sloth)

PLANE 4

4–7 (Lack of Love of others)
  4.9 Emotional self-acceptance and contentment (giving others appeasement/relief of grief)
  4.8 Need for appeasement and attachments (emotional affirmation, comfort) or relief of discomfort

4–5 (Lack of Fellowship or Friendship)
  4.7 Concentration with empathy/pragmatism
  4.7 Tender-minded sentimentality (sensitivity to social cues)/tough-minded (insensitivity to social cues)
  4.6 Sensibility to details and relations/disinterest in details and relations
  4.6 Need for intimacy (warmth)/detachment (coldness)

4–4 (Lack of Calmness)
  4.5 Considerate and reassuring/not depending on reassurance of others
  4.5 Security-giving/not needing security from others
  4.4 Seeking support and commitment/convenience (declining support)
  4.4 Social dependence (dependently demanding, need for social protection)/independence (resisting social pressure)

4–3 (Lack of Interdependence or Mutual Support)
  4.3 Feeling appreciated by others/feeling unappreciated by others
  4.3 Attachment (trying to please, courteous)/disloyalty
  4.2 Social vulnerability (feeling hurt, wounded, rejected)/social aloofness
  4.2 Need for recognition (openness to warm communication)/privacy-seeking (need to hide feelings)

4–2 (Lack of Benevolence or Good Will)
  4.1 Yearning for sympathetic companionship/disgust
  4.1 Concern about approval or loneliness/being unloved
  4.0 Self-abasing dependence and need for protection/resentful independence
  4.0 Complaints of succorance or approval and protection-seeking/rejection of others

PLANE 5

5–7    (Lack of Faith)
  5.9  Resourcefulness, creativity or self-actualization (faithful gratitude for inspiration/sense of individual creativity and wholeness)
  5.8  Integrity or oceanic feelings: in states of ecstasy, happy and peaceful participation in what is indivisible and limitless), but perfectionistic

5–5    (Lack of Perseverance)
  5.7  Self-transcendence (growing awareness of transpersonal inseparability and selfless caretaking and preservation of what is meaningful to all)
  5.7  Nonsuppression of what is true and resisting censorship of what is natural
  5.6  Generative service to others, eagerness of effort, or acts of morality and resistance to laziness, moral relativism or autocratic control (respecting the freedom of others within your influence)
  5.6  Self-forgetful (mindful) meditation and letting go of judging and despair

5–4    (Lack of Prudence)
  5.5  Tranquil feelings with meaningful achievement and conscientious judging
  5.5  Persistence (determined attainment of happiness) and resisting underachievement
  5.4  Conscientiousness and avoidance of any manipulation
  5.4  Determination to succeed and little reaction to frustration or nonreward

5–3    (Lack of Justice)
  5.3  Intention to be cooperative/striving to be better than others
  5.3  Career consolidation and ambitious overachievement/underachievement
  5.2  Capable of intimacy and helpful sharing/minimizing others depending on self
  5.2  Tolerance/avoiding prejudice toward others
5–2    (Lack of Moderation)
  5.1  Self-directedness (purposeful, executive)/striving for leadership
  5.1  Ambition (wanting to achieve)/striving for dominance
  5.0  Need to maximize rationality (work-hardened)/minimizing spoiled emotionality
  5.0  Need for self-sufficiency and sense of identity/ minimizing ineptness

PLANE 7

7–7  Coherence (Virtue, Holiness)
  7.9  Wisdom (coherent understanding of faith, hope, and charity)
  7.9  Well-being (full range of positive emotions, no negative emotions)
  7.8  Creative acts of compassionate service
  7.8  Unshakable confidence and love of truth

7–5  Patience
  7.7  Integrated Intelligence (awakened rational intuition)
  7.7  Understanding of faith (spiritual awareness)
  7.6  Restfulness (accepting correction easily)
  7.6  Renewal (spontaneity, fruitfulness)

7–4  Compassion (Conciliation)
  7.5  Impartiality
  7.5  Understanding of harmony (fluidity)
  7.4  Trust in divine mercy
  7.4  Anticipation of peace

7–3  Reverence of God (Piety)
  7.3  Understanding of charity (charitable principles)
  7.3  Reverent and loving prayer giving thanks and glory
  7.2  Gentleness or acts of kindness
  7.2  Commitment to virtuous living

7–2  Awe of God
  7.1  Understanding of hope (enlightened second nature, hopefulness) or self-
       recollection of divinity of being
  7.1  Humility or consciousness of God
  7.0  Acts of repentance and perfectionistic deliberation
  7.0  Spiritual perfectionism and mastery-seeking

# INDEX

Page numbers followed by "f" and "t" indicate figures and tables, respectively.